Practical Immunology

Practical Immunology

LESLIE HUDSON

Department of Immunology,
St George's Hospital Medical School,
London, UK;
Present address:
Division of Cellular and Molecular Sciences,
Glaxo Group Research Ltd,
London, UK

FRANK C. HAY

Departments of Immunology and Rheumatology Research,
University College and Middlesex School of Medicine,
London, UK

THIRD EDITION

BLACKWELL SCIENTIFIC PUBLICATIONS

OXFORD LONDON

·EDINBURGH BOSTON MELBOURNE

©1976, 1980, 1989 by
Blackwell Scientific Publications
Editorial offices:
Osney Mead, Oxford OX2 0EL
  (*Orders*: Tel: 0865 240201)
8 John Street, London WC1N 2ES
23 Ainslie Place, Edinburgh EH3 6AJ
3 Cambridge Center, Suite 208
  Cambridge, Massachusetts 02142, USA
107 Barry Street, Carlton
  Victoria 3053, Australia

First published 1976
Second edition 1980
Third edition 1989

Set by Setrite Typesetters, Hong Kong;
Printed and bound in Great Britain
by Mackays of Chatham Plc.

DISTRIBUTORS

USA
  Year Book Medical Publishers
  200 North LaSalle Street
  Chicago, Illinois 60601
  (*Orders*: Tel: (312) 726–9733)

Canada
  The C.V. Mosby Company
  5240 Finch Avenue East
  Scarborough, Ontario
  (*Orders*: Tel: (416) 298–1588)

Australia
  Blackwell Scientific Publications
  (Australia) Pty Ltd
  107 Barry Street
  Carlton, Victoria 3053
  (*Orders*: Tel: (03) 347–0300)

British Library
Cataloguing in Publication Data

Hudson, Leslie
  Practical Immunology.
  3rd ed.
  1. Medicine. Immunology. Laboratory
  techniques
  I. Title II. Hay, Frank C. (Frank Charles),
  1944–
  616. 07'9'028

ISBN 0–632–01491–1

Contents

V

Foreword to the First Edition

Immunology might well claim to be the most popular and the most glamorous of biological sciences today. I suspect that there has been a sharper increase in the number of research workers in immunology over the last two decades than in any other scientific discipline.

Applied immunology, plus the intangibles we lump together as the rising standard of living, has virtually rid the world of smallpox, yellow fever, diphtheria and poliomyelitis and has helped in many other fields. Its prestige lingers on as the major tool of preventive medicine but, as one whose first immunological paper was published more than 50 years ago, I have seen a complete switch in the contemporary importance of immunology — but not a diminution.

Immunology today is a science in its own right. The enthusiasm of younger workers, like the authors of this book, is primarily directed toward understanding; medical applications of the new knowledge will be wholeheartedly welcomed but they are not central. For me, and to some extent all of us in immunology, the excitement is in the lead that our subject is giving toward a real understanding of the form and strategy of living process. Thanks to the *recognisability* of the significant molecules, antibody, antigen and the like, we have been able to apply the new techniques of molecular biology to the elucidation of one of the essential bodily functions. We are leading the field, for nowhere else have genetics, biochemistry and every other basic science that can help, been so effectively applied to living function. It is the first step toward a sophisticated understanding of what we are and how we became so.

This book is basically an introduction to the techniques and ideas on which immunology is based; to one who grew up with the older, predominantly medical approach, the new version can be sensed everywhere in the authors's approach.

I wish them every success.

F.M. BURNET
Basel, Switzerland
1976

Acknowledgements to the Third Edition

Immunology is a discipline in its own right. Equally, however, it provides essential tools and approaches for many other disciplines — molecular biology, biochemistry, cell biology, pharmacology, microbiology, clinical and veterinary medicine, pathology, forensic science, etc. — thus creating a challenging and rewarding environment for experimental immunologists who are able to traverse the whole of modern biology in the furtherance of research.

The blurring of intellectual demarcation has created an intellectually rich environment but provided us with a problem in the compilation of this third edition — how complete does it need to be to justify its place on the laboratory bench? Fortunately, our original principles for the selection of material for the first two editions have been useful guides: describe techniques that we know work, reflect current trends and provide a source of methods, not of references.

We have been very fortunate to receive help and advice from our friends and colleagues: Kikki Bodman, Angela Bond, Debbie Bridge, Callum Campbell, Laura Davis, Brian DeSousa, Brian Fenton, Jean-Marc Gallo, Tracy Hatton, Meinir Jones, John Kirby, Gurdip Kour, Vera Malkovska, Carlos Moreno, Sara Jane Morgan, Bill Newman, Veronica Newton, Scott Pereira, Andy Soltys, Nazira Sumar, Pochun Tai, Garry Takle and Jenny Tooze. The initial impetus that enabled us to convert from the format of Caxton to that of IBM was provided by Wendy Appelby — we will be enduringly grateful.

Anyone familiar with the layout of the first two editions of this book will readily appreciate the ideas and effort contributed to this new edition by Edward Wates and Emmie Williamson, both of Blackwell Scientific Publications.

Acknowledgements to the Second Edition

Our original notion in the compilation of this book was based on the lazy hope that such a small collection of 'core' techniques would change little, and so would entail little future revision. How wrong we were! In addition to a general revision, we have had to re-write many of the sections dealing with the isolation of immunoglobulins, affinity chromatography, ELISA and, of course, add a complete new chapter on hybridomas and monoclonal antibodies.

We are extremely grateful to our many friends and colleagues who have suggested or discussed our revisions. In particular, we wish to thank Roger Budd, Hansha Bhayani, Janette Flint, Jens Jansenius, Alan Johnstone, Meinir Jones, David Male, Alison Mawle, Lynn Nineham, Graham Rook, Colin Shapland, Yasmin Thanavala and John Whateley.

Our special thanks are due to Margaret Williams and Queenie Jaywardena for their excellent secretarial assistance.

Acknowledgements to the First Edition

This book was started while we were carrying out research for our doctorates in the department of Professor Ivan M. Roitt, FRS. He both encouraged and, indeed, stimulated us to become interested in the teaching of immunology. Our grateful thanks are also due to Dr Giorgio Torrigani for initiating us into the world of immunochemistry.

We wish to thank our colleagues Siraik Zakarian, Harald von Boehmer, Andrew Kelus, Hansruedi Kiefer, Clive Loveday, Jan Obel, Marcus Nabholz, Richard Pink and Jonathan Sprent both for their helpful discussions and in many cases for allowing us to use their unpublished material. We are particularly grateful to Sir Macfarlane Burnet for writing the foreword to this book.

Without the valuable assistance of Lynn Nineham and Anthony Finch it would have been impossible for us to gather all the information and data required for this book. In addition, we wish to acknowledge the tenacity with which Penny Hamilton-Jones converted our pages of hieroglyphs into typewritten sheets.

We have written this book for the use of those individuals, from the undergraduate to post-doctoral level, with a sound theoretical knowledge of immunology, who wish to extend their knowledge by experimentation.

We have been made painfully aware of the interdependence of the branches of immunology in writing this book. It proved extremely difficult to find a point at which to begin. The approach finally adopted was one from the view of cellular biology rather than the classical approach which starts with antibody, a mediator produced half-way through the immune response, and leads to the logical gymnastics of proceeding backwards, to the cellular basis of this response, and forwards, to the secondary mechanisms, initiated by antibody−antigen interaction. We believe that the development of the book from the basic 'lymphocyte unit' to the complete immune system avoids the fast approaching dichotomy between cellular immunology and immunochemistry.

1 The Basic Techniques

The 'immunology research support industry' has grown enormously over the past 8 years and now offers products which combine quality and reproducibility with sophistication and diversity. Even so, the basic techniques, such as antigen preparation and polyclonal antiserum production, are essential tools for the research immunologist. The techniques described in this chapter use common materials that are cheap to purchase or easy to prepare. However, the basic methods are the same for rare or exotic research materials.

1.1 Antigens

Antigens based upon human or animal serum proteins are usually inexpensive because of industrial manufacturing processes used in their production. More sophisticated antigens such as chemically derivatised proteins (hapten–carrier conjugates, see Section 1.6) can be based on these cheap molecules.

1.2 Erythrocytes

Sheep erythrocytes (SRBC) are used widely in immunology both as antigens and indicator cells. They should be purchased in Alsever's solution (See Appendix II), and have a shelf life of 3–4 weeks at 4°. Horse RBC are sold commercially as oxalated whole blood (Appendix II). Their shelf life at 4° is only 2 weeks.

1.3 Soluble antigens (ammonium sulphate precipitation)

Fowl γ-globulin is a very powerful antigen (a strong immunogen) in mammalian species, because of phylogenetic distance, and is prepared as an ammonium sulphate precipitate of whole chicken serum. It is not strictly the serum γ-globulin fraction alone but is essentially serum depleted of albumin.

1.3.1 Preparation of chicken γ-globulin

Materials and equipment
Ammonium sulphate
Dilute ammonia solution
Chicken (adult)

1

UV spectrophotometer
0.14 M sodium chloride solution (saline)
Phosphate-buffered saline, PBS (Appendix I)

Method

1 Dissolve 1000 g ammonium sulphate in 1000 ml distilled water at 50°, allow to stand overnight at room temperature and adjust to pH 7.2 with dilute ammonia solution.
2 Bleed chicken by cardiac puncture (Section 1.11) and separate the serum from the clotted whole blood (Section 1.12.1).
3 Dilute serum 1:2 with saline and add saturated ammonium sulphate solution (prepared in 1) to a final concentration of 45% saturated (v/v).
4 Stir at room temperature for 30 min.
5 Spin off precipitate (1000 g for 15 min at 4°).
6 Wash precipitate with 45% saturated ammonium sulphate and re-centrifuge.
7 Re-dissolve the precipitate in the same volume of PBS as the original serum.
8 Centrifuge to remove any insoluble material.
9 Re-precipitate the γ-globulin using a final concentration of 40% saturated ammonium sulphate.
10 Spin off the precipitate and wash with 40% saturated ammonium sulphate.
11 After centrifuging the washed precipitate, re-dissolve in a minimum volume of PBS.
12 Dialyse the fowl γ-globulin against five changes of PBS at 4° (typically five changes of 1 litres). Centrifuge to remove any precipitate.
13 Prepare a 1:20 dilution of the fowl γ-globulin and determine the absorbance at 280 nm using a UV spectrophotometer.

Calculation of protein content

At 280 nm, an absorbance of 1.0 (1 cm cuvette) is equivalent to a fowl γ-globulin concentration of 0.74 mg ml^{-1}.

Example: if absorbance of sample diluted 1:20 = 0.95

fowl γ-globulin concentration = 0.95 × 0.74 × 20
$$= 14.1 \text{ mg ml}^{-1}.$$

Technical notes

1 Use cockerel blood as this has a low lipid content.
2 Calculation of volume of saturated solution required to achieve a required concentration of ammonium sulphate:

$$V_r = \frac{100\,(S_f - S_i)}{1 - S_f}$$

where:

V_r = volume saturated solution (ml) to be added per 100 ml volume protein solution,

S_f = final saturation (fraction, not per cent),
S_i = initial saturation (fraction, not per cent).

To minimise excessive volumes of solution when working in bulk, add solid ammonium sulphate according to the nomogram on the front inside cover.

3   Determination of protein concentration by UV spectrophotometry is accurate down to about 0.05 mg ml^{-1}.

4   Use of protein solutions containing residual ammonium sulphate can interfere with some of the chemical reactions described in this book. It is good practice to test for residual ammonium sulphate by adding 1 drop of dialysate to 0.5 ml acidified barium chloride solution (use 1 M HCl to acidify a 10 mg ml^{-1} solution of barium chloride in water). If a precipitate forms, continue the dialysis of the protein solution.

1.3.2   Preparation of mouse γ-globulin

Materials and equipment
20 mice, any in- or outbred strain (Section 1.19.1 and Appendix II)
Ether
Saturated ammonium sulphate solution, pH 7.2
UV spectrophotometer

Method
1   Anaesthetise the mice and exsanguinate by severing the axillary vessels under the arm with a pair of scissors.
2   Collect the blood into glass tubes and allow it to clot.
3   Free the clot from the walls of the tube to aid retraction.
4   Collect the exuded serum and remove any contaminating cells by centrifuging at 150 g for 15 min and then at 350 g for 15 min.
5   Precipitate the γ-globulin with ammonium sulphate as described in Section 1.3.

After dialysis determine the protein content of the solution using the following conversion factor: at 280 nm, absorbance of 1.0 (in a 1 cm cuvette) = 0.69 mg ml^{-1} γ-globulin.

1.4   Estimation of protein concentration

Proteins containing tryptophan, tyrosine or phenylalanine residues absorb UV light at 280 nm in a concentration-dependent manner. Consequently, a spectrophotometer may be used to determine the increased absorption obtained when a protein is dissolved in a buffer (the buffer alone is used to 'zero' the spectrophotometer, so this 'difference' is obtained directly) and this value used to calculate the concentration of a pure solution using a published extinction coefficient ($E_{1\,cm}^{1\%}$ — the absorbance at 280 nm due to a 10 mg ml^{-1} solution measured in a quartz cuvette with a 1 cm light path; values for commonly used proteins are given in a table in Appendix III) or, if the solution contains more than one protein, to estimate their total concentration.

Materials and equipment
Protein solution, of unknown concentration
Buffer solution, used for dissolving the protein
Spectrophotometer, capable of operating at UV wavelengths
Quartz cuvettes, typically with 1.0 or 0.5 cm light path

Method
1 Turn on the spectrophotometer and allow it to stabilise for 15 min at 280 nm, in the absorbance rather than transmission mode.
2 Add buffer to the cuvette and use it to adjust the absorbance to zero.
3 Replace the buffer with protein solution (or use another cuvette if you have a matched set) and read the absorbance.
4 Using its extinction coefficient (Appendix III) calculate the concentration of protein, remembering to allow for any dilutions made and standardise for a 1 cm cuvette.

Technical notes
1 To ensure that the relationship between concentration and UV absorption is linear, the absorbance should be below 2.0, ideally between 0.1 and 1.5 absorbance units.
2 If the extinction coefficient of the protein is not known, or if the solution is a mixture of several proteins, total protein concentration may be calculated according to the following equation:

Protein concentration, mg ml^{-1} = $1.55 \times A_{280} - 0.77 \times A_{260}$

where:

A_{280} = absorbance value at 280 nm
A_{260} = absorbance value at 260 nm.

3 Protein solutions frequently show much greater absorbance at wavelengths below 280 nm; however, so do many other materials. The ratio of the A_{280} and A_{260} readings should be below 0.6 for protein solutions; higher ratios usually indicate contaminants such as nucleic acids, peptides, detergents and preservatives such as sodium azide. If you know this to be a problem, use a colorimetric method (Section 1.4.1).
4 The technique is accurate for protein solutions at concentrations greater than 0.1 mg ml^{-1}.

1.4.1   Lowry technique

Although the estimation of protein concentration by UV absorption is simple, direct and allows recovery of the material, many detergents and some buffers absorb light strongly in these wavelengths. It is possible to overcome these problems by the judicious selection of chemicals with low UV absorption; for example, the substitution of the non-ionic detergent Renex 30 for Nonidet NP-40. More often, however, it is necessary to use a different principle for estimation of protein content; for example, the colorimetric method developed by Lowry.

In this technique, a standard curve of colour versus protein concentration is constructed by reacting different concentrations of a known protein with Folin and Ciocalteu's phenol reagent. The blue colour generated by the unknown protein solution can then be converted into concentration units by reference to the standard curve. Although the accuracy of this technique is enhanced if the known and unknown proteins are structurally related, it is common practice to use bovine serum albumin as a ubiquitous standard.

PREPARATION IN ADVANCE

Materials and equipment
As Section 1.4, but in addition:
Protein for use as standard
Phosphate-buffered saline, PBS (Appendix I)

Method
1 Dissolve the standard protein in PBS to 1 mg ml^{-1}.
2 Centrifuge or filter to remove any undissolved material.
3 Determine the 280 nm absorbance of the protein solution and calculate its precise concentration using the extinction coefficient (Section 1.4).
4 Dispense in small aliquots and store at -20° for use.

ESTIMATION OF UNKNOWN PROTEIN SOLUTION

Materials and equipment
Standard and unknown protein solutions
Sodium carbonate, 2.0% w/v in 0.1 M sodium hydroxide
Cupric sulphate, 1.0% w/v in distilled water
Sodium potassium tartrate, 2.0% w/v in distilled water
Folin and Ciocalteu's reagent (Appendix I)
Spectrophotometer, visible light

Method
1 Prepare a dilution series of the standard protein solution in five steps between 0 and 500 µg ml^{-1} in 100 µl (final volume).
2 Prepare a series of dilutions of the unknown protein solution so that at least one tube falls within the range of the standard series. (As a first approximation, prepare a 1 : 5 dilution series through three steps and use 100 µl of each.) Include also a tube containing only the buffer used to dissolve the unknown protein, if this differs from that used to dissolve the protein standard.
3 Mix an equal volume of copper sulphate and sodium potassium tartrate solutions, remove 1 ml and mix with 50 ml sodium carbonate solution (this mixture must be

freshly prepared for each assay). Add 1 ml of this final mixture to each of the tubes containing standard or unknown protein solutions.

4 Add 100 µl of Folin and Ciocalteu's reagent to each tube and mix vigorously.

5 Incubate the tubes at room temperature for 15 min and quantitate the colour reaction in a spectrophotometer at 650 nm.

6 Plot absorbance against protein concentration for the standard solution (the curve deviates slightly from linearity) and from this determine the protein concentration equivalent to the colour reaction of the unknown.

Technical notes

1 As a guide, a protein solution of 250 µg ml^{-1} initial concentration yields a colour reaction with an absorbance of approximately 0.4. The lower limits of detection are about 5 µg ml^{-1}.

2 If the buffer used to prepare the unknown solution gives a colour reaction in the absence of protein, this value should be subtracted from the absorbance of the unknown solution. In addition, it is not uncommon to find that buffer molecules or non-ionic detergents react with the phenol reagent to form a precipitate, without affecting the validity of the colour reaction in the supernatant.

3 If a blue reaction is seen in the tube containing only the buffer used to prepare the standard curve, this indicates protein contamination, usually of the phenol reagent.

4 The cupric sulphate and sodium potassium tartrate should be dissolved independently before mixing, to avoid precipitation.

1.5   Buffer exchange and de-salting of protein solutions

Dialysis is often used to remove small molecular contaminants or to change the buffering conditions of a macromolecular solution. The same effect can be achieved rapidly by the use of a Sephadex G-25 column. Small molecules, such as free dinitrophenol, as well as the ions of the original buffer, are retarded by the Sephadex while protein molecules are excluded from the gel and can be collected in the effluent, already equilibrated in the column buffer. Rapid 'dialysis' by this means is often important when the protein is under harsh conditions, where conventional dialysis would be too slow and would allow irreversible denaturation.

The technique described here is similar in principle to that used for size fractionation of proteins by molecular sieving (Section 8.2). However, because the required molecules are excluded from the gel, and so cannot be size fractionated, filtration through the gel is faster and the whole procedure is less critical.

1.5.1   Preparation of exchange column

Materials and equipment

Sephadex G-25, fine (swollen in water containing sodium azide, Appendix II)
Chromatography column (Appendix II)

Blue dextran, 1% w/v in water (Appendix II)
Peristaltic pump for column

DETERMINATION OF COLUMN VOID VOLUME
1   Pour the Sephadex into a chromatography column and pack under pressure.
2   Ensure that the surface of the gel is level, open the flow-control valve and allow the water to completely enter the column. (With Sephadex G-25, the gel bead size is sufficient to support the column of water inside the gel by surface tension; consequently, liquid flow stops as the meniscus comes into contact with the top of the gel. With fine grades of Sephadex this does not happen. The column may dry out and crack if left to flow unattended.) Close the column outflow.
3   Add 1 ml of blue dextran solution to the surface of the gel. Allow this to enter the gel completely while collecting the effluent into a graduated cylinder. Close the column.
4   Add water to the surface of the gel and continue collecting the effluent until the blue dye just appears. The liquid collected represents the *void volume* of the column.

Repeat the void volume determination for different heights of the gel. Plot a graph of void volume against column height. If you use the same diameter column each time then the void volume may be read off from the graph using the column height.

Molecules in the excluded fraction of Sephadex G-25, for example proteins, leave the gel just after the void volume, and their volume is expanded to approximately 1.5 times the original sample volume.

1.5.2   Use of column for buffer exchange

Materials and equipment
Sephadex G-25 column (Section 1.5.1)
1% w/v blue dextran solution (Appendix II)
Peristaltic pump
Protein solution to be dialysed

Method
1   Determine void volume of the column.
2   Equilibrate the gel with buffer; equivalent to three times the void volume of the column.
3   Apply the sample in a volume not greater than half the void volume.
4   Allow the void volume of buffer to leave the column and collect up to 1.5 times the original sample volume.

If you are using small sample volumes and mini-columns, for example during radio-iodination of protein, it is advisable to determine the volume of the final sample more precisely by using a test volume of blue dextran equal to the original sample volume. This avoids unnecessary dilution.

After one run, the column may be re-equilibrated with three times the void volume of buffer, provided the retained material has not irreversibly bound to the column, for example as with fluorescein isothiocyanate, or has not altered the gel chemically.

1.6 Chemical derivatisation of protein

Many of the early insights into antibody specificity came from chemical studies of antigens, both natural and artificial. More recently, entirely synthetic antigens and chemically modified proteins have been used to investigate the nature of the lymphocyte surface receptor for antigen and to uncover the intricacies of T- and B-lymphocyte cooperation. The techniques described in this section have had wide application in immunology.

1.6.1 Dinitrophenyl–fowl γ-globulin or KLH

A hapten is a small molecule which will bind to B cells or pre-formed antibody. However, the hapten alone is too small to cross-link lymphocyte cell-surface receptors and so will not stimulate B-cell differentiation to plasma cells and antibody production. In addition, the B-cell response to antigen, in the majority of cases, requires co-operation by T cells. Again because of its small size, around $400-800$ Da, the hapten cannot stimulate two lymphocytes simultaneously. However, if the hapten is conjugated to an immunogenic protein, the T cells will recognise this protein, or carrier molecule, and so cooperate with B cells to produce anti-hapten antibody (anti-carrier antibody is also produced). These defined antigens are powerful tools for investigating cell interactions in the immune response.

Probably the most commonly used hapten is dinitrophenyl (DNP) which is conjugated to protein via one of its two reactive forms shown in Fig. 1.1. Dinitrofluorobenzene is highly reactive with the amino groups of proteins under alkaline conditions where the peptide bond is quite stable. It is used when high substitution ratios are required.

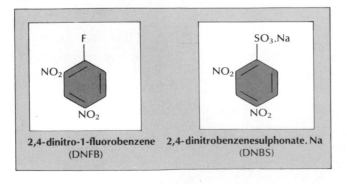

2,4-dinitro-1-fluorobenzene (DNFB)

2,4-dinitrobenzenesulphonate.Na (DNBS)

Fig. 1.1 Chemicals used for dinitrophenyl derivatization of protein carriers. DNFB is much more highly reactive than DNBS and is used when rapid and higher molar substitution ratios are required. Both chemicals are extremely potent skin sensitisers so avoid personal contamination.

High substitution ratios

Materials and equipment
Keyhole limpet haemocyanin, KLH (Appendix II)
1 M sodium bicarbonate
2,4-dinitrofluorobenzene, DNFB (Appendix II)
Sephadex G-25 column (Section 1.5.1)
UV spectrophotometer

Method

1 Dissolve 100 mg KLH in 1 M sodium bicarbonate (minimum initial concentration $10-20$ mg ml^{-1}).
2 Add 0.5 ml DNFB (*take care as DNFB is an extremely potent skin-sensitising agent*).
3 Mix vigorously on a magnetic stirring platform for 45 min at 37°.
4 Separate the DNP-KLH conjugate from the free DNFB on a Sephadex G-25 column (Section 1.5.2).
5 Determine the number of DNP groups per KLH molecule using the conversion:

   DNP: at 360 nm, absorbance of 1.0 (1 cm cuvette) is equivalent to 0.067 mmol DNP.
   KLH: at 278 nm, absorbance of 1.0 (1 cm cuvette) is equivalent to 0.00018 mmol KLH.

   The presence of dinitrophenyl groups on the protein accounts for approximately 40% of the absorbance at 278 nm. This is allowed for in the conversion.

Technical notes
1 KLH tends to self associate so it is not possible to assign an accurate molecular weight. The above calculations assume an average molecular weight of 3×10^6.
2 Removal of KLH molecular complexes by ultracentrifugation tends to reduce its immunogenicity.

Low substitution ratios

Materials and equipment
Fowl γ-globulin, FγG (Section 1.3.1)
0.15 M potassium carbonate
Dinitrobenzene sulphonate, DNBS, sodium salt re-crystallised (Appendix II)
Sephadex G-25 column
UV spectrophotometer

Method

1 Dissolve 100 mg FγG in 5 ml 0.15 M potassium carbonate.
2 Add 20 mg Na DNBS and mix overnight at 4°.

3 Prepare a column of Sephadex G-25 and equilibrate against phosphate-buffered saline (PBS) (Section 1.5.1).

4 Add the DNP−FγG mixture to the column and pump through, adding more PBS when required.

5 Collect the first visible band to elute from the column. This is the DNP−FγG conjugate. The free DNP is retained at the top of the column.

6 Collect 1.5 times the original sample volume.

7 Dilute DNP−FγG solution 1:20 with PBS, and read absorbance in the spectro-photometer at 280 and 360 nm.

Calculation of DNP:FγG ratio

DNP: At 360 nm, absorbance of 1.0 (1 cm cuvette) is equivalent to 0.067 mmol DNP. FγG: At 280 nm, absorbance of 1.0 (1 cm cuvette) is equivalent to 0.0029 mmol FγG. (The DNP interferes with the absorbance reading at 280 nm. This is allowed for in the conversion factor.)

The chemical and antigenic properties of carrier proteins are often altered after hapten substitution. FγG, for example, is irreversibly denatured and becomes insoluble at ratios greater than DNP_{40} FγG. With the method described for dinitrophenylation of FγG you should obtain DNP_{3-4} FγG. There is good hapten and carrier priming when mice are immunised with conjugates with these molar ratios. With DNP_{15-20} FγG, carrier priming is greatly reduced, whereas with DNP_{30-35} FγG, direct (IgM) plaques alone are detected; there is no switching to indirect (IgG) plaque formation in the antibody response to the hapten (cf. Section 4.5).

The KLH molecule can accept up to 100 hapten groups before carrier priming is affected.

1.6.2   Penicilloylation of protein

Materials
Penicillic acid
95% ethanol
Protein solution (5−10 mg ml^{-1})
0.1 M phosphate buffer, pH 7.5 (Appendix 1)
Phosphate-buffered saline, PBS (Appendix I)

Method

1 Prepare a 1 mM solution of penicillic acid in 95% ethanol and add 1 ml to 7 ml of protein solution.

2 Leave to mix overnight at room temperature.

3 Dialyse against five changes of PBS to remove unreacted penicillic acid or to achieve this more rapidly as in Section 1.5.

Estimation of penicilloyl substitution

Materials and equipment
p-(hydroxymercuri) benzoate
0.1 M sodium hydroxide
0.1 M carbonate buffer, pH 7.0 (Appendix I)
Derivatised protein solution
UV spectrophotometer

Method
1 Dissolve p-(hydroxymercuri) benzoate in minimum volume of 0.1 M sodium hydroxide.
2 Dilute with 0.1 M carbonate buffer, pH 7.0 to obtain a stock solution of approximately 1.5×10^{-2} M.
3 Determine the precise concentration of this solution spectrophotometrically (molar extinction coefficient, $E^{1cm}M$, through a 1 cm light path at 232 nm is 1.69×10^4).

This solution will keep for months if stored in the dark at 4°.

Titration of penicilloyl groups

1 Dilute the stock solution of p-(hydroxymercuri) benzoate with carbonate buffer, to obtain a 2×10^{-3} M solution.
2 Dilute the derivatised protein solution 1:10 with carbonate buffer and add 1.0 ml to a spectrophotometer cuvette.
3 Read absorbance at 280 nm.
4 Add 0.1 ml of diluted p-(hydroxymercuri) benzoate solution to the same cuvette, mix and leave at room temperature for 10 min. Determine the new absorbance value.

The difference in the two spectrophotometer readings is due to the p-(hydroxymercuri) benzoate reacting with the penicilloyl groups to form a penamaldate derivative which absorbs at 280 nm. The molar extinction coefficient of penamaldate at 280 nm, 1 cm light path, is 2.38×10^4.

Calculation of substitution ratio

Protein: the interference of the penicilloyl groups with the estimation of protein absorbance at 280 nm is insignificant. The extinction coefficients given for underivatised proteins in Appendix I may be used without correction.

Penicilloyl: at 280 nm, absorbance of 1.0 (1 cm cuvette) is equivalent to 0.0526 mM penamaldate. (An average molar extinction coefficient of 1.9×10^3 has been used for this calculation as the relationship between an increase in the molar substitution ratio and absorbance is not linear.)

Technical notes

1 The *p*-(hydroxymercuri) benzoate stock solution might form a slight precipitate when carbonate buffer is added to the original solution in sodium hydroxide. This should be removed by centrifugation.

2 Remember to allow both for the original dilution of the derivatised protein solution and the dilution due to benzoate addition when calculating the final penamaldate absorbance value.

3 The rate of substitution varies with pH and protein concentration. At pH 11.0 and a 30–50 molar excess of penicillic acid with respect to the free amino groups on the protein, there is an almost quantitative substitution of the protein lysyl groups.

1.7 Polyclonal antisera

Although monoclonal antibodies (Chapter 12) offer distinct advantages, the potential diversity of epitopes recognised by polyclonal antisera, even against a single molecular species of antigen, can yield enormous benefits in immunoassays. Every laboratory has its own methods for raising antisera. Those we describe below are known to work and are rapid.

There is considerable variation in the route and frequency of immunisation as well as the choice of adjuvant depending on the species being immunised. Surprisingly, there is little variation in amount of antigen: both mice and goats can be immunised effectively with 100–200 µg of foreign protein.

Antigens are more immunogenic when presented in an insoluble form (Section 1.8) or with an adjuvant (Section 1.7.1). The most commonly used adjuvant is Freund's complete adjuvant into which soluble antigen is combined as a stable water-in-oil emulsion. The mode of adjuvant action is unclear but it is probable that the slow release of the antigen from the emulsion 'depot' acts as a prolonged series of small injections. In addition, a proportion of the subsequent antibody production occurs within the granuloma induced by the *Mycobacterium tuberculosis* in the adjuvant.

1.7.1 Adjuvants

Freund's complete adjuvant is a mixture of oil (Bayol F) and detergent (mannide mono-oleate) containing *Mycobacterium tuberculosis*. The incomplete adjuvant is a mixture of oil and detergent alone. The complete and incomplete adjuvant may be purchased commercially (Appendix II).

For obvious reasons, this adjuvant is not clinically acceptable for human use and indeed care should be taken to avoid personal contamination during its experimental use. Although Freund's complete adjuvant was first described almost 40 years ago, it is still the most effective non-specific immunopotentiator known.

Saponin is a safer immunostimulating agent and is used in a variety of veterinary vaccines. It consists of a mixture of water-soluble triterpene glycosides extracted from the bark of a South American tree *Quillaia saponaria* and when purified is known as

Quill A. Saponin is highly surface active and forms stable complexes with proteins released from the viral envelopes of viruses such as para-influenza, influenza, measles and rabies. The complexes are about 30 nm in diameter and are referred to as ISCOMS — immunostimulating complexes.

1.7.2   Rabbit anti-mouse γ-globulin

The general methods described in the next few sections are applicable for polyclonal antisera against any protein or glycoprotein antigen.

Materials and equipment
Mouse γ-globulin (Section 1.3.2 or Appendix II)
Freund's complete adjuvant (Appendix II)
Glass syringe with Luer lock
Large rabbits

Method
1   Dissolve 500 μg of mouse γ-globulin in 1 ml saline.
2   Add protein dropwise to 1 ml of Freund's complete adjuvant. Homogenise with a syringe and needle to a white cream after each addition.
3   Continue homogenising until a stable water-in-oil emulsion is obtained. Check this by gently placing 1 drop from the syringe onto saline. If the emulsion is stable the first or second drop will not disperse.
4   Inject approximately 1 ml of the emulsion intramuscularly into each hindquarter of the rabbit. (Many investigators favour a foot-pad injection regime. Theoretically this is advantageous as there is good lymphatic drainage to the local nodes. In practice, however, it is not advisable, especially if the rabbits are housed over wire grilles.)
5   Two weeks later repeat the injections. (If the granuloma ulcerates after the second injection of antigen in Freund's complete adjuvant, we suggest you omit the *M. tuberculosis* from this second injection in your general immunisation schedule.)
6   After 2 further weeks take a 5 ml sample bleed from the central ear artery.
7   Transfer the blood to a glass tube and allow it to clot at room temperature for 1 h. Loosen the clot from the sides of the tube to aid retraction.
8   Leave at 4° until serum is expressed, and harvest as in Section 1.12.1.
9   Test the antiserum in an interfacial ring test (Section 1.8.1).

1.8   Alum precipitation of proteins

Materials and equipment
Protein antigen
1 M sodium bicarbonate

0.2 M aluminium potassium sulphate
Phosphate-buffered saline, PBS (Appendix I)

Method
1 For each 10 ml of protein solution add 4.5 ml of 1 M sodium bicarbonate.
2 Add 10 ml of 0.2 M aluminium potassium sulphate while stirring. Add slowly to minimise frothing.
3 Leave for 15 min.
4 Spin off precipitate (300 g for 15 min) and wash three times with PBS by centrifugation.
5 Re-suspend the insoluble protein to the required concentration.

1.8.1 Interfacial ring test

This assay provides a rapid check on the efficacy of immunisation.

Materials and equipment
Test serum
Durham tubes (Appendix II)
Antigen solution (10−20 mg ml^{-1} protein solution)

Method
1 Place 0.1 ml of serum into the small rimless (Durham) test tube.
2 Carefully layer over 0.1 ml of the solution of immunising antigen.

If a visible interfacial precipitate is not formed within 1−2 min you must continue boosting the animal.

1.9 Immunisation schedules

Commonsense and experience provide the best guide to effective immunisation. For example, if the object of immunisation is to obtain antibody-secreting plasma cells or an antiserum, then the interval between immunisation and use will be much shorter than if the intention is to generate memory B lymphocytes.

It is good practice to obtain serum from the animal(s) prior to immunisation. If the animal is large (rabbit, goat, etc.) then a blood sample of 50 ml or more will yield a useful quantity of normal or pre-immunisation serum. If the animal is small (mouse, guinea pig, etc.) then it is not usually feasible to pre-bleed the same individual intended for immunisation. In this case a pool of serum is a practical alternative, derived from non-immunised animals of the same strain, the same colony (i.e. same environmental antigens) and of approximately the same age.

1.9.1 ## Rabbits

1 Use between 50 and 500 μg foreign protein antigen, in Freund's complete adjuvant (Section 1.7.1), injected intramuscularly into the thigh muscle.

2 Repeat the inoculation after 2 weeks, being careful to inject into the opposite flank to that previously used.

3 If a good precipitating antiserum is not obtained 2 weeks after the second inoculation of antigen, continue boosting with 300 μg of alum-absorbed antigen (Section 1.8) given into the marginal ear vein. To avoid systemic anaphylaxis the animals should be given intravenous promethazine hydrochloride, at the recommended dose rates, prior to intravenous boosting.

SAMPLE BLEED

It is relatively easy to obtain a 10−20 ml blood sample (under aseptic conditions) by bleeding from the central ear artery using a hypodermic syringe and needle. Larger volumes (up to 50 ml) can be obtained more conveniently on a weekly basis by the use of a vasodilating agent.

Materials and equipment
Xylene
Butterfly needle (Appendix II)
Glass Universal container, 20 ml
Ethanol
Cotton-wool swabs

Method
1 Shave the fur from the region over the central ear artery using a new scalpel blade or razor blade (take care not to abrade the skin).

2 Apply a drop of xylene over the shaved area to stimulate the supply of blood.

3 Insert a 21 gauge butterfly needle and allow the blood to flow freely, without suction, into a glass container. Between 20 and 50 ml of blood may be collected every 2 weeks by this method.

4 Apply pressure to the proximal end of the artery, remove the needle and swab the area with ethanol to remove the xylene.

5 Apply firm pressure to the artery until bleeding stops.

When required, exsanguination can be accomplished by cardiac puncture under phenobarbital anaesthesia. A 2.5 kg rabbit should yield 100−120 ml blood, equivalent to 70−80 ml serum, when killed.

1.9.1 ## Rats and mice

Good B-cell responses in mice can be obtained by intraperitoneal immunisation with 0.1 ml alum precipitated protein (400 μg) mixed with 0.1 ml of standard 'whooping cough' vaccine (equivalent to 4×10^9 killed *Bordetella pertussis* organisms). IgG and IgM plaque-forming cells (Section 4.3) can be detected in the spleen after 8 days and the serum antibody levels are maximal by 10–14 days (slight variations, depending on antigen used). If memory B cells are required then at least 2–3 months should be allowed to elapse after the last immunisation.

If T-cell priming is required then immunisation in Freund's complete adjuvant is advised. Use 10–100 μg of antigen in 200 μl Freund's complete adjuvant and inject the emulsion subcutaneously near the nape of the neck.

Immunisation of mice against membrane antigens is particularly effective when saponin (Quill A purified extract) is used as an adjuvant. Mix 15–20 μg of saponin with 10–100 μg of antigen in phosphate-buffered saline and inject the mixture subcutaneously near the nape of the neck. The adjuvant effects of saponin are highly dose dependent — 20 μg is about the maximum subtoxic dose that can be given to a mouse.

Although it is generally recognised that good non-specific immunostimulators (adjuvants) are the key to effective immunisation, there has been relatively little research attention given over to it. Recently, two developments have engendered considerable practical interest: (a) the synthesis and use of muramyl dipeptide (a synthetic dipeptide originally identified in the cell wall of *Corynebacterium parvum*) as an adjuvant chemically conjugated to peptide vaccines; and (b) the claim that combination of lysed malaria organisms with recombinant interferon-γ produces an immune response equivalent to that obtained with saponin immunostimulation. The potential use of defined chemicals as adjuvants is of great practical importance.

Mice can be selectively immunised for an IgE response by immunisation with the antigen of choice and infection with the nematode *Nippostrongylus brasiliensis*.

Animals are primed with alum-precipitated antigen, followed 2–3 weeks later with infection with 300–500 *N. brasiliensis* larvae. On further boosting with antigen, pronounced IgE responses are induced. Exsanguinate mice either by cardiac puncture or by severing the underarm vessels (Fig. 1.2) under ether anaesthesia.

Rats may be immunised by subcutaneous or intramuscular injection of 10–100 μg antigen in 500 μl Freund's complete adjuvant, distributed at three sites. Exsanguinate by cardiac puncture under general anaesthesia.

1.9.3   Goats, sheep and pigs

These large animals can be immunised easily and provide relatively large volumes of serum (up to 1.5 litres even when done commercially as a customer request). The animals can be immunised by intramuscular injection with up to 1 mg of foreign protein antigen in Freund's complete adjuvant and boosted for repeated bleeding. Test bleeds can be taken from the jugular vein and exsanguination accomplished by insertion of an arterial shunt. The size of these animals puts the inexperienced immuniser at a considerable disadvantage. It is wise to seek expert help or a commercial supplier.

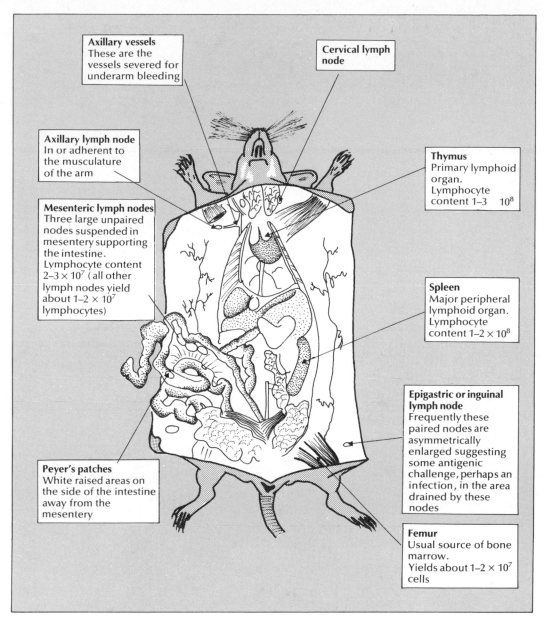

Axillary vessels
These are the vessels severed for underarm bleeding

Cervical lymph node

Axillary lymph node
In or adherent to the musculature of the arm

Thymus
Primary lymphoid organ. Lymphocyte content 1–3 $\times$ 10^8

Mesenteric lymph nodes
Three large unpaired nodes suspended in mesentery supporting the intestine. Lymphocyte content 2–3 $\times$ 10^7 (all other lymph nodes yield about 1–2 $\times$ 10^7 lymphocytes)

Spleen
Major peripheral lymphoid organ. Lymphocyte content 1–2 $\times$ 10^8

Epigastric or inguinal lymph node
Frequently these paired nodes are asymmetrically enlarged suggesting some antigenic challenge, perhaps an infection, in the area drained by these nodes

Peyer's patches
White raised areas on the side of the intestine away from the mesentery

Femur
Usual source of bone marrow. Yields about 1–2 $\times$ 10^7 cells

Fig. 1.2 The major lymphoid organs of the mouse. One of the major lymphoid organs not obvious in the drawing is the blood; it contains about $3-10\times10^6$ lymphocytes ml^{-1} in a total leucocyte count of $4-12\times10^6$ ml^{-1}. As a guide, the differential leucocyte count of mice is approximately: neutrophils 25%, eosinophils 2%, basophils <0.1%, lymphocytes 65% and monocytes 8%. The data for lymphocyte content of the various organs were derived from an SPF stock of CBA mice aged about 4–8 weeks old. At this age the total blood volume is about 6.3 ml per 100 g body weight. The change in blood volume with weight (age) shows a curvilinear relationship probably due to an enhanced fat deposition after 20 g. It follows the general form:

$$y = 0.097x - 0.002x^2$$

where: y = blood volume (ml)
$\quad\quad\quad x$ = body weight (g).

Other strains of mice, particularly if they are outbred, show a linear relationship between body weight and blood volume. For example, the relationship for Swiss mice is:

$$y = 0.072x$$

unknowns as above.

The cell content of each lymphoid organ is known to vary with age (especially the thymus), strain, sex, health and immune status of the individual.

1.10 ## Sites for intravenous inoculation and bleeding

If blood samples or their products are required for sterile use, aseptic precautions and a different site for bleeding and exsanguination may be needed. The alternatives are given in the table below:

Animal	i.v. inoculation	Blood sampling	Exsanguination
Mouse	Tail vein after warming under light	Small samples by clipping end from tail	Cardiac puncture or underarm bleeding
Rat	Tail vein	Cardiac puncture with care	Cardiac puncture
Guinea-pig	Lateral vein of penis	Cardiac puncture with care	Cardiac puncture
Chicken	Underwing vein	Cardiac puncture	Cardiac puncture
Rabbit	Marginal ear vein	Central ear artery or marginal vein after swabbing with vasodilator	Cardiac puncture
Goat/sheep	Jugular vein	Jugular vein	Shunt in carotid artery

Immunisation and bleeding of large animals such as sheep or goats will require specialist advice and the aid of an assistant. Insertion of a carotid shunt is a major undertaking.

1.11 ## Exsanguination of chickens

Small volumes of blood may be obtained from the underwing vein of chickens. However, the vessel is flimsy, poorly supported by the surrounding tissue and tends to haemorrhage easily. In contrast, exsanguination is relatively straightforward, but is best carried out with the aid of an assistant.

Materials and equipment
2–4-month old white leghorn cockerel
Heparin (25 000 iu ml^{-1})
50 ml syringe
19 gauge hypodermic needle

Method
1 Invert the chicken over the edge of the bench with its head pointing downwards.
2 Extend the bird's wings and grasp the wing feathers and legs with one hand and its head with the other.
3 Take 0.1 ml heparin into the syringe.
4 Use the forefinger to locate the internal apex of the clavicles ('wishbone') and insert the syringe needle through this area, keeping the syringe horizontal.

5 Exert a slight negative pressure on the syringe so that blood enters rapidly when the heart is pierced.

6 Exsanguinate the chicken and mix the blood and heparin in the syringe. (A bird of this age and type should yield in excess of 50 ml of blood.)

7 Kill the chicken by cervical dislocation.

1.12 Serum and plasma

Serum is to be preferred to plasma for any immunoassay due to the tendency of the clotting factors in plasma to form spontaneous clots and so mimic or mask antigen—antibody reactions.

1.12.1 Collection of serum

Materials and equipment
Blood without anticoagulant
Glass containers (test tubes or conical flasks)
Low-speed centrifuge

Method

1 Collect the blood into a glass container and allow it to clot at room temperature for 1 h.

2 Once the clot has formed, loosen it from the walls of the container to aid retraction.

3 Transfer to 4° and leave overnight if necessary.

4 Collect the expressed serum and centrifuge at 150 g for 5 min (to sediment the erythrocytes) and then at 350 g for 15 min.

5 Transfer the serum (straw-coloured supernatant) to containers suitable for long-term storage and heat at 56° for 30 min to destroy the heat-labile components of complement.

Technical notes

1 Blood clots better in glass compared to plastic containers.

2 Although heating to destroy the complement components is largely of historical interest, it is still good practice as the unrecognised activation of complement in an antiserum can have far-reaching consequences in some immunoassays.

3 Serum may be frozen at −20° for long-term storage but repeated freezing and thawing should be avoided. Protein denaturation at room temperature is minimal, if serum is sterilised by filtration (0.22 μm pore size). For filter sterilisation of volumes of serum greater than 20 ml use a combination of filters; 0.45 μm pre-filter pad, 0.22 μm filter. A single 0.22 μm filter will block very rapidly. Alternatively storage at 4° is possible after the addition of merthiolate (0.01% w/v, final concentration) as a preservative. Preservation of non-sterile serum for transport without refrigeration can be achieved by the addition of 50% v/v glycerol with no interference with its immune reactivity.

1.12.2 ## Serum preparation from plasma

Pooled plasma is frequently the only source of human serum for use as a tissue culture supplement or for the isolation of plasma proteins. Although the action of the anticoagulant used to prevent clotting can be successfully reversed, some of the plasma proteins are degraded during the preparation.

Citrate—dextrose anticoagulant

Materials
Plasma with citrate anticoagulant
Thrombin solution (Appendix II)
1 M calcium chloride solution

Method
1　Prepare thrombin solution for use by diluting to 100 iu ml^{-1} in calcium chloride solution.
2　Warm plasma to 37°, add 1/100 volume of thrombin solution and mix vigorously to promote clot formation during 5—10 min.
3　Leave at room temperature for 60 min and collect supernatant.
4　Centrifuge at 20 000 *g* for 20 min at 4° and collect the supernatant.
5　Filter sterilise (0.22 μm), if required, and heat inactivate at 56° for 45 min.
6　Store at −20° until used.

Technical note
For filter sterilisation of volumes of serum greater than 20 ml use a combination of filters; 0.45 μm pre-filter pad, 0.22 μm filter. A single 0.22 μm filter will block very rapidly.

Heparin anticoagulant

Materials
Plasma with heparin anticoagulant
Protamine sulphate (Appendix II)
Thrombin solution (Appendix II)
1 M calcium chloride solution

Method
1　Prepare thrombin solution for use by diluting to 100 iu ml^{-1} in calcium chloride solution and adding 5 mg ml^{-1} protamine sulphate.
2　Warm plasma to 37°, add 1/100 volume of thrombin solution and mix vigorously to promote clot formation during 5—10 min.
3　Leave at room temperature for 60 min and collect supernatant.

4 Centrifuge at 20 000 g for 20 min at 4° and collect the supernatant.
5 Filter sterilise (0.22 μm), if required, and heat inactivate at 56° for 45 min.
6 Store at −20° until used.

Technical note
Additional protamine sulphate may be added if a clot does not form.

1.13   ## Basic cell techniques

The techniques described in the following sections are basic to the manipulation and study of cell populations and are aimed at the rapid preparation of uniformly viable cell populations in sterile suspension. In many cases, more sophisticated or more discriminatory variations of these basic techniques are described in later chapters.

1.14   # Preparation of lymphocytes from blood

Many different methods have been described for separating white cells from erythrocytes. Differential centrifugation on a density gradient gives high-purity lymphocyte preparations and is rapid.

1.14.1   ## Mouse and human lymphocytes

Blood is layered onto a density gradient formulated such that only the red cells form a pellet.

Materials
Triosil 75 (available commercially, and is sterile) (Appendix II)
Ficoll (Appendix II)

Method
1 Prepare a 9.2% w/v Ficoll solution in distilled water and autoclave.
2 Mix 43.4 ml of Ficoll solution and 6.6 ml of Triosil 75 under sterile conditions.
3 Dilute the blood 1:1 with sterile tissue culture medium without serum.
4 Layer 5 ml of diluted blood onto 2 ml of the gradient mixture and centrifuge at 300 g for 15 min at 4°. The white cells should not enter the gradient, but remain at the plasma−density gradient interface as a white band.
5 Remove and discard the medium above the white lymphocyte band.
6 Recover the lymphocyte band and wash three times by centrifugation (150 g for 10 min at 4°).

Technical notes
1 This technique works with heparinised blood.
2 Discarding the supernatant above the lymphocyte band removes much of the

platelet contamination. Washing in tissue culture medium will reduce the numbers of remaining platelets. The supernatant of the first wash will appear turbid because of unsedimented platelets; consequently, it is good practice to check by eye that a well-defined pellet has formed before discarding the wash supernatant.

3   Do not collect too much of the density gradient; this contains neutrophils.

4   Lymphocyte yield $1-2\times10^6$ ml^{-1} of venous blood.

Commercial preparations of the density gradient are prepared gravimetrically and give more reproducible results. There are many suppliers; for example, Lymphoprep (Appendix II).

1.14.2   Defibrination of blood

Materials and equipment
100 ml bottles
Glass balls (Appendix II)
Blood without anticoagulant
1 M HCl

PREPARATION IN ADVANCE

1   Wash the glass balls overnight in 1 M HCl then wash three times with a free rinsing detergent; for example, Deconex.

2   Wash the balls thoroughly with distilled water and dry them in an oven.

3   Add 3 g of the glass balls to each 100 ml bottle and autoclave at 138 kPa for 20 min.

A 100 ml bottle, prepared as above, can be used to defibrinate 50 ml of blood.

Method

1   Add blood to bottles and mix by inverting until the clot has completely formed (10−20 min). Do not allow the blood to clot without mixing.

2   Allow the clotted blood to stand for 30 min and remove the serum which will contain free cells.

Virtually pure lymphocytes may be prepared from this cell suspension using density gradient centrifugation. Overall yield of lymphocytes is approximately $0.25-0.5\times10^6$ ml^{-1} of original blood.

1.14.3   Chicken lymphocytes

Although dextran sedimentation techniques are available to prepare chicken leuco-cytes, they give poor cell yields. Fortunately chicken erythrocytes are much larger than the white cells and so separation by differential centrifugation is possible without a density gradient. In addition, chicken polymorphonuclear cells tend to clump readily under normal conditions and so these are also removed from the plasma.

Material
Chicken blood containing heparin

Method
1 Cool the blood to 4°.
2 Centrifuge at 150 *g* for 3 min at 4°.
3 Reduce the centrifugal force to 35 *g*, and continue spinning for a further 10 min at 4°.

The supernatant plasma will contain lymphocytes virtually free of all other cells, lymphocyte yield $3-5\times10^6$ ml^{-1} whole blood. It is essential to use blood containing heparin, as citrated saline reduces the viscosity of the plasma and reduces cell yield and purity. As cockerel blood has a lower viscosity than hen blood due to its lower lipid content, a loose buffy coat often forms during centrifugation. This should be re-suspended by gentle stirring.

1.15 Preparation of lymphocytes from solid lymphoid organs

Lymphocyte suspensions may be prepared from solid lymphoid organs, for example spleen, lymph nodes, bursa, thymus, etc. by teasing the organs apart using forceps or

Organ	% T lymphocytes	%B lymphocytes	% 'null' cells
Thymus	97	1	2
Lymph node	77	18	5
Spleen	35	38	27
Blood	70	24	6
Thoracic duct lymph	80	19	1

Fig. 1.3 Percent lymphocyte subpopulations of murine lymphoid organs. Definition of cells in the table: T lymphocyte — thymus-derived small lymphocyte, with Thy-1-positive, surface immunoglobulin-negative phenotype. B lymphocyte — in chickens B lymphocytes are simply bursa-derived (i.e. from the bursa of Fabricius, a sac-like organ ventral to and communicating with the rectum); however, this primary lymphoid organ is only anatomically distinct in the avian species. In mammals, B lymphocytes are primarily derived from the bone marrow and may be defined serologically by their expression of surface immunoglobulin but not Thy-1 antigens. 'Null' cells resemble small lymphocytes morphologically, but do not have Thy-1 or surface immunoglobulin surface markers. This is a mixed cell lineage some members of which are undoubtedly of the lymphoid series and can express antibody-dependent cell cytotoxicity (ADCC) as they have IgG Fc receptors (Section 4.14). These cells have some of the characteristics of monocytes and can even express some T-lymphocyte markers. Typically, these have the morphology of large granular lymphocytes (Fig 3.1c). Natural killer cells (NK) also belong to this population and are thought to be important in non-specific killing of tumour and virally infected cell targets.

needles, over fine nylon gauze to retain the connective tissue capsule of the organ. The gauze should be wetted with a few ml of tissue culture medium. Lymphocyte viability tends to vary with the amount of fibrous tissue in the organ and the 'deftness of touch' of the operator. Approximate cell yields from each of the organs are given in Fig. 1.2 — cell viability should be as follows: thymus 95%, spleen 80—90% and lymph node 70—80%. The lymphocyte subpopulations of each organ are summarised in Fig. 1.3.

If uniformly viable cell suspensions are required, for example for antibody-mediated cytotoxicity assays, dead cells may be removed as described in Section 1.16.

Sterile cell suspensions may be prepared from solid lymphoid organs by pressing the organ through autoclaved nylon gauze in tissue culture medium (Appendix II) using the piston from a 5 or 10 ml disposable syringe. The debris adheres to the nylon gauze and the cell suspension may be dispersed by aspiration with a pasteur pipette.

1.16 Removal of dead cells

The surface charge difference between dead and viable cells is very great when they are suspended in media with a low ionic strength (isotonicity is maintained by the addition of glucose). Filtration of such cell suspensions through a column of hydrophilic cotton wool results in the retention of dead cells; cells in the effluent volume will then be uniformly viable.

Materials and equipment
Phosphate-buffered saline, PBS (Appendix I)
0.308 M glucose in water
Siliconised Pasteur pipettes
10 ml conical centrifuge tubes, siliconised
Absorbent cotton wool
Fetal bovine serum

All steps in this procedure should be carried out with solutions equilibrated on ice or at 4°.

Method
1   Mix 1 volume of PBS with 19 volumes of the glucose solution (low ionic strength buffer).
2   Spin down lymphocytes and re-suspend to $2-4 \times 10^7$ ml^{-1} in low ionic strength buffer.
3   Cut end from a siliconised Pasteur pipette just below the drawn-out shoulder, and pack with cotton wool (to about 5 mm in height).
4   Add up to 4 ml of cell suspension to each pipette, allow the suspension to flow through under 1 g and collect the effluent in a siliconised tube.
5   Wash through with 0.5 ml of low ionic strength buffer, underlay the cell suspension with 1 ml of fetal bovine serum and centrifuge at 220 g for 15 min at 4°.

6 Re-suspend the cells in tissue culture medium and perform a viability count (Section 3.4).

Technical notes

1 This method of dead-cell removal is often of crucial importance in micro-scale assays, where the sensitivity of the assay depends on high initial cell viability.
2 If a sterile cell suspension is required, autoclave PBS, glucose and pre-packed columns. Using solutions pre-cooled on ice, the columns may be run in a laminar flow hood at room temperature.
3 Siliconising of plastic and glassware. Large containers may be coated with a thin film of silicone by rinsing them with one of the proprietary siliconising solutions in heptane (Appendix II). Small items, such as pipettes, etc., may be treated in bulk with dichlorodimethylsilane vapour (*this chemical is highly volatile and extremely toxic. Handle it only inside a fume hood*).

SILICONISING PLASTIC AND GLASSWARE

Materials and equipment
Items for siliconising
Dichlorodimethylsilane
Large glass desiccator

Method
1 Load the plastic or glass items into the desiccator, place in a fume hood and add 1 ml of dichlorodimethylsilane.
2 Evacuate the desiccator through a trap for 5 min and then release the vacuum to disperse the dichlorodimethylsilane vapour.
3 Re-evacuate the desiccator and leave overnight (minimum 2 h).

All items of glassware should be baked at 180° for 2 h before use, and all plasticware should be rinsed five times with distilled water.

1.17 Removal of phagocytic cells

Macrophages can be removed from a cell suspension using either their adherence or phagocytic properties.

1.17.1 Adherence to Sephadex

Materials and equipment
Cells for depletion
Sephadex G-10 (Appendix II)
Tissue culture medium (Appendix I) containing 10% fetal bovine serum, FBS
Syringe barrel, 20 ml

Method

1 Hydrate the Sephadex in PBS and settle for 10 min to remove 'fines'.
2 Autoclave in glass bottles at 138 kPa for 15 min.
3 Pack 10 ml of sterile Sephadex into a 20 ml syringe barrel fitted with a sintered plastic disc, and wash with 10 ml of warm tissue culture medium.
4 Add a maximum of 3×10^8 cells in 1 ml and allow them to become included into the column bed.
5 Wash out the non-adherent cells with 20 ml of warm tissue culture medium, collect the effluent and concentrate the cells by centrifugation (150 g for 10 min at 4°).

Technical notes

1 Sephadex G-10 filtration is known to remove rat dendritic cells, even though they are not adherent to glass or plastic surfaces. Human and mouse suppressor T cells are also adherent to Sephadex.
2 Although adherent cells may also be removed by filtration through glass beads or fibres, the resulting cell suspensions show a greater depletion of B lymphocytes compared with the technique described above.

1.17.2 Phagocytosis of iron powder (for removal of actively phagocytic cells)

Materials and equipment
Iron powder (Appendix II)
Samarium cobalt magnet (Appendix II)
Cell suspension in medium containing 5% fetal bovine serum
10 ml conical plastic tubes

Method

1 Wash the iron powder in ethanol and then in distilled water; autoclave at 138 kPa for 15 min if required for sterile cell separation.
2 Adjust the cell suspension to $2-3 \times 10^7$ lymphocytes ml^{-1}.
3 Add 4 mg of iron powder and mix thoroughly.
4 Incubate at 37° for 30 min, mixing occasionally.
5 Stand the plastic tube on one of the poles of the magnet and leave at 4° for 10 min.
6 Remove the cells in suspension (with the tube still standing on the magnet) and transfer to a second plastic tube.
7 Re-settle the cells on the magnet for a further 10 min at 4°.

These are not preparative techniques. Phagocytic cells attached to Sephadex or containing iron powder are not functional.

1.18 Peritoneal cells

Macrophages containing up to 50% lymphocytes may be prepared by washing the peritoneal cavity of normal mice or guinea-pigs. For many purposes it is possible to elicit larger numbers of macrophages by producing a local inflammatory response; for example, with starch, sodium trioleat, paraffin oil, etc. You must remember, however, that macrophages elicited in this wash will contain engulfed particles and will not be normal.

1.18.1 Isolation of normal peritoneal macrophages

Materials
Mice or guinea-pigs
Tissue culture medium containing 10% fetal bovine serum
1% w/v neutral red in saline

Method
1 Kill the mouse or guinea-pig by cervical dislocation.
2 Inject 8.0 ml of tissue culture medium into the mouse's peritoneal cavity (80 ml for guinea-pigs).
3 Knead the abdomen gently to bring the cells into suspension.
4 Open the abdominal skin to expose the peritoneum.
5 Using a syringe with 21 gauge needle, push the needle into the peritoneum, roll the mouse on its side and aspirate the medium. Alternatively, insert the needle into the peritoneal cavity towards the xiphisternum with the needle bevel directed downwards. The ventral peritoneal wall can be raised slightly with the syringe needle and the internal organs tend to settle, this reduces the possibility of the fat bodies blocking the needle during withdrawal of the fluid.
6 Collect the peritoneal exudate cells by centrifugation (150 g for 10 min at room temperature) using siliconised glassware or plastic.
7 Estimate the number of phagocytes using a haemocytometer by the uptake of a 1% neutral red solution.

Technical notes.
1 A normal mouse will yield 5×10^6 peritoneal exudate cells, up to 50% of which will be lymphocytes.
2 Although more of the peritoneal infusion can be collected by using a pipette after opening the peritoneum, care is needed if the cells are intended for sterile use.

1.18.2 Eliciting peritoneal exudate cells

Materials
Mice or guinea-pigs
1% starch in saline
Tissue culture medium (Appendix I)
1% w/v neutral red in saline

Method
1 Inject 2 ml of starch suspension into the peritoneal cavity of the mouse (25 ml with guinea-pigs).

2 Kill the animals after 3 days.

3 Inject 2—5 ml of tissue culture medium into the peritoneal cavity and gently press the abdomen to bring the cells into suspension (100 ml for guinea-pigs).

4 Open the abdominal skin of the mouse and hold up the centre of the peritoneum with forceps.

5 Make a small hole in the peritoneum and remove the medium with a pipette.

6 Finally, open the mouse fully and suck out all the medium. To handle these peritoneal exudate cells you must either use siliconised glassware or plastic.

7 Estimate the number of phagocytes by the uptake of a 1% neutral red solution (haemocytometer count).

The exudate should contain approximately 75% phagocytes and 25% leucocytes, this may be confirmed by non-specific esterase staining. Although more cells are obtained after starch treatment, remember that some of them will be activated as the starch induces a mild inflammatory response.

1.18.3 Non-specific esterase staining of macrophages

Although peritoneal macrophages stain more strongly for non-specific esterase activity (particularly if they have been elicited by an inflammatory stimulus) than macrophages and monocytes elsewhere in the body, the latter types of cells are still easily distinguished by this staining reaction.

PREPARATION IN ADVANCE

1 Prepare a stock solution of the stain by mixing 1 g pararosaniline with 5 ml concentrated HCL (10 M) and 20 ml distilled water.

2 Heat to 70°, allow to cool to room temperature, filter and store at 4° in the dark.

Materials and equipment
Source of macrophages or monocytes
Pararosaniline stock solution, prepared as above
Phosphate buffers (Appendix I)
Acetone
Formaldehyde solution
Sodium nitrite, 4% w/v in water, freshly prepared
0.1 M Sodium hydroxide
α naphthyl acetate
Methyl green dye, 0.4% w/v in water
DePeX artificial mountant (Appendix II)
Equipment for smear preparation, as Section 3.2.2 or 3.2.3

Method

1 Prepare a smear of the cells on a microscope slide, either manually (Section 3.2.2) or using a cytocentrifuge (Section 3.2.3).

2 Fix the cells for 30 sec at 4° in 30 ml of 0.1 M phosphate buffer, pH 6.6 (Appendix I) mixed with 45 ml acetone and 25 ml formaldehyde solution.

3 Wash three times with distilled water and air dry.

4 Immediately prior to use, prepare the active diazonium salt, hexazotised pararosaniline by mixing 6 ml of 4% w/v sodium nitrite (freshly prepared) with an equal volume of the above stock solution and dilute to 200 ml with 0.067 M phosphate buffer, pH 5.0 (Appendix I).

5 Adjust the activated dye solution to pH 5.8 with 0.1 M sodium hydroxide, this is the optimum pH for esterase activity.

6 Dissolve 50 mg α naphthyl acetate in 2 ml acetone and add to the staining solution.

7 Incubate the smears in the stain for 4 h at room temperature or 45 min at 37°, rinse in distilled water and counterstain for 1–2 min in a 0.4% aqueous solution of methyl green dye.

8 Wash the smears in distilled water, air dry and mount with DePeX.

1.19   Experimental animals

Many of the protocols described in this book can be performed with material from outbred animals. However, *in vivo* experimental work, especially that which involves cell transfer, tissue or organ transplantation and the use of animal models of human disease, relies crucially on the availability of inbred animal strains. In these strains reproducibility and genetic homogeneity is guaranteed by brother–sister mating through many generations. Although a wide range of rat and mouse inbred strains are available, those of rabbit, guinea-pig and pig origin are more limited in genetic range and availability.

1.19.1   Mice

The common strains of inbred mice are widely available from commerical breeders (Appendix II) and are listed in Fig. 1.4. This figure and Fig. 1.5 list useful immunological characteristics of these strains. Several strains of congenic mice have now been developed where each strain is identical to the next except for a single gene and short stretch of associated chromosome. The B10 series, for example, was derived by the introduction of different H-2 loci onto a C57BL/10 genetic background (different strains representing more than 18 different loci are commercially available) and has been used extensively for the investigation of the linkage of various immunological phenomena to different regions of the H-2 gene complex.

Spontaneous mutations with immunological consequences have also been identified in inbred mice or introduced into inbred mice by backcrossing and progeny selection. The best known example of this is the mutation which arose in about 1960 in an outbred stock of mice and was observed to result in both hairlessness and a congenital failure of thymus development. The mutated gene is referred to as *nu* and

Inbred strain	Coat colour	H-2 haplotype (17)*	Lymphocyte-surface alloantigens		
			Ly-I (19)	Ly-2, -3 (6)	Thy-I (9)
AKR	White	k	b	a,a	a
BALB/c	White	d	b	b,b	b
CBA	Agouti	k	a	a,b	b
C57BL	Black	b	b	b,b	b
C3H	Mahogany	k	a	a,b	b
SJL	White	s	b	b,b	b

Fig. 1.4 **Common inbred strains of mice used in immunological research**. Inbred strains are derived by brother–sister mating for more than 20 generations. Consequently, individual members of each strain should be genetically homogeneous and show only the minor phenotypic differences determined by differential response to environmental conditions. Although C57BL is by far the commonest strain used for immunological research, BALB/c is the oldest. It has been inbred since 1923.

Histocompatibility antigens, which are associated with tissue rejection, were discovered as a result of the generation of inbred mouse strains. The most important set of these antigens is determined by closely linked genes in the so-called H-2 or major histocompatibility complex (MHC). The term haplotype is used to indicate alternative forms of the entire H-2 complex which consist of several regions and subregions. This gene family is very complex (highly polymorphic) and so the number of loci in each subregion of the entire H-2 complex has yet to be determined. *The H-2 complex is carried on chromosome 17, other chromosomal locations also in brackets.

Isotype H-chain locus	Immunoglobulin allotypes							Haplotype
	IgM Igh-6	IgD Igh-5	IgG1 Igh-4	IgG2b Igh-3	IgG2a Igh-1	IgE Igh-7	IgA Igh-2	
AKR	b/a	a	d	d	d	a	d	d
BALB/c	a	a	a	a	a	a	a	a
CBA	a	a	a	a	j	a	a	j
C57Bl	b	b	b	b	b	b	b	b
C3H					j			
SJL					b			

Fig. 1.5 **Immunoglobulin allotypes of commonly used mouse strains.** There are many polymorphic forms of both human and mouse (shown here) immunoglobulin heavy chains. In mice, antisera are generally raised to these so-called immunoglobulin allotypes by immunising between strains which differ at the locus of interest, using purified immunoglobulin of a single isotype.

When referring to the whole immunoglobulin or isotypic class one speaks of IgM, IgD, etc. For isolated heavy chains the corresponding Greek letter is used — μ, δ, etc. and for the allotype one refers to the heavy-chain locus — Igh-6b, Igh-5a, etc. These loci were numbered in the order in which they were discovered to be polymorphic. Within each Igh locus there may be several different alleles, expressed as minor differences in amino acid sequence of the polypeptide chain, which can be recognised by monoclonal antibodies. Further details of these, and allotypes in other mouse strains, may be found in Parsons M, Herzenberg LA, Stall AM and Herzenberg LA (1986) Mouse immunoglobulin allotypes. In 'Genetics and Molecular Immunology', Chapter 97, *Handbook of Experimental Immunology*, Volume 3, Weir DM (Editor). Blackwell Scientific Publications, Oxford.

a homozygous *nu/nu* mouse is 'nude'. This mutation has now been introduced into the BALB/c, CBA/Ca and C57BL/10ScSn inbred lines and has virtually replaced the experimental counterpart of thymectomy, irradiation and bone marrow reconstitution. Other inbred strains have been developed as experimental models of human auto-immune and lymphoproliferative disease as described below.

GENETIC DEFECTS OF THE IMMUNE SYSTEM

C57BL/6-bg/bg. Beige mutant of previously black strain. Deficiencies in NK-cell activity and lysosomal function.

AKR. Over 90% of either sex develop spontaneous thymomas and leukaemias by 6–8 months.

SCID. Although these mice have a severe combined immunodeficiency (hence SCID) they can be kept alive in a clean, but not necessarily germ-free, environment. They are ideal recipients for cells from histocompatible strains of mice, for example in reconstitution experiments, and also will support the growth of xenogenic human lymphoid and tumour cells. It seems likely that they will augment the 'nude' mouse in future studies on the function of the immune system.

MODELS OF AUTOIMMUNE DISEASE

NZB. Autoimmune haemolytic anaemia with Coombs' test positive erythrocytes (autoantibodies binding to, but not agglutinating, erythrocytes).

(NZB×NZW) F_1. Develops a lupus-like syndrome with glomerulonephritis and anti-DNA antibodies.

MRL/Mp–lpr/lpr. Model for human systemic lupus erythematosus and rheumatoid arthritis, with enlarged lymph nodes due to generalised lymphoproliferation. This strain shows an early production of anti-DNA antibodies and rheumatoid factor (anti-immunoglobulin antibody).

MRL/Mp–+/+. Develops chronic glomerulonephritis and anti-DNA antibodies late in life but no lymphadenopathy.

C57BL/KS–db/db. Obese mouse strain which develops severe diabetes due to decreased insulin secretion at about 4 months.

NOD. Non-obese diabetic mouse strain. Its genetically based disease is thought to parallel human diabetes more closely than other murine models.

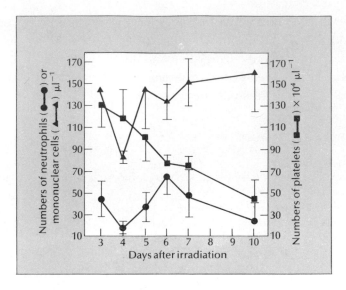

Fig. 1.6 Response of peripheral blood cells to whole-body irradiation. Male C57Bl mice were given 6.0 Gy whole-body irradiation and the numbers of peripheral blood cells determined at various days thereafter. Initial values of cells: neutrophils 1300 ± 340 μl^{-1} (●), mononuclear cells 8900 ± 1500 μl^{-1} (▲) and platelets 1200 ± 180×10^{-3} μl^{-1} (■), each population showed marked variation in their response to irradiation. At 4–5 days maximum leucocyte suppression was seen, with only minimal depression of platelet numbers. Lower doses of irradiation produced much less dramatic effects on cell numbers; for example, the 4 day neutrophil count in response to 4.0 and 5.0 Gy was 170 ± 46 and 180 ± 31 μl^{-1}, respectively. Whole-body irradiation has no acute effects on the plasma levels of the complement components.

X-irradiation of mice

Mice may be immunosuppressed by 6.0–8.0 Gy whole-body irradiation; the precise dose being dictated by the degree of immunosuppression required and the 'cleanliness' of the environment. Under these conditions you should have only the occasional death by 7 days post-irradiation without bone marrow therapy. Early X-ray death is usually due to gut damage; accordingly, X-ray resistance may be increased by starving the mice 24 h before irradiation. If infection-associated deaths are noted after routine immunosuppression the following antibiotic regime may be used: in drinking water, *ad libitum* 1 *g* neomycin and 400 mg polymixin B to 10 litres distilled water.

Figure 1.6 shows the variation in numbers of peripheral blood mononuclear cells, neutrophils and platelets measured at various times after irradiation, in C57Bl mice given 6.0 Gy whole-body irradiation. A dose–response curve of X-ray-induced immunosuppression may be determined as in Section 11.1.

1.20
Further reading

Harlow E and Lane D (1988) *Antibodies: A Laboratory Manual*. Cold Spring Harbour Laboratory, New York.

Hood LE, Weissman IL, Wood WB and Wilson JH (1984) *Immunology*, 2nd edition. Benjamin/ Cummings, Wokingham, Berks.

Johnstone A and Thorpe R (1987) *Immunochemistry in Practice*, 2nd edition. Blackwell Scientific Publications, Oxford.

Lefkovits I and Pernis B (editors) (1979) *Immunological Methods*. Academic Press, London.

Rickwood D and Hames BD (Series editors) *Practical Approach* series, IRL/Oxford University Press. An excellent series of monographs edited by specialists, many of interest to experimental immunologists.

Roitt IM (1988) *Essential Immunology*, 6th edition. Blackwell Scientific Publications, Oxford.

Rosen F, Steiner L and Unanue E (editors) (1988) *Dictionary of Immunology*. Macmillan, London.

Weir DM (editor) (1986) *Handbook of Experimental Immunology*, 4 volumes, 4th edition. Blackwell Scientific Publications, Oxford.

Reviews and updates

Advances in Immunology. Academic Press, London.

Contemporary Topics in Microbiology and Immunology. Springer-Verlag, London.

Immunological Reviews, Moller G (editor). Munksgaard, Copenhagen.

Immunology Today (the immunologist's tabloid). Elsevier/North Holland.

Recent Advances in Clinical Immunology, Thompson RA (editor). Churchill Livingstone, Edinburgh.

Key journals

Immunological articles appear in a vast array of journals so that broad coverage is only possible through an abstracting or indexing service. The key primary sources of research publishing for the working immunologist are:

Nature, Science, Clinical and Experimental Immunology, Immunology, Journal of Experimental Medicine, Journal of Immunology, Molecular Immunology, European Journal of Immunology, Journal of Immunological Methods, Scandinavian Journal of Immunology, Transplantation.

2 Antibody as a Probe

The techniques in this section have been selected not only to describe the labelling and detection of antibody molecules, but also to illustrate the discriminatory power of antibody when used as a probe, often in very complex biological systems. This latter point can be readily appreciated if one considers, for example, the importance of antibodies in screening plasmid or bacteriophage expression libraries. One cannot help but be impressed by the perseverance of an antibody which is able to find its complementary antigenic determinant when the determinant is present as only a partial sequence in a completely unnatural fusion protein, expressed as a trace contaminant, in a sea of irrelevant bacterial proteins.

Although most of the techniques described in this section can be used for the labelling of macromolecules other than immunoglobulin, the reaction conditions may have to be adjusted to achieve optimal substitution.

2.1 Preparation of fluorochrome-conjugated antisera

Although a wide diversity of good quality conjugates are commercially available, the techniques in the following sections will be invaluable if you have to prepare and standardise your own conjugates for specialist applications.

2.1.1 Fluorescein conjugation technique

Materials and equipment
Antiserum
Saturated ammonium sulphate, pH 7.2
0.25 M carbonate buffer, pH 9.0 (Appendix I)
Sephadex G-25 column
UV spectrophotometer
Fluorescein isothiocyanate

Method
1 Precipitate the antiserum with 40% saturated ammonium sulphate as described in Section 1.3.1.
2 Dialyse the γ-globulin fraction of the antiserum against 0.25 M carbonate buffer, pH 9.0, using a Sephadex G-25 column (Section 1.5).
3 Determine the protein concentration of the solution (Section 1.4) and adjust to 20 mg ml^{-1}.
4 Add 0.05 mg fluorescein isothiocyanate per mg of total protein.
5 Mix overnight at 4°.

6   Separate the conjugated protein from the free fluorochrome by passing the mixture down a Sephadex G-25 column equilibrated with PBS (Section 1.5).

Conjugation with tetramethylrhodamine isothiocyanate (Appendix II) is done under the same conditions but it is necessary to separate rhodamine-conjugated antisera from free rhodamine on a DEAE (diethylaminoethyl) ion-exchange column (Section 8.5).

2.1.2   Calculation of fluorochrome : protein ratio

This should be done routinely every time a new conjugate is made. The presence of the fluorochrome interferes with the absorbance of the protein at 280 nm; this is allowed for in the formula

$$\text{Fluorescein : protein ratio} = \frac{2.87 \times \text{abs}_{495\,\text{nm}}}{\text{abs}_{280\,\text{nm}} - 0.35 \times \text{abs}_{495\,\text{nm}}}.$$

Unless you use crystalline rhodamine for conjugation, which we do not recommend, it is not possible to make the same correction when calculating the rhodamine : protein ratio.

$$\text{Rhodamine : protein ratio} = \frac{\text{abs}_{515\,\text{nm}}}{\text{abs}_{280\,\text{nm}}}.$$

If you intend to use the conjugate to stain fixed material the fluorochrome : protein ratio should be low (2 : 1); however, antisera used to stain viable cells, where the specific and non-specific fluorescence is much weaker, should have a higher conjugation ratio (2–4 : 1).

2.1.3   Conjugation with phycoerythrin

Phycoerythrin is one of a family of phycobiliproteins which are crucial to the light-harvesting apparatus of blue–green algae, red algae and the cryptomonads. It contains multiple bilin chromophores and so can absorb efficiently over a relatively wide spectral range and emits with a high quantum yield of fluorescence. Comparison of the useful absorption and emission wavelengths of fluorescein and phycoerythrin illustrates the advantages of this dye combination, particularly for flow cytometry:

	Fluorescein	Phycoerythrin
Excitation	488	488
Emission	515	576

Wavelengths shown in nm.

The two dyes may be excited at the same wavelength and their emissions resolved by the appropriate combination of long- and short-pass filters.

Phycoerythrin can be conjugated to immunoglobulin and protein A using the heterobifunctional cross-linking agent SPDP (Section 2.3.3). Although crystalline phycoerythrin is commercially available, the chemistry of derivatisation and purification is sufficiently arduous for us to strongly recommend the purchase of commercial conjugates (Appendix II).

2.1.4 Fractionation of fluorochrome-conjugated antisera

The fluorochrome:protein ratio calculated above is only an average determination; some protein molecules will have more fluorochrome and others less. As each fluorochrome molecule is added to the protein molecule there is a net decrease in charge. Consequently, conjugated antisera may be fractionated according to molar their substitution ratio by ion-exchange chromatography using an elution gradient of increasing ionic

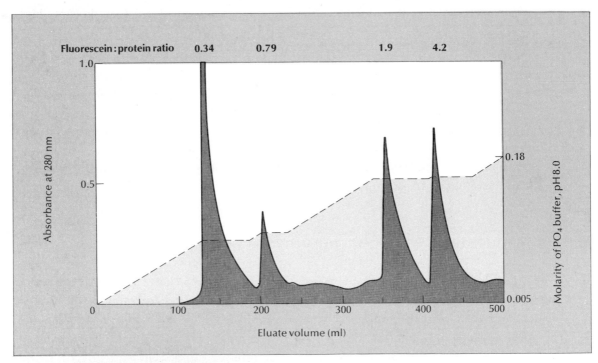

Fig. 2.1 Elution of homogeneously conjugated fluorescein−anti-rabbit IgG from DEAE-cellulose. Fluorescein-conjugated goat anti-rabbit IgG was applied to an ion-exchange column of DEAE-cellulose equilibrated with 0·005 M, pH 8.0 phosphate buffer and eluted with a stepwise gradient of increasing buffer molarity (_ _ _ _). Limit buffer 0·18 M, pH 8.0 phosphate. Antibody activity against rabbit IgG was detected in each peak.

The stepwise gradient was established using an Ultrograd gradient device and level sensor (Appendix II). The molarity of the eluting buffer is increased by the Ultrograd until eluted protein is detected by the level sensor. At this point, the molarity of the buffer is maintained automatically until elution is complete when the molarity is once more increased to obtain the second and subsequent peaks.

strength. For fluorescein-conjugated proteins, adsorb the conjugate to a DEAE ion-exchanger in 0.005 M phosphate buffer, pH 8.0, and elute with a linear gradient, limit 0.2 M, phosphate buffer, pH 8.0 (Section 8.5.2). A typical result is shown in Fig. 2.1.

2.1.5 Indirect versus direct immunofluorescence

Indirect immunofluorescence using an unlabelled antiserum detected by a second, fluorochrome-conjugated antiserum is much more sensitive than direct immuno-fluorescence where one antiserum alone is used. The direct technique gives excellent results with an incident light UV microscope (Appendix II) or flow cytometric analysis and can save a lot of time. However, in the indirect technique, binding of a single first antibody can act as a target for up to eight second antibodies. This amplification is not always all gain, as the background due to non-specific binding can also increase.

The techniques of fluorochrome conjugation can be used with human, goat, sheep and rabbit antisera. They are, however, unsatisfactory for the conjugation of mouse antisera because of excessive denaturation of the antibody molecules. Biotinylation (Section 2.4.1) offers better prospects for 'in house' labelling of mouse antibodies, especially as the same biotin-derived antibody can then be detected with avidin molecules conjugated with fluorochrome, radioisotope or enzyme labels. In addition, mouse alloantisera and monoclonal antibodies can only be used as direct conjugates when staining mouse lymphocytes, as the anti-immunoglobulin second antibody would react directly with the B-cell receptors for antigen. This problem has been circumvented using hapten sandwich labelling, whereby monoclonal antibodies required for single- or double-fluorochrome immunofluorescence may be chemically derived with different haptens (Section 2.2) and antibody binding visualised using anti-hapten sera conjugated with different fluorochromes.

2.1.6 Standardisation of conjugated antisera

This should be done before attempting to use immunoconjugates in detection systems, even if you are using a commercially prepared conjugate. Determine the titration range over which the antiserum gives a plateau of staining values and then work within this titration range.

PROTOCOL FOR RABBIT ANTI-MOUSE Ig INDIRECT IMMUNOFLUORESCENT STAINING
The details of the staining technique are given in Section 3.5.1. A similar protocol may be used for the standardisation of any immunoconjugate, provided appropriate antigen substrates are used.

1 Incubate mouse thymocytes and lymph node cells with a series of dilutions of the unconjugated antiserum starting at 1 : 5 (Fig. 2.2).

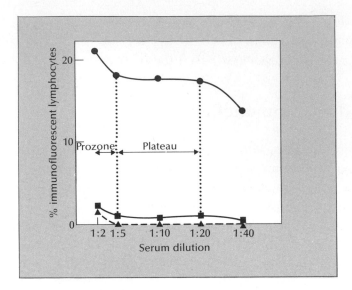

Fig. 2.2 Indirect immunofluorescent staining of mouse thymus and lymph-node lymphocytes.
●———●Lymph-node cells with rabbit anti-mouse Ig.
■———■Thymus cells with rabbit anti-mouse Ig.
▲___▲Thymus cells with normal rabbit serum.
Lymph-node cells showed no prozone with normal rabbit serum. The binding of the rabbit antiserum was detected by a fluorescein-conjugated goat anti-rabbit IgG serum.

2   Detect the antibody with fluorescein-labelled goat or sheep anti-rabbit γ-globulin (1 mg ml^{-1}).

Remember to include a pre-immunisation bleed or pooled normal serum as control (normal rabbit serum, NRS).

If you are using a monoclonal as the first antibody then it is essential to use a monoclonal with an unrelated antigen-binding specificity, but the same isotype, as a negative control.

Evaluation of results
Plot a graph of percentage staining for each antiserum dilution as shown in Fig. 2.2. As can be seen from Fig. 2.2, at low dilutions there is an elevated percentage staining, or prozone, before the plateau. This is probably caused by non-specific sticking of serum proteins at high concentration (cf. staining with NRS). Obviously the best dilution at which to use this antiserum would be between 1 : 10 and 1 : 15. One can be sure that the immunoconjugate is not limiting, but still economise in the use of antiserum (see also Section 3.5.1 for details of immunofluorescent staining).

2.1.7   Specificity of immunofluorescent staining

Antisera, their subfractions and even purified monoclonal antibodies are biological materials and not chemical reagents. Accordingly, many antibodies do not behave as expected. You should be aware of the limitation on the use of these conjugates, especially in a sensitive system such as immunofluorescence. We have listed some of the pitfalls of this technique and their correction. For maximum sensitivity you should use an epi-fluorescent microscope in the dark and, of course, ensure that the microscope has the correct filter combinations for the fluorochrome in use.

EVERYTHING STAINING EVERYWHERE

It is probable that one of the antisera is recognising species or cell-surface determinants other than immunoglobulin. If both control and anti-Ig slides show total staining then the lack of specificity is probably due to the conjugate. If only one of the slides shows high staining it is probably one of the unconjugated sera. We suggest that you absorb the offending serum with liver membranes as follows:

1 Force chopped mouse liver through a tea-strainer or a 63 μm steel sampling sieve into tissue culture medium on ice.
2 Wash the membrane suspension 10–15 times by centrifugation (500 g for 20 min at 4°) until the absorbance of the supernatant is below 0.1 ($E_{280nm}^{1.0cm}$.)
3 Mix a volume of the packed cell membranes with an equal volume of the serum to be absorbed.
4 Leave the suspension to mix at 4° overnight.
5 Spin off the cell membranes (500 g for 20 min at 4°) and re-test the antiserum.

Technical note

If problems of non-specific staining are encountered these can be due either to non-specific adsorption (due to the forces which can cause any two protein molecules to interact) or inappropriate antibody binding. Inappropriate binding can apply to the first or second (conjugated) antibody but only in the case of a polyclonal serum can this be removed by absorption. Similar absorption of a purified monoclonal antibody might leave only phosphate-buffered saline! Non-specific absorption is more frequently a problem with the fluorochrome-conjugated antibody, not only because it is usually used at higher concentration than the first (these forces of non-specific interaction are concentration dependent, as determined by the law of mass action, Section 6.3.1) but also because it is more highly charged than a native molecule.

NO STAINING ANYWHERE

Almost certainly you have forgotten to add the conjugate. If you are sure you added the conjugate, then you have forgotten the positive unconjugated antibody or it does not bind in any case. It is rare for conjugates to become completely inactive during storage.

This may also be due to the UV microscope — a transmitted light microscope is acceptable for stained sections but epi-illumination is essential for cell-surface immunofluorescence. Finally, ensure that the eye-pieces are of the correct magnification for the lens system; the intensity loss with ×12.5 compared with ×6.3 eye-pieces often makes the difference between nothing and superb fluorescence.

EVERYTHING STAINING WITH BRIGHT STARS

Your conjugated antiserum is either contaminated with bacteria or has been frozen or thawed too many times thus producing immune complexes. Ultracentrifuge the conjugate to remove the contamination.

Whenever possible, store antisera at 4° with a preservative (either 0.02% w/v sodium azide or 0.01% merthiolate, final concentration). If it is not desirable to use a preservative, store at −20° in small aliquots.

NEGATIVE-CONTROL SERUM GIVING POSITIVE STAINING
Strictly, the negative-control serum must be taken from the animal before immunisation. Staining either indicates non-specific binding (perhaps due to a high protein concentration, see Technical note above) or the presence of antibodies not elicited by immunisation. It is not valid to attempt to absorb out this reactivity. You must purchase or prepare another serum and review the specificity of the whole system with care.

UPTAKE OF EXOGENOUS PROTEINS ONTO CELL SURFACES
In later sections, cells will be cultured in medium containing a serum supplement. Serum supplements can absorb to the surface of cultured cells and as a consequence might give rise to spurious staining reactions. If required, we suggest that you ensure that your conjugates stain specifically by absorbing them in the manner described below.

2.1.8 Absorption of antisera with insolubilised antigens

Materials
Saturated ammonium sulphate, pH 7.2
Phosphate-buffered saline, PBS (Appendix I)
Fetal bovine, human or rat serum (whichever serum supplement is giving problems)
0.14 M sodium chloride (saline)
2.5% v/v glutaraldehyde in aqueous solution

Method
1 Precipitate the serum with 50% saturated ammonium sulphate (Section 1.3.1) and re-dissolve the precipitate in a minimum volume of PBS.
2 Dialyse against PBS (Section 1.5) to remove ammonium sulphate.
3 Measure the protein concentration of the sample and adjust to 20 mg ml^{-1}.
4 Add glutaraldehyde dropwise to the protein solution while stirring (use 0.5 ml of a 2.5% aqueous solution of glutaraldehyde for each 100 mg of protein to be insolubilised). A gel should form almost immediately.
5 Allow the gel to stand for 3 h at room temperature and then disperse in PBS using a Potter homogeniser.
6 Wash the gel with PBS by centrifugation (500 g for 20 min) until protein cannot be detected in the undiluted supernatant by UV spectroscopy (absorbance less than 0.01, $E_{280nm}^{1.0cm}$).
7 Mix an equal volume of the immunoadsorbent gel with the anti-Ig serum. Mix at 4° overnight.
8 Spin off the immunoadsorbent (500 g for 20 min) and store the antiserum at −20° until used.

It is obviously necessary to ensure specificity of the antiserum under these conditions as one may simply be examining the uptake of proteins from the serum supplement of the tissue culture medium. It is important to use an insoluble immunoabsorbent to avoid the formation of soluble complexes in the absorbed antiserum.

2.2 Hapten sandwich labelling

Two monoclonal antibodies from the same species can be used in the same binding reaction either as direct conjugates or, if an increased sensitivity is essential, after chemical manipulation to permit visualisation by distinct immunoconjugates. In Section 1.6, methods are given for the addition of dinitrophenyl (DNP) or penicilloyl (Pen) to the lysyl groups of proteins. If two monoclonal antibodies are derivatised with DNP or Pen, they may be detected independently using, for example, fluorescein-conjugated anti-DNP and rhodamine- or phycoerythrin-conjugated anti-Pen. To obtain reliable results from this system, considerable time and care is required for standardisation; however, the method can yield considerable amplification in systems where the epitopes to be detected by the first antibodies are at low density.

2.2.1 Chemical derivatisation of first antibodies

Materials
Monoclonal antibodies
Materials for DNP labelling (Section 1.6.1)
Materials for Pen labelling (Section 1.6.2)
Sephadex G-25 mini-columns (packed in Pasteur pipettes)
Mini-concentrator for multiple samples (Appendix II)

Method
1 Isolate the antibody protein either by ammonium sulphate precipitation (Section 1.3.1), if using tissue culture supernatant, or by protein A affinity chromatography (Section 9.1) if using ascitic fluid.
2 Prepare the derivatisation mixture for DNP (Section 1.6.1) or Pen (Section 1.6.2) labelling using 20 mg antibody protein in a total volume of 2 ml, and the other chemicals pro rata.
3 Remove 0.2 ml of sample at each of the following time points: 0, 0.25, 0.5, 1.0, 1.5 and 2.0 h and re-isolate the antibody by chromatography through a Sephadex G-25 column. (Use a fresh equilibrated column for each sample.)
4 At the end of the time course determine the molar substitution ratios for DNP or Pen as in Section 1.6.
5 Plot a graph of molar substitution ratio against time, as in Fig. 2.3.

The hapten-conjugated antibodies tend to work best at a substitution ratio of between 15 and 25 moles mol^{-1}. Having determined the time and conditions for optimum

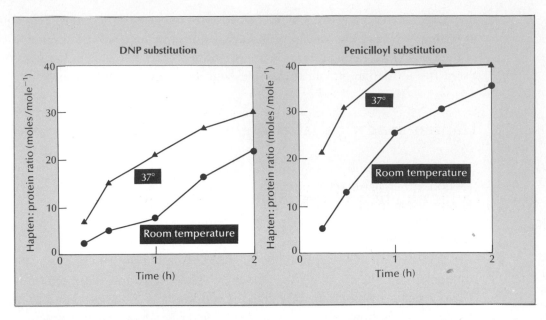

Fig. 2.3 Time course of dinitrophenyl and penicilloyl substitution of mouse IgG1 monoclonal antibodies. Each time point shows the hapten : protein molar ratio determined for derivatisation reactions carried out at room temperature (●) or 37° (▲).

substitution, repeat the derivatisations for a single time point using sufficient antibody protein for the intended use.

Technical notes

1 These chemically modified antibodies are very stable if stored at −20° in the dark.
2 The rate of reaction is temperature dependent. If greater control over derivatisation is required, perform the reaction at 4°. It will take about 16 h to obtain the maximum values shown in Fig. 2.3.
3 If the monoclonal antibodies are against pure antigens, it is possible to carry out the derivatisation reactions while the antibody is bound to an affinity column, thus protecting the binding site. Subsequent washing of the column with buffer prior to elution of the bound antibody (Section 9.2) eliminates the need for dialysis to remove unreacted hapten.

2.2.2 Preparation of anti-DNP and anti-Pen fluorescent conjugates

Materials

Two cheap proteins, available in pure form; for example, ovalbumin and bovine serum albumin, BSA (Appendix II)

Materials for DNP and Pen labelling (Section 1.6)

Materials for fluorochrome conjugation (Section 2.1)

Method

1 Prepare two hapten—carrier conjugates; for example, DNP—ovalbumin and Pen—BSA (Sections 1.6.1 and 1.6.2).

2 Immunise rabbits, or larger animals, with the conjugates independently, to obtain good antisera (Section 1.9).

3 Isolate the IgG fraction of each antiserum (Section 8.5) and conjugate one with fluorescein, FITC, and the other with rhodamine, RITC, or phycoerythrin, PE (Section 2.1).

2.2.3 ## Determination of optimum reaction conditions

Materials
DNP- and Pen-labelled monoclonal antibodies (Section 2.2.1)
Fluorochrome-labelled anti-DNP and anti-Pen (Section 2.2.2)
Target cells or tissues carrying antigens of interest

It is necessary to determine the optimum reaction conditions for the most intense specific staining and the lowest non-specific background. The major variables will be: (a) molar substitution ratio of hapten : antibody; (b) concentration of antibody protein; and (c) dilution of fluorescent conjugates. In practice, a molar substitution ratio of 20 : 1 (hapten : antibody protein) and a dilution of 1 : 20 to 1 : 40 of fluorescent conjugate has been found to give generally acceptable results. More precise refinements can be introduced as experience with the system increases. The concentration of first antibody will vary widely, both with the quality of the monoclonal and the epitopes to be detected.

Carry out standardisation as described in Section 2.1.6, according to the Protocol below. Remember to use a concentration range of haptenated antibodies to obtain optimum results.

Protocol

Tube number	1	2	3	4	5	6	7
Cells carrying antigens A and B	+	+	+	+	+	+	+
DNP_{20} anti-A monoclonal	+	−	+	−	−	−	+
Pen_{20} anti-B monoclonal	−	+	−	+	−	−	+
FITC anti-DNP (1 : 30 dil.)	+	−	−	+	+	−	+
RITC (or PE) anti-Pen (1 : 30 dil.)	−	+	+	−	−	+	+

Technical notes

1 As a guide, use 5—50 µg DNP or Pen antibody protein as an initial concentration range.

2 Tubes 3—6 are specificity controls; 3 and 4 to ensure that the haptens and

conjugates do not cross-react, 5 and 6 to ensure that the fluorescent conjugates do not react directly with the target cells.

3 Tube 7 contains the full set of reactants — add the first antibodies as a mixture, but then wash thoroughly before adding the fluorescent conjugates. Remember to increase the volume of reactants to maintain the same protein concentration throughout. An increase in the protein concentration (as opposed to total protein) in tube 7 could give a higher non-specific background than with tubes 1–6.

This method can work well when sensitive double labelling is required either for microscopy or flow cytometry (Section 3.9). The same general approach can be used with other detection systems; for example, enzyme immunoconjugates (Section 2.3).

2.3 Enzyme labelling of immunoglobulins

The technology of derivatisation and detection of enzymes has improved enormously over the past 10 years, such that their sensitivity has come to match that of radio-isotopes for many applications and their safety has been greatly improved, beyond that of radioisotopes, by the replacement of the commonly used carcinogenic substrates. In technical terms, enzyme labels compare favourably with fluorescent probes in that they do not require special microscopes and darkened rooms for visualisation, and offer both speed and simplicity in detection compared to radioisotopes.

2.3.1 Conjugation of horse radish peroxidase

Peroxidase is a glycoprotein with about 18% carbohydrate which is not necessary for its enzymic activity. This carbohydrate can be converted to aldehyde groups by oxidation with sodium periodate. The periodate aldehyde can then form Schiff bases with immunoglobulin.

Materials
Horse radish peroxidase (Appendix II)
IgG fraction of antiserum or monoclonal antibody (8 mg ml^{-1} in carbonate buffer) (Appendix II or Section 8.5)
0.1 M sodium periodate
0.001 M acetate acetic buffer, pH 4.4 (Appendix I)
0.1 M sodium carbonate buffer, pH 9.5 (Appendix I)
Sodium borohydride (4 mg ml^{-1} in distilled water)
0.1 M borate buffer, pH 7.4 (Appendix I)
Glycerol
Bovine serum albumin

Method
1 Dissolve 4 mg horse radish peroxidase in 1 ml distilled water.

2　Add 200 µl freshly prepared sodium periodate solution and stir gently for 20 min at room temperature. The mixture should turn greenish brown.

3　Dialyse overnight at 4° against sodium acetate buffer.

4　Add 20 µl of sodium carbonate buffer to raise the pH to approximately 9–9.5 and immediately add 1 ml (8 mg) of the protein to be conjugated.

5　Leave at room temperature for 2 h with occasional stirring.

6　Add 100 µl of freshly prepared sodium borohydride solution (4 mg ml^{-1} in distilled water) and leave for 2 h at 4°. This reduces any free enzyme.

7　Dialyse against borate buffer.

8　Add an equal volume of 60% glycerol in borate buffer and store at 4°. (Carrier protein such as bovine serum albumin may be added to 1% w/v if required.)

Technical notes

1　This conjugate should be stable for at least 1 year.

2　Although it is not usually necessary to separate conjugated immunoglobulin from unconjugated immunoglobulin or enzyme, this may be done by gel filtration on G-200 Sephadex (Section 8.2.6).

2.3.2　Conjugation of alkaline phosphatase

Alkaline phosphatase can generally be successfully conjugated to immunoglobulin with glutaraldehyde.

Materials and equipment

Alkaline phosphatase (Appendix II)

Phosphate-buffered saline, PBS (Appendix I)

IgG fraction of antiserum (minimum initial concentration 2 mg ml^{-1} in PBS) (Appendix II or Section 8.5)

Glutaraldehyde, 25% v/v in PBS

0.1 M Tris–HCl buffer, pH 7.4

Bovine serum albumin

Sodium azide

Dialysis tubing

PREPARATION IN ADVANCE

If alkaline phosphatase is supplied as an ammonium sulphate precipitate, the salt must first be removed by dialysis.

Method

1　Place 5 mg alkaline phosphatase in a test tube, centrifuge and discard supernatant.

2　Add 2 mg of the IgG fraction of antiserum to the enzyme pellet.

3　Dialyse overnight at 4° against PBS.

4　Adjust to 1.25 ml with PBS.

5　Add 10 µl of 25% v/v glutaraldehyde. Mix and allow to stand for 2 h at room temperature.

6 Dialyse exhaustively against PBS; five changes of 1 litre at 4°.

7 Dialyse for 8 h against two changes of Tris—HCl buffer.

8 Adjust volume to 4 ml with Tris—HCl buffer containing 1% bovine serum albumin and 0.02% sodium azide.

2.3.3 SPDP conjugation of enzymes

Very effective conjugates between antibody and enzymes can be made using the heterobifunctional cross-linking reagent *N*-succinimidyl-3-(2-pyridylthio) propionate (SPDP). This reagent can be coupled separately to both antibody and enzyme through free amino groups on the proteins. The resultant antibody—pyridyldithio groups can then be reduced to thiol groups and disulphide-linked to the enzyme—pyridyldithio groups with the release of 2-pyridinethione (Fig. 2.4).

Materials and equipment
0.2 M phosphate—saline coupling buffer, pH 7.5 (Appendix I)
IgG fraction of antiserum (2 mg ml^{-1} in coupling buffer)
Horse radish peroxidase (1.0 mg ml^{-1} in coupling buffer)
N-succinimidyl-3-(2-pyridylthio) propionate, SPDP (Appendix II)
Methanol
1 M dithiothreitol
Iodoacetamide
Sephadex G-25 column for rapid buffer-exchange (Section 1.5)
Rotator
Bovine serum albumin

Method

1 Dissolve 3 mg of SPDP in 0.3 ml methanol. This solution must be prepared freshly each time

Carry out procedures 2—4 **A** and **B** in parallel.

A

2 Add 50 µl SPDP solution to the horse radish peroxidase (0.5 mg in 0.5 ml coupling buffer).

3 Rotate gently for 1 h at room temperature.

4 Isolate the labelled enzyme on the Sephadex G-25 buffer-exchange column equilibrated with coupling buffer.

B

2 Add 8 µl of SPDP solution to the antibody (1 mg in coupling buffer).

3 Rotate for 1 h at room temperature.

4 Isolate the labelled antibody on the Sephadex G-25 buffer-exchange column equilibrated in coupling buffer.

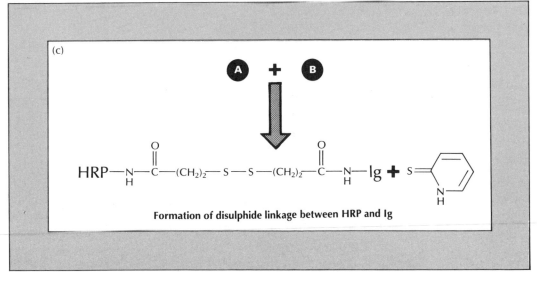

Fig. 2.4 Disulphide coupling of enzyme−immunoglobulin conjugates. The amino groups of a protein may be reacted with SPDP to form a PDP derivative, which in turn may be reduced with dithiothreitol to form sulphydryl groups. This modified protein may be reacted with other PDP-bearing proteins and coupled via disulphide linkages.

5 Measure the volume of antibody solution and add 1 M dithiothreitol to a final concentration of 50 mM.

6 Incubate at room temperature for 15 min.

7 Re-equilibrate one of the Sephadex G-25 columns with coupling buffer.

8 Remove the dithiothreitol by passing sample down the Sephadex buffer-exchange column equilibrated in coupling buffer.

9 Mix the labelled enzyme with the reduced labelled antibody.

10 Rotate gently for 5–8 h.

11 Measure volume and alkylate any remaining thiol groups by adding iodoacetamide to a final concentration of 30 mM.

12 Incubate at room temperature for 15 min.

13 Isolate protein by passing down the Sephadex buffer-exchange column in coupling buffer. Store at 4° with bovine serum albumin added to 1% w/v.

2.4 The biotin–avidin system

Biotin is synthesised by plants and many microorganisms; in particular, large amounts are formed by the intestinal flora. It is essential for warm-blooded animals and acts as a coenzyme in CO_2 fixation and transcarboxylation reactions. Many years ago it was found that feeding animals a diet rich in raw egg white provoked a serious biotin deficiency. This has been shown to be due to a protein present in egg white which has an extremely high affinity ($>10^{15}$ mol^{-1}) for biotin. This small glycoprotein was thus named avidin. Avidin binds so strongly to biotin that for most purposes the binding can be treated as though it was covalent. There are four sites on the avidin molecule at which biotin may be bound. Biotin is a small molecule (MW 244) which can be easily coupled to proteins, including antibodies, enzymes and many antigens without significant loss of the protein's biological activity. The loss of activity is much less than the damage done by coupling a large enzyme directly or following exposure to oxidising agents, as in radiolabelling. Sandwich assays may then be performed in which antibodies bound to solid-phase antigen may be revealed by adding, in sequence, biotinylated anti-immunoglobulin, avidin and then biotinylated enzyme.

The avidin may itself be conjugated with enzyme, thus eliminating one step in the assay. A recent development, which considerably amplifies the resultant signal, is to use pre-formed complexes of avidin and biotinylated enzyme — formed such that a few biotin-binding sites are still free on the avidin molecules.

A big advantage of this system is that the avidin may be labelled with enzyme, fluorochromes, radiolabels, ferritin, etc. so that the same biotinylated antibody may be used with the different avidin conjugates in enzyme immunoassay, radioimmunoassay, immunofluorescence and electron microscopy, without the need for preparing separate labelled antibodies. Egg-white avidin was originally introduced for these assays but some preparations had rather high non-specific binding. Purified preparations are now available (Appendix II) which do not suffer from this problem. Streptavidin from *Streptomyces avidinii* is also used. Although there are no problems with non-specific binding, the biotin-binding site is thought to be less accessible which sometimes necessitates coupling the biotin via a spacer arm.

The technique described below may be used with proteins and carbohydrates; however, in our hands, the biotinylated proteins tend to retain more of their activity after conjugation. Many different biotin-linked antibodies are commercially available (Appendix II). Similarly, avidin may be purchased already substituted with a wide variety of fluorochrome, enzyme or radioisotope labels (Appendix II).

2.4.1 Biotinylation

Materials
Biotin-*O*-succinimide ester (Appendix II)
IgG fraction of antiserum (Section 8.5)
Enzyme; for example, horse radish peroxidase (Appendix II)
Sephadex G-25 buffer-exchange column (Section 1.5) or dialysis tubing
0.1 M bicarbonate buffer, pH 8.4 (Appendix I)
Dimethyl sulphoxide, DMSO
0.1 M Tris—HCl buffer, pH 8.4

Method
1 Equilibrate IgG and enzyme in bicarbonate buffer using the Sephadex G-25 column or by dialysis.
2 Adjust each protein concentration to 1 mg ml^{-1} in bicarbonate buffer.
3 Dissolve 1 mg biotin ester in 1 ml DMSO just before use.
4 Add 75 μl biotin solution to each 1 ml of protein solution.
5 Mix immediately and rotate for 4 h at room temperature.
6 Re-equilibrate the column with 0.1 M Tris—HCl buffer, pH 7.4, and buffer-exchange the two samples on this column (or dialyse against this buffer).

2.5 Radiolabelling of soluble proteins

The methods in this section vary in the harshness (potential for alteration of the conformation of the labelled material) of the reaction required to achieve the desired result. Chloramine T and iodogen labelling involve tyrosyl residues predominantly; if they inactivate antibody binding then try labelling onto lysyl residues (Section 2.6).

2.5.1 Chloramine T method

In alkaline conditions, chloramine T is slowly converted to hypochlorous acid which acts as an oxidising agent. At pH<8.0, oxidation results in iodine incorporation into tyrosine residues, but at a higher pH histidine also becomes labelled. The method is simple and usually the best one to try first for the labelling of antigens or antibodies, either in solution or bound to a solid-phase immunoadsorbent to protect the active site.

Materials and equipment
All reagents should be prepared just before labelling.

0.1 M Tris—HCl, pH 7.4 buffer (Appendix I)
Protein for iodination (500 μg ml^{-1} in Tris—HCl buffer)
Chloramine T (1 mg ml^{-1} in Tris—HCl buffer)
Sodium metabisulphite (2 mg ml^{-1} in Tris—HCl buffer)
Potassium iodide (5×10^{-5} M in Tris—HCl buffer)
Sodium ^{125}I, carrier free (Appendix II)
Phosphate-buffered saline, PBS (Appendix I), containing 0.25% w/v gelatin (Appendix II)
Sephadex G-25
Disposable chromatography column (made from glass tubing or a disposable pipette)
γ spectrometer

Method
1 Mix 100 μl of protein (500 μg ml^{-1} initial concentration) with 18.5×10^6 Bq ^{125}I and 10 μl of chloramine T (1 mg ml^{-1} initial concentration).
2 Incubate for 2—4 min at room temperature.
3 Add 10 μl of sodium metabisulphite solution (2 mg ml^{-1} initial concentration) and mix thoroughly.
4 After 2 min, add 10 μl of potassium iodide solution.
5 Separate the labelled protein from the free iodine using a column of Sephadex G-25 equilibrated with PBS containing 0.25% gelatin (Section 1.5).
6 Elute the column with PBS containing gelatin and collect 0.5 ml fractions.
7 Determine the c.p.m. of each fraction using a γ spectrometer. Identify the first peak of radioactivity, this contains the labelled protein.
8 Store at 4° for use.

Technical notes
1 Proteins denature readily at low concentration, therefore gelatin is incorporated in the elution buffer. The gelatin is also necessary to prevent non-specific binding of protein to the Sephadex. If labelled proteins without carrier protein are needed, the column can be pre-cycled with gelatin to block non-specific uptake and the column used with buffer alone.
2 Although the Sephadex G-25 column is adequate to rapidly separate the protein from the harmful reaction reagents and the free iodine, the labelled protein often needs further purification. Frequently, labelled proteins show some non-specific 'stickiness' due to protein aggregates. These can be removed by gel filtration on Sephadex with an appropriate fractionation range (Appendix III). The nascent formation of unrelated immune complexes at equivalence within the labelled

protein solution is also an effective way of removing non-specific binding, but must be used with care in case the complex components interfere with the subsequent assay.

3   This labelling technique may be used to iodinate antibodies attached to an antigen immunoadsorbent (this protects the antigen binding site). The free iodide is removed by washing with buffer, and the labelled antibody is recovered by acid elution (Section 9.2).

2.5.2   Determination of specific activity of radiolabelled protein

The protein concentration of the labelled material changes during radiolabelling and one cannot assume that all of the radioactive iodine is covalently bound to the protein. Total radioactivity (in c.p.m.) is, therefore, a less useful measure of the efficiency of labelling than specific activity, c.p.m. mg^{-1} protein. It is necessary, therefore, to determine the new protein concentration, either by its UV absorbance if it is a pure protein (Appendix III, for extinction coefficients of common immuno-chemicals) or by the Lowry method if it is a mixture of proteins (Section 1.4).

Materials and equipment
Radioiodinated sample
Glassfibre filter discs; for example, Whatman GF/A (Appendix II)
Large mapping pins in a cork board
Automatic pipette, 1–5 μl (Appendix II)
10 ml glass test tubes
Ice-cold 10% w/v trichloroacetic acid, TCA
Absolute ethanol
γ spectrometer

Method
1   Mount each filter on a map pin (or hypodermic syringe needle) so that it is held clear of the cork board.
2   Dispense between 1 and 5 μl of each sample (this should correspond to approximately 10–50 000 c.p.m. of total radioactivity) onto two separate filter discs and transfer one into a 10 ml test tube.
3   Add 2 ml of ice-cold TCA to the tube, mix by vortexing and leave for 10 min.
4   Decant the TCA and replace with 2 ml of ethanol.
5   Mix by vortexing and leave for 10 min.
6   Transfer each pair of TCA treated and untreated filters to separate small plastic tubes and determine their radioactive content in a γ spectrometer.

Calculation of labelling efficiency

$$\% \text{ protein-bound radioactivity} = \frac{\text{c.p.m. TCA-treated sample}}{\text{total c.p.m. in untreated sample}} \times 100.$$

$$\text{Specific activity,} \atop \text{c.p.m. } \mu g^{-1} = \frac{\text{c.p.m. TCA-treated sample}}{\text{volume of treated sample } (\mu l)} \times \frac{1000}{\text{protein concentration } (\mu g \text{ ml}^{-1})}.$$

Technical notes

1 Proteins labelled to a very high specific activity (for example, for autoradiography or immunoprecipitation) can give problems in this procedure: often it is not possible to measure accurately a sufficiently small aliquot to obtain a c.p.m. within the spectrometer range and the protein concentration can be too low for efficient TCA precipitation. Both these problems can be overcome by prior dilution of an aliquot of the labelled protein in bovine serum albumin (1 mg ml^{-1}) dissolved in phosphate-buffered saline.

2 The same principles apply for the measurement of any radioactive label bound to a protein molecule, with modifications to take account of the nature of the isotope. Clearly, if the radioisotope is a low-energy emitter (^{3}H, ^{14}C or ^{35}S) then a β spectrometer should be substituted for the γ spectrometer.

3 Treating the filter with ethanol not only serves to aid the removal of TCA-soluble material but also speeds drying. Low-energy emitters need liquid scintillants, many of which will not tolerate water.

2.5.3 Iodination of proteins with iodogen

The main damaging reaction in the chloramine T method is the exposure of proteins to the oxidising agent. The use of the insoluble chloroamide 1,3,4,6-tetrachloro-3a, 6a-diphenylglycoluril (Iodogen) coated onto the surface of the reaction tube, or a plastic bead (Appendix II), reduces denaturation of antigen or antibodies during iodination.

PREPARATION IN ADVANCE

Materials and equipment
Iodogen (Appendix II)
Dichloromethane
Test tube, 10×75 mm solvent-resistant plastic (for example, polypropylene)
Water bath
Nitrogen cylinder

Method

1 Prepare a solution of Iodogen (0.1 mg ml^{-1}) in dichloromethane.
2 Add 0.2 ml of this solution (20 µg Iodogen) to a test tube.
3 Evaporate the methylene chloride in a stream of nitrogen, while rotating the tube slowly in a water bath at 37°, to leave a thin film of Iodogen in the bottom of the tube.
4 Store in the dark at −20°. The stored tubes may be used for several weeks.

IODINATION TECHNIQUE

Materials and equipment
Protein for iodination (1 mg ml^{-1}) in borate–saline buffer, pH 8.3,
   ionic strength 0.1 (Appendix I)
Sodium ^{125}I, carrier free (Appendix II)
Iodogen-coated tubes, prepared as above

Method
1 Place the Iodogen-coated tube on ice and add 0.2 ml of protein solution (1 mg ml^{-1} initial concentration).
2 Initiate the reaction by the addition of 10 μl of sodium ^{125}I solution (37×10^6 Bq ^{125}I).
3 Incubate for 5 min with gentle stirring.
4 Terminate the reaction by decanting the protein solution and leave for 10 min to allow reactive iodine to decay.
5 Separate the labelled protein from the free iodine by gel filtration as for the chloramine T method (Section 2.5.1).
6 Determine the protein-bound radioactivity and specific activity as in Section 2.5.2.

Technical notes
1 This method has been found to be more efficient than the chloramine T reaction for some proteins but is inferior for others. The labelling technique of choice must be determined by experimentation.
2 A similar method may be used for the iodination of cells. Typically, use 4×10^6 cells, 6.6 μg of potassium iodide and 37×10^5 Bq ^{125}I in a total volume of 400 μl of phosphate-buffered saline (Appendix I). Add mixture to a tube coated with 50 μg Iodogen. Incubate for 15 min on ice with gentle stirring. Terminate the reaction by decanting the cells and wash three times in phosphate-buffered saline by centrifugation (150 g for 10 min at 4°). This technique does not alter cell viability, as assessed by the uptake of trypan blue.

2.5.4 Biosynthetic labelling of hybridoma-derived antibody

Secreted proteins, as well as cellular components, can be labelled biosynthetically by incorporating labelled amino acids into a culture medium. Immunoglobulins, and many cell-surface and secreted molecules, are glycoproteins; therefore, radio-active sugars, as well as amino acids, can be used as labelled precursors. A culture medium deficient in the particular amino acid must be used to support cell culture during the incorporation of the labelled residue. Culture medium normally contains glucose as the sole sugar as cells biosynthesise the other sugars. If another sugar, such as labelled galactose is added, little conversion to other sugars occurs. To optimise the utilisation of the labelled sugar the level of glucose may be lowered, but cannot be omitted completely as cell viability and therefore incorporation of the label will be adversely affected.

Materials and equipment
Hybridoma cells (or other cells in tissue culture)
Horse or fetal bovine serum, dialysed against phosphate-buffered saline, PBS (Appendix I)
Selective culture medium deficient in leucine (Selectamine is ideal — Appendix II) containing: either ^{3}H-leucine (74−740×10^3 Bq ml^{-1}) (Appendix II), or ^{14}C-leucine (37−185×10^3 Bq ml^{-1}) (Appendix II), and/or ^{14}C-galactose (37−185×10^3 Bq ml^{-1}) (Appendix II), in each case with 5% dialysed serum
Plastic culture tubes, sterile

Method
1 Count the cell suspension (Section 3.4).
2 Add 2×10^5 cells to a sterile culture tube and centrifuge at 150 *g* for 10 min at room temperature.
3 Remove the supernatant and add 0.2 ml of the labelling medium.
4 Incubate overnight at 37° in a humid incubator gassed with 5% CO_2 in air.
5 After incubation, centrifuge (150 *g* for 10 min at room temperature) and remove the supernatant.
6 Determine the protein-bound radioactivity and specific activity as in Section 2.5.2.
7 Store at −20°.

Technical notes
1 ^{14}C-leucine gives a higher energy emission than ^{3}H-leucine and so is counted more efficiently in a scintillation counter, but ^{14}C-amino acids are produced at a lower specific activity than the ^{3}H form and they are more expensive.
2 ^{14}C and ^{3}H have far longer half lives than ^{125}I; therefore, antibodies labelled with these radioisotopes have a longer potential lifetime for use.
3 ^{35}S methionine is another amino acid frequently used for biosynthetic labelling of proteins. It is available at very high specific activity and has a higher energy of emission than ^{14}C or ^{3}H, but a shorter half life. This amino acid is less frequent in the average protein, about one in 20 residues, so the protein is usually labelled to a lesser specific activity. The higher energy of emission is an advantage when this label is used in fluorography (Section 2.10.2). Seleno-methionine (^{75}Se-methionine) is a γ emitter and so is very easy to detect, especially in whole-body systems. It has the significant disadvantage that the radioactive moiety may be cleaved *in vivo* and so is not always a reliable tracer for the original amino acid.
4 Sufficient incorporation of labelled precursor may be achieved by incubation times of only 3−4 h. This might be necessary if the tissue culture conditions are not ideal for cell maintenance.
5 Tissue culture media prepared for biosynthetic labelling by the omission of an

amino acid should not be used for the determination of the rate of protein synthesis by incorporation of isotopically labelled amino acids as the rate of uptake and incorporation is often crucially dependent on the external concentration of amino acids.

6 *In vivo* biosynthetic labelling may be achieved by injecting mice intraperitoneally with 18.5×10^6 Bq of a ^{3}H labelled amino acid mixture: inject once daily on days 7–10 after the initial inoculation of hybridoma cells (Section 12.7). Collect the ascitic fluid by drainage and dialyse against phosphate-buffered saline until no ^{3}H is detectable in the dialysis fluid. For an IgG monoclonal antibody, all of the radioactivity should be TCA precipitable (Section 2.5.2), approximately 30% should be retained by a protein A column and the specific activity of the protein A purified material should be approximately 3.7 GBq mmol^{-1}. *Remember that the mice will excrete ^{3}H after day 7, so appropriate precautions to contain the radioactivity and prevent personal contamination must be taken.*

2.6 Conjugation labelling

Most proteins can be labelled easily by one of the direct methods, but some antibodies, particularly those with many tyrosines within the combining site, can be damaged by these methods. To avoid this, Bolton and Hunter designed a compound, *N*-succinimidyl-3-(4-hydroxyphenyl) propionate, which can be labelled easily by the chloramine T method. The labelled ester is isolated by gel filtration (Section 1.5.2) and then mixed with the protein so that conjugation occurs via an amide linkage to lysine residues on the protein. The ester (Bolton and Hunter reagent) is also available commercially ready labelled with ^{125}I (Appendix II).

2.7 Antibody-based analytical and preparative techniques

The techniques in this section form a basic set of powerful analytical tools for the analysis of complex antigenic systems, including detergent-solubilised cells. The techniques are also sufficiently flexible and compatible to be capable of improvement and modification to facilitate novel experimental applications.

2.7.1 Radiolabelling of cells and their secreted products

Radiolabelling of cell components (proteins, glycoproteins, phosphoproteins, phospholipids, etc.) can provide convenient markers for analytical and preparative techniques.

Endogenous or biosynthetic labelling of secreted proteins is described in detail for monoclonal antibodies and hybridoma cell lines (Section 2.5.4). Precisely similar techniques can be used for the labelling of other proteins or glycoproteins; for example, cytokines secreted from cell lines *in vitro* or, indeed, for any constitutive cell protein which undergoes significant turnover during the labelling period.

Chemical or exogenous labelling of the surface of a viable cell has been a common starting point for many studies on cell-surface antigens. Similarly, differential exogenous labelling of the surface of intact, viable cells, compared with labelling of the cells of the same type after detergent solubilisation, can provide valuable information on the relative distribution of an antigen between the cytoplasm and exterior of the surface membrane. External labelling is usually achieved by confining the chemical coupling reaction to the outer surface of the membrane, for example by using a molecule too large to cross the membrane (often a protein, as in lactoperoxidase labelling), or by binding one of the essential components of the reaction to an insoluble support (the surface of a plastic macro-bead or tube, as in iodogen labelling). The success of this procedure relies crucially on a population of cells with high (preferably uniform) viability and intact surface membranes.

2.7.2   ## Cell-surface iodination: lactoperoxidase technique

Lactoperoxidase, in the presence of hydrogen peroxide, catalyses the incorporation of iodine into tyrosine residues. Rather than adding the hydrogen peroxide directly, a more gentle and efficient method utilises the action of glucose oxidase on glucose to generate hydrogen peroxide continuously during the reaction. As the enzymes are too big to be able to cross the plasma membrane the addition of iodine is confined to the cell surface.

Materials and equipment
Phosphate-buffered saline, PBS (Appendix I)
Cells for iodination (10^8 ml^{-1} in PBS)
Lactoperoxidase (Appendix II) (0.2 mg ml^{-1} in PBS)
Glucose oxidase (Appendix II) (2.0 iu ml^{-1} in PBS)
50 mM glucose in PBS
Sodium ^{125}I, carrier free (Appendix II)

Method
1   Wash the cells three times in PBS by centrifugation (150 g for 10 min at room temperature) to remove exogenous material, count and adjust to 10^8 cells ml^{-1}.
2   To 100 μl of cell suspension add 10 μl lactoperoxidase (0.2 mg ml^{-1} in PBS initial concentration), 10 μl glucose oxidase (2 iu ml^{-1} in PBS, initial concentration) and 18.5×10^6 Bq ^{125}I.
3   Initiate the reaction by the addition of 10 μl of 50 mM glucose in PBS and incubate for 10 min at room temperature.
4   Add 10 ml of ice-cold PBS to stop the reaction.
5   Wash the cells three times in PBS by centrifugation (150 g for 10 min at 4°).
6   If required, the cells may be detergent solubilised as in Section 2.8, and their radioactive incorporation determined.

Technical notes

1 Because the lactoperoxidase cannot cross the plasma membrane of viable cells, only surface proteins are iodinated. However, internal and external proteins are labelled if the cells are dead; therefore, good cell viability is essential. See Section 1.16, for dead-cell removal.

2 The method is also useful for soluble proteins, but the enzymes will contaminate the protein preparation. To avoid this, enzymes coupled to a solid phase should be used. Polyacrylamide beads coupled with lactoperoxidase and glucose oxidase are available commercially (Enzymobeads, Appendix II). The reaction may then be terminated by removal of the beads.

3 Lactoperoxidase may be 'poisoned' by the addition of 10 mM sodium azide and the reaction terminated precisely. In addition, be sure that the PBS does not contain sodium azide as a preservative, otherwise the reaction will never start.

4 Lactoperoxidase catalyses its own iodination. In some systems, iodination artifacts have been reported due to the adsorption of this material to surface of the cell being labelled. If this is a problem, cells may be iodinated with insolubilised Iodogen (Section 2.5.3, Technical note 2) but with reduced efficiency.

2.7.3   Tritium labelling of cell-surface glycoproteins

Low concentrations of sodium metaperiodate induce specific oxidative cleavage of sialic acids. The aldehydes thus formed can be reduced easily with ^{3}H-sodium borohydride. At 0° the periodate anion only penetrates the cell membrane very slowly and so oxidation will be restricted mainly to cell-surface sialic acid residues.

Materials
Phosphate-buffered saline, PBS (Appendix I)
Lymphocytes (3×10^7 ml^{-1} in PBS)
1 M sodium metaperiodate in PBS
0.1 M glycerol in PBS
Tritiated sodium borohydride (Appendix II)
Ice

Method

1 Wash lymphocytes (3×10^7) twice with PBS by centrifugation (150 g for 10 min at 4°).

2 Re-suspend in 1 ml PBS and place on ice.

3 Add 0.1 ml 1 M sodium metaperiodate and incubate on ice for 5 min.

4 Quench the reaction by adding 0.2 ml glycerol (0.1 M).

5 Wash the cells three times with PBS by centrifugation.

6 Re-suspend cells in 0.5 ml PBS.

7 Add 18.5×10^6 Bq sodium ^{3}H-borohydride.

8 Incubate for 30 min at room temperature.

9 After washing in cold PBS, the cells may be solubilised in detergent according to

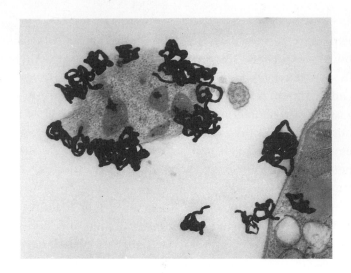

Fig. 2.5 Electron microscopic autoradiography of ¹²⁵I-labelled Trypanosoma cruzi organisms. Trypomastigotes of the protozoan *Trypanosoma cruzi* were labelled with ¹²⁵I by the lactoperoxidase technique (Section 2.7.2) and processed for ultramicrotome sectioning. Ultrathin sections were dipped in K5 nuclear emulsion, allowed to expose and finally processed photographically before viewing in a transmission electron microscope. The photograph shows individual silver grains at or near the cell membrane, confirming that the majority of the radioiodine has indeed conjugated to cell-surface residues. Final magnification ×31 000.

Section 2.8, if required and their radioactive incorporation determined (Section 2.5.2).

2.7.4 Specificity of the labelling reaction

In early studies of cell-surface labelling, it was usual to demonstrate that the addition of the radiolabel was indeed limited to the surface membrane; for example, by electron microscope autoradiography (Fig. 2.5). These techniques are now sufficiently established so that, unless you are working with a totally novel or bizarre system, this type for evidence of the localisation of labelling is not sought. However, it is necessary to bear in mind that cells can adsorb exogenous proteins (particularly from dead and dying cells) on to their surface and so have a well-developed propensity to trap the unwary.

2.8 Detergent solubilisation of cells

Ionic detergents such as sodium dodecyl sulphate (SDS, anionic detergent) or cetyltrimethyl ammonium bromide (cationic detergent) are very efficient at solubilising cells but, except at low concentrations (for SDS <0.1%), they tend to disrupt proteins by destroying their secondary, tertiary or quaternary structure. Non-ionic detergents, such as Nonidet P-40, Triton X-100 or Renex 30, tend to be less efficient solubilisers; however, they preserve not only protein structure but also protein–protein interaction. Many multi-chain cell-surface macromolecules have their non-covalent interchain binding preserved when cells are solubilised in detergent excess and lipids and membrane proteins transfer from the membrane into the detergent micelles. The configuration of most of the protein molecules and the external orientation of many is sufficiently preserved that antibodies are still able to react with antigens from solubilised cells for radioimmunoassay, immunoprecipitation, etc.

Under the conditions described in the following method, non-ionic detergents are able to solubilise the surface membranes of cells but leave the nuclear membrane intact, the intact nuclei are removed by centrifugation. Consequently, it is possible to solubilise cells without the viscosity changes due to released DNA. For most purposes, the aliphatic polyoxyethylene isoalcohol Renex 30 (Appendix II) is preferable to either Nonidet P-40 or Triton X$-$100 (aromatic detergents of the polyoxyethylene *p-t*-octyl phenol series) as it does not absorb at 280 nm (and so may be used for application where UV monitoring of protein content is required), does not interfere with the Lowry estimation of protein and is not labelled during the iodination procedures described above.

Materials and equipment
Radiolabelled viable cells (10^7 lymphocytes, use pro rata and adjust for significant variations in cell-surface area)
Phosphate-buffered saline, PBS (Appendix I), containing 5×10^{-7} M potassium iodide
Renex 30 (Appendix II), 1% v/v in PBS
Protease inhibitors (Section 2.8.1)
High-speed centrifuge, Sorval (Appendix II)

Method
1 Wash the cells three times in PBS by centrifugation (150 *g* for 10 min at 4°) and re-suspend the dry pellet by vortexing.
2 Add 100 µl of Renex solution and mix by vigorous vortexing while adding the protease inhibitors.
3 Leave solubilised cells for 20 min on ice, vortex and then centrifuge at 250 *g* for 10 min at 4° to remove the intact nuclei (and unsolubilised cell membranes, if the detergent was not in excess).
4 Clarify the solubilised membranes by centrifugation at 100 000 *g* for 20 min at 4°.
5 Determine the fraction of total radioactivity associated with protein and also the specific activity, if required, as in Section 2.5.2.
6 Store at $-80°$ until use. The low temperature is preferable to retard proteolytic degradation.

Technical notes
1 During cell-surface iodination, up to 10% of the apparent coupling of ^{125}I is through non-covalent interaction with membrane lipids. A significant proportion of this unwanted label can be exchanged back into the medium during the 20 min incubation on ice.
2 If a gel forms during solubilisation the nuclei have been disrupted, usually because one of the solutions is not isotonic. Ideally start again. However, if the cells are very valuable vortex very violently to try to reduce the viscosity by

shearing the DNA and then add 40 μg ml^{-1} DNAse II and 20 μg ml^{-1} phosphodiesterase (both final concentrations) per 10^7 cells and incubate at room temperature for 30 min. Some proteolytic degradation is inevitable as most nucleases are contaminated with proteinases.

3   Some cells, particularly exotic protozoan parasites, tend to contain membrane-partitioned proteolytic enzymes which can significantly degrade proteins from solubilised cells. In the case of *Trypanosoma cruzi* epimastigotes, the released proteinases can produce a Cleveland peptide map without the need to add V8 proteinase. Consequently, it is advisable to use a good range of proteinase inhibitors (Section 2.8.1), add them with the aid of an assistant while vortexing the cell-detergent mixture, keep everything cold and generally complete the whole procedure as rapidly as possible, prior to storage at −80°.

4   The final protein concentration may be measured by the Lowry technique (Section 1.4.1) as Renex 30, unlike Nonidet P-40 and Triton X-100, does not induce precipitation with the Folin−phenol reagent.

5   Incorporated radioactivity may be measured as in Section 2.5.2. However, lipids, which still might be carrying unexchanged ^{125}I, are precipitated by treatment with trichloroacetic acid (TCA). It is good practice at the beginning of a series of labelling experiments to determine the amount of residual lipid-bound radioactivity by soaking an additional TCA/ethanol-treated filter in 2 ml of a 2 : 1 mixture of chloroform−methanol for 10 min at room temperature prior to drying.

6   Significant losses can occur during washing of the cell pellet. If the cells are destined for immunoprecipitation it is acceptable to reduce the number of washes because of the rigorous washing procedure after the adsorption of the immune complex onto the immunoabsorbent. Even so, the protein-associated radioactivity should be >60% for iodinated cells and >85% for metabolically labelled cells.

7   Renex 30 is often semi-solid at room temperature; if so, warm in 60° water bath prior to use.

2.8.1   Inhibitors of proteolytic degradation

There are four classes of proteolytic enzymes:

serine proteinases
cysteine proteinases
aspartic proteinases
metalloproteinases.

Unless you have detailed knowledge of the range of proteinases present in the cells lysed with detergent, or are attempting to work within a system which relies on one of the classes of protease for its action (for example, blood clotting or complement activation), it is usual to choose a cocktail made up of a range of non-specific inhibitors with activity against each of the above classes of enzymes. The information below will help you to choose a useful combination of inhibitors.

SERINE PROTEINASES

Aprotinin (Trasylol) inhibits plasmin, kallikreins, trypsin and chymotrypsin with high activity; it does not inhibit thrombin or Factor Xa. Phenylmethane sulphonyl-fluoride (PMSF) inactivates a wide variety of enzymes including chymases, tryptases, elastases and serine proteinases of the plasma; for example, the blood coagulation proteinases. The sulphonyl−enzyme derivative is stable at neutral pH but may hydrolyse at non-neutral pH. The reaction of PMSF with enzyme can be slow, and the PMSF can itself undergo spontaneous hydrolysis. Other inhibitors of trypsin-like enzymes are TLCK, an irreversible chloromethyl ketone inhibitor, and soya bean trypsin inhibitor.

CYSTEINE PROTEINASES

p-chloromercuriphenyl sulphonic acid (CMPS) is more soluble than p-chloro-mercuribenzoate (PCMB), but both inhibit sulphydryl-dependent enzymes. N-ethylmaleimide and sodium tetrathionate are less commonly used inhibitors.

ASPARTYL PROTEINASES

Pepstatin is usually employed in inhibitor cocktails to nullify the effects of aspartyl proteinases such as pepsin and cathepsin D. Lysosomal cathepsin D can be a problem in cell homogenates especially if buffers with a pH <7.0 are used.

METALLOPROTEINASES

Ethylenediamine tetra-acetic acid (EDTA) tends to be rather non-selective in cation binding and will chelate Ca, Mg, Cu, Fe, Mo, Zn, etc. Ethylene glycol-bis [β-aminoethyl ether] N, N, N', N'-tetra-acetic acid (EGTA) is more selective than EDTA for Ca. Consequently EGTA can be used to inhibit Ca-dependent enzymes in the presence of Mg-dependent ones; for example, treating serum with EGTA while supplementing the Mg^{2+} levels will inhibit the classical pathway of complement activation but leave the alternative pathway intact. O-phenanthroline shows selectivity towards the chelation of Zn, Fe and to a lesser extent other cations, but does not chelate Ca. Therefore a cocktail with both phenanthroline and EGTA would be more selective than EDTA, and would be Mg sparing.

Greater detail is available in Barrett and Salvensen (1986). See Appendix II for commercial availability of inhibitors from Sigma.

2.9 Immunoprecipitation

The technique of immunoprecipitation may be used to analyse antigens in complex protein mixtures. The combination of antibody specificity and the discrimination of SDS-PAGE fractionation of proteins by molecular weight (Section 2.10) permits an impressive resolution of antigenic moieties. The technique has found many analytical applications because of its relative ease of use and wide applicability. For example, it is possible to determine the molecular weight and distribution of an antigen in various cell populations using a monoclonal antibody. Conversely, the range of antigens recognised during the development of a humoral immune response may be determined by carrying out an immunoprecipitation reaction between the immunising antigen and timed sample bleeds. The technique is usually used to gain quantitative information about the apparent size of polypeptides (Fig. 2.6a) but rarely about their relative abundance (see Section 2.10.2, Technical note 6, p. 72). The resolution of the analysis of antigen in the immune complex can be greatly increased by the combination of isoelectric focusing (Section 6.12) and SDS-PAGE separation (Section 2.10) as illustrated in Fig. 2.6d.

In immunoprecipitation the antigen mixture of interest is usually radioactively labelled, either by exogenous or endogenous (biosynthetic) labelling (Section 2.5) and, if cell associated, is solubilised by the addition of a non-ionic detergent. After high-speed centrifugation to remove aggregates and insoluble material, the antigen of interest may be delineated by the addition of a specific antiserum or monoclonal antibody. Although immune complexes are formed, there is usually no precipitation because of the low concentration of the reactants. Isolation of the complex is achieved by the addition of an affinity particle or bead (for example, whole fixed *Staphylococcus aureus* (Cowan strain) or protein A or anti-immunoglobulin antibody covalently bound to Sepharose 4B followed by centrifugation). After thorough washing, the immune complexes are released by denaturation induced by boiling in the presence of SDS and a reducing agent; for example, dithiothreitol.

Fig. 2.6 (*Facing page*) **SDS-PAGE fractionation of immunoprecipitated cell-surface polypeptides in one- and two-dimensional gels**.
(a) to (c) show the use of different autoradiograph exposure times to gain maximum information from the powerful combination of immunoprecipitation, polyacrylamide gel electrophoresis under denaturing conditions (SDS-PAGE) and autoradiography. In the experiment, a single antiserum and its control were reacted with detergent-solubilised, ^{125}I-labelled polypeptides from three different cell types. After 24 h exposure there was a clear image of the distribution of the polypeptides in the track containing the original mixtures — photograph (a) — but virtually nothing else visible. After 3 days exposure the photographic images of labelled polypeptides were visible in the other lanes — photograph (b) — but the starting material was then overexposed. Photograph (c) shows the result of a collage of both exposures, labelled to identify the tracks and sizes of the molecular weight (MW) standard proteins. It is remarkably difficult to balance the initial loading of each lane in the SDS-PAGE gel, even using c.p.m. per sample. It is not usually possible to predict in advance whether the radioactivity will be associated with few or many polypeptide bands.
(d) The combination of isoelectric focusing and SDS-PAGE results in an analytical technique with exquisite discrimination between polypeptide chains separated both on the basis of their size and charge. In photograph (d) radioactive polypeptides were precipitated by a polyclonal antiserum against the blood stage of the malaria parasite, *Plasmodium yoelii*, and electrofocused under non-reducing conditions in a pH 4.0–7.0 gradient. A strip from this first gel was sealed onto an 12.5% SDS-polyacrylamide gel under denaturing conditions and separated by size. This combined technique resolves mixtures of polypeptide chains which otherwise would run at the same isoelectric point or migrate to the same position in a sizing gel.

Although the tremendous complexity of the protozoan antigens shown in this Figure might seem bewildering and unnerving at first sight, remarkable advances in the characterisation of functionally important molecules have been made by the combination of molecular biological techniques with monoclonal antibodies and also the analysis of the antigen specificity of T-lymphocyte cloned lines and hybridomas (Chapter 12). In this way, a spot on two-dimensional gel can be related not only to the functional protein in the intact organism but also its DNA sequence.

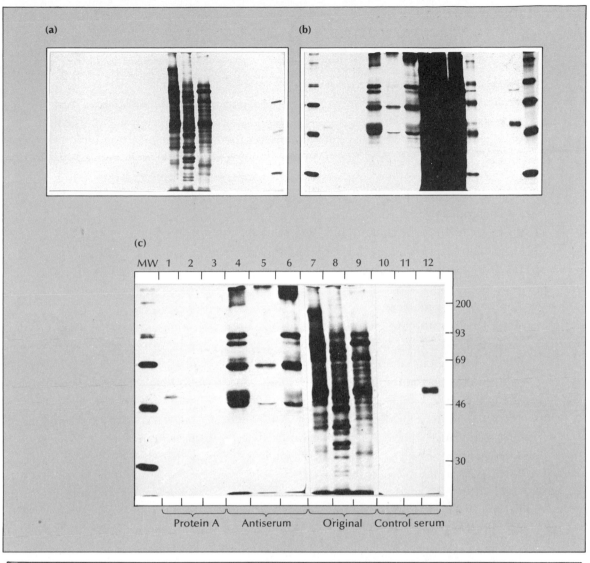

(a)

(b)

(c)

MW 1   2   3   4   5   6   7   8   9   10   11   12

200

93

69

46

30

Protein A   Antiserum   Original   Control serum

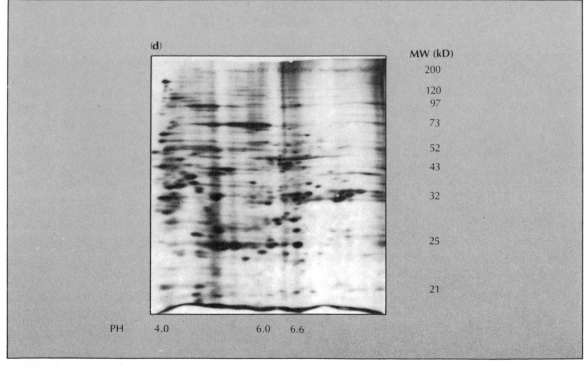

(d)

MW (kD)

200

120
97

73

52

43

32

25

21

PH   4.0   6.0   6.6

PREPARATION IN ADVANCE

1 Radiolabel the antigen mixture or cells using one of the techniques described in Sections 2.5—2.7.

2 If the antigen is cell associated, solubilise the cell pellet in a non-ionic detergent, for example 1% w/v Renex 30 (alternatively Triton X-100 or Nonidet P-40, Section 2.8), in the presence of a cocktail of proteinase inhibitors (Section 2.8.1).

3 Centrifuge at high speed (100 000 g for 20 min) to remove aggregated and insoluble material.

4 Recover the supernatant and determine its content of protein-bound radioisotope (Section 2.5.2).

5 Store at $-80°$ until used.

Materials and equipment

Radiolabelled antigen mixture

Affinity beads; for example, protein A—Sepharose (Appendix II)

Poly- or monoclonal antibody, with relevant control

Affinity-purified anti-immunoglobulin and control antibodies, if required

Sodium dodecyl sulphate, SDS, in water, 20% w/v

Non-ionic detergent; for example, Renex 30

Microcentrifuge tubes, 1.5 ml (Appendix II)

Microcentrifuge; for example, Microcentaur (Appendix II)

Mixing rotor for microcentrifuge tubes

Method

1 Dissolve 220 mg of EDTA in a minimum volume of water and adjust the pH of the solution to neutrality with 0.1 M sodium hydroxide.

2 Weigh 8.7 g of sodium chloride into a 500 ml measuring cylinder, add 30 ml of 10-fold concentrated PBS and 3 ml of Renex 30. Wash the EDTA solution into this mixture and adjust the final volume of the solution to 300 ml (high-salt buffer).

3 Dissolve 100 mg of bovine serum albumin, BSA, in 100 ml of high-salt buffer (BSA buffer).

4 Add 0.25 ml of 20% w/v SDS to 100 ml of high-salt buffer (SDS buffer).

5 Mix the detergent-solubilised radiolabelled antigens with a half-packed volume of Sephadex immunoadsorbent (previously washed with phosphate-buffered saline containing 2% w/v Renex and 2 mg ml^{-1} BSA) and mix for 30 min at 4° on a rotor.

6 Recover the supernatant by microcentrifugation and dispense aliquots containing approximately 10^6 c.p.m. into each assay tube to be used.

7 Add an aliquot of the first antibody (5 µl of a polyclonal antiserum or ascitic fluid containing a monoclonal antibody, alternatively 100 µl of tissue culture supernatant from a hybridoma line) and incubate on ice (5 min for a monoclonal antibody or 15 min for an antiserum).

8 If required, add 2 µl of affinity-purified anti-immunoglobulin antibody (10 mg ml^{-1}) (Section 9.2) and incubate on ice for 5 min.

9   Add 30 µl of 50% v/v protein A—Sepharose to each tube, mix by vortexing and incubate for 30 min at 4° on a mixing rotor.

10 Wash the Sepharose free of unbound proteins by two cycles of centrifugation and re-suspension in each of the following buffers: BSA buffer, high-salt buffer, SDS buffer and finally PBS alone.

11 The dry pellet may be stored at −80° or processed immediately for SDS-PAGE analysis (Section 2.10).

Technical notes

1   It is essential to include appropriate controls for each antibody used in this assay. Although normal serum is acceptable as a control for unfractionated polyclonal serum, it is essential to match a monoclonal antibody with an irrelevant monoclonal antibody of the *same isotype*. Similarly, the appropriate control for affinity-purified anti-immunoglobulin antibodies is affinity-purified irrelevant antibodies

2   If the first antibody used in this reaction binds directly to the affinity bead or particle, then an anti-immunoglobulin second antibody is not required.

3   Three main parameters influence the apparent difference between specific and non-specific adsorption: the length of the incubation period with antibody, the amount of total protein present (purified antibody versus whole serum, or whether a second anti-immunoglobulin is used or not) and the stringency of the washing procedure. If the antisera used are weak, incubation periods may be extended up to 24 h. The washing cycle needs to be particularly thorough because of the fine point of the microcentrifuge tube; it is advisable to re-suspend the dry cell pellet prior to the addition of washing buffer.

4   Renex is often semi-solid at room temperature — warm in a 60° water bath prior to dispensing.

5   If *Staphylococcus aureus* is used as the affinity particle, it is important to note that some proteins react directly with the bacterial cell wall. Consequently, pre-absorption of the radiolabelled proteins with a strain of the bacterium not producing protein A is necessary.

6   No matter what affinity particle is used, it is good practice to wash a portion of the pre-absorption pellet in parallel with the rest of the assay and analyse any bound protein in the same SDS-PAGE gel as the antibody-treated samples. The results do not necessarily merit publication, but might save embarrassment.

2.10 SDS polyacrylamide gel electrophoresis

In electrophoresis the migration of proteins is dependent upon the charge, size and shape of the molecules. However, in the presence of sodium dodecyl sulphate (SDS), proteins bind the SDS, all become negatively charged and have similar charge: weight ratios. When SDS-coated proteins are placed in an electric field, their spatial separation will depend only upon their size and shape. By varying the concentration of the polyacrylamide gel, used as the medium for the electrophoretic separation, different resolution ranges of molecular weights may be obtained. Proteins may be fractionated in the native state, but better resolution is usually obtained if the disulphide bonds are first reduced, allowing separation of the individual peptide chains. After heating to 100° in the presence of reducing agents and SDS, the proteins unfold and bind about 1.4 g SDS g^{-1} protein. The strong negative charge on the proteins thus means that their electrophoretic mobility will be inversely proportional to the logarithm of their molecular weight. There are exceptions to this behaviour: (a) heavily glycosylated proteins bind less SDS than unglycosylated molecules of similar molecular weight; (b) some proteins, such as J chains, do not unfold completely and retain some of their native configuration.

In practical terms, a stacking gel is cast on the top of the separating gel, this has both a lower percentage polyacrylamide concentration (typically, between 3 and 5%) and is prepared using a buffer with a slightly different composition. The different mobilities of chloride and glycine and the slow rate of entry into the separating gel relative to the rate of progression through the stacking gel are exploited to concentrate the proteins in a narrow band at the interface between the stacking and separating gels. This allows the loading of variable volumes of sample.

Originally the technique was performed in gel tubes but these have almost entirely been replaced by flat gel slabs. Many manufacturers now produce apparatus for casting and running the gels.

A large improvement in resolution can be obtained by running a two-dimensional gel in which the proteins are first separated by isoelectric focusing in the absence of reducing agents (Section 6.12) and then electrophoresed in a second direction, at right angles to the first, under reducing conditions (Fig. 2.6d). This allows the determination of the molecular weight of a protein in its multi-chain structure and also the composition and weight of its individual chains.

Materials and equipment
Vertical slab gel system (Appendix II)
Acrylamide
N,N′-methylenebis acrylamide
3.0 M Tris—HCl buffer, pH 8.7 (Appendix I)
1.0 M Tris—HCl buffer, pH 6.8 (Appendix I)
EDTA
Sodium dodecyl sulphate, SDS
N,N,N′,N′-tetramethylethylene diamine, TEMED
Water-saturated butan-3-ol
Ammonium persulphate
Bromophenol blue
Sucrose

Solutions	Separating gels				Stacking gel 5%
	15%	10%	7.5%	6%	
40% acrylamide	11.25	7.5	5.6	4.5	1.25
1% bis acrylamide	7.8	7.8	7.8	7.8	1.3
3 M Tris−HCl pH 8.7	3.75	3.75	3.75	3.75	1.25*
10% ammonium persulphate	0.2	0.2	0.2	0.2	0.1
Distilled H_2O	6.84	10.35	12.25	13.35	5.0
20% SDS	0.15	0.15	0.15	0.15	0.05
TEMED	0.02	0.02	0.02	0.02	0.01
100 mM EDTA	—	—	—	—	1.0
Molecular weight range	8000−50 000	20 000−100 000	40 000−150 000	55 000−175 000	

* Use 1 M Tris−HCl buffer for the stacking gel.

CASTING THE GEL

1 Wash thoroughly plates, spacers, etc., rinse in distilled water, air dry. Rinse in 70% ethanol and dry.

2 Assemble the slab gel mould, check it is vertical.

3 Mix the solutions for the separating gel according to the table above, but omit the SDS and TEMED at this stage. The precise final volume of reagents needed will depend on the type of equipment being used, but the table gives a guide to the proportions required to produce gels for separation in various molecular weight ranges.

4 De-gas the solution under vacuum.

5 Add the SDS and TEMED and run the solution between the plates; within 4 cm of the top of the plates. Take care to avoid air bubbles.

6 Overlay the top of the separation gel with aqueous isobutanol (butan-3-ol saturated with distilled water). This reduces surface tension and ensures that the polymerised gel will have a flat surface.

7 Leave to polymerise for about 30−60 min and then wash off the butanol with three changes of distilled water and dry the surface carefully with filter paper. Alternatively, prepare an excess of stacking gel solution and use this to rinse away all traces of the isobutanol.

8 Mix the stacking gel and de-gas under vacuum prior to the addition of TEMED and SDS, pour into the mould over the separating gel and insert the plastic comb to form the sample wells. Leave the stacking gel to polymerise for 30 min.

SAMPLE PREPARATION

Materials
Polyacrylamide sample buffer (Appendix I)
Dithiothreitol
Bromophenol blue
Molecular weight standards; for example, rainbow markers (Appendix II)

Method

1 If the sample to be analysed is in a strong buffer, dialyse it against sample buffer, otherwise proceed to step 2.
2 Add 40 μl sample (containing 2–20 μg protein) to 20 μl of sample buffer (containing 31 mg ml^{-1} dithiothreitol) and 3 μl bromophenol blue (1 mg ml^{-1} in water). For unreduced samples omit the dithiothreitol.
3 Prepare the molecular weight standards in the same way.
4 Heat for 3 min in a boiling water bath.

RUNNING THE GEL

Materials and equipment
Power supply (Appendix II)
Gas-tight glass syringe (50 μl) (Appendix II)
Plastic capillary tubing (Appendix II)
Polyacrylamide running buffer: Tris–glycine, pH 8.3, containing 3 ml 20% sodium dodecyl sulphate, SDS, per 600 ml buffer (Appendix I)

Method

1 Carefully remove the comb from the polymerised gel, clean wells of any unpolymerised acrylamide with running buffer, mount the gel plate in the electrophoresis apparatus and fill with running buffer.
2 Add samples to wells using a 50 μl syringe with plastic capillary tubing or a fine pipette. Do not forget the molecular weight standards.
3 Connect to power supply with anode at the bottom. Run at constant current: 20 mA while the sample is in the stacking gel and 40 mA after it enters the separating gel. The precise power requirements will vary with the length and thickness of gel and whether the apparatus has a cooling plattern.
4 Once the bromophenol blue marker dye is approximately 1 cm from the bottom of the gel, turn off the power and remove the gel either for fixation and staining (Section 2.10.1) or electrophoretic transfer to nitrocellulose (Section 2.11).

Technical notes

1 Although this is a relatively robust technique, it is prone to artifacts from various sources. If too much current is applied to speed separation, then heating effects can distort the separation pattern and are seen as a horizontal wave pattern after protein staining. Either use cooling or reduce the current across the gel. Individual tracks are sometimes seen to give vertical streaks, this is due to a high salt content in the initial sample allowing a local increase in the current. This may be corrected by sample dialysis against the running buffer.
2 Samples in the outside tracks may show an upward curve in their polypeptide bands due to greater electrical resistance at the edge of the gel. This is usually only a problem if the gel is being run to analyse and compare complex protein mixtures. This may be eliminated by running a sample of an irrelevant protein, such as bovine serum albumin, in the outside tracks.
3 It is possible to prepare an 'in-house' mixture of molecular weight standards by

buying pure proteins from one of the chemical suppliers. In addition, these can be radiolabelled using ^{14}C-formaldehyde (Appendix II). However, commercial mixtures are now available which contain intensely dyed proteins. It is therefore possible to monitor the progress of polypeptide bands across the whole gel during electrophoresis.

2.10.1 Staining and molecular weight estimation

If you wish to locate and recover a particular polypeptide band; for example, for use in T-lymphocyte stimulation assays, we recommend the use of Aurodye (Appendix II) rather than the methods described below. This procedure is said to be as sensitive as silver staining and yet does not affect mitogenesis assays (Section 12.16).

Proteins (minimum detection limit 1 µg)

Materials
Methanol
Acetic acid
Coomassie blue

Method
1 Fix the gel in a mixture of 40% methanol, 10% acetic acid for 4 h.
2 Stain in 0.1% w/v Coomassie blue in methanol—acetic acid for 5 h.
3 De-stain in 30% methanol, 10% acetic acid for 2 h.
4 Complete the de-staining in 10% methanol, 10% acetic acid.
5 Re-swell and store in 7% acetic acid.

Carbohydrates (minimum detection limit 5 µg)

Materials
Methanol
Acetic acid
Periodic acid
Schiff's reagent
Sodium metabisulphite

Method
1 Fix gel in 40% methanol, 20% acetic acid for 4 h.
2 Re-swell in 7% acetic acid.
3 Oxidise in a mixture of 1% periodic acid in 7% acetic acid for 1 h in the dark.
4 Wash in 7% acetic acid for 24 h, changing the wash several times.
5 Stain with Schiff's reagent at 4° for 1 h in the dark.
6 Differentiate in 1% w/v sodium metabisulphite in 0.1 M hydrochloric acid.

The apparent relative molecular weight (app. MW$_r$) of unknown polypeptide or glycopeptide bands may be determined by reference to the set of internal standards which should be run in each gel.

1 Identify each polypeptide band in the track of molecular weight standards and measure its migration distance from the interface between the stacking and separating gels.
2 Plot a graph of log molecular weight against distance travelled and use this to read back from the distance travelled by the unknown band to its log molecular weight.

Technical notes
1 The molecular mass estimate determined by this technique is an apparent relative molecular weight as it is obtained by comparison with the set of molecular weight marker proteins run in the same gel. The value thus obtained should be expressed as a simple number, without units.
2 Size determination by this technique can produce surprising and dramatic deviations from reality, due to artifacts produced by unexpected behaviour or unrecognised peculiarities of the unknown protein, for example:
(a) Unfolding of a protein mixture to random coils may occur to different degrees.
(b) Inactivation of proteinases from cell-based assays may be incomplete, thus permitting protein degradation during sample preparation. Some proteinases are poorly inactivated by boiling and SDS treatment; consequently, the unfolded proteins are likely to be even more susceptible to proteolytic cleavage than in their native state.
(c) The unknown proteins might be heavily glycosylated or phosphorylated and so not show the full charge for weight gain expected after SDS treatment. When some glycophosphoproteins have been compared as native proteins and *in vitro* translation products by this technique, the latter show increased app. MW$_r$, even though the molecular mass of the unglycosylated and unphosphorylated *in vitro*-derived protein is smaller.
3 A reducing agent, dithiothreitol or 2-mercaptoethanol, is included to reduce both inter- and intrachain disulphide bonds. Remember to include unreduced samples when analysing unknown proteins by this technique.

2.10.2 Autoradiography and fluorography

Although direct visualisation of proteins and glycoproteins in SDS-PAGE gels has many applications, the utility and sensitivity of the technique can be greatly increased by the use of radioactively labelled molecules, particularly in combination with immunoprecipitation (Section 2.9). It is also possible to convert this essentially qualitative technique into a quantitative one, as explained in Technical note 6.

DIRECT AUTORADIOGRAPHY

Materials and equipment
SDS-PAGE gel, containing radioactively labelled proteins
X-ray film (Appendix II)
Polyacrylamide gel drier (Appendix II)
3MM paper (Appendix II)
Cling film or Saran wrap
Intensifying screen (Appendix II)
Metal X-ray cassette (Appendix II)

Method
1 Remove the polyacrylamide gel from the electrophoresis apparatus and cut away the stacking gel with a scalpel blade.
2 Fix the gel for 4 h in an aqueous solution of 40% v/v methanol and 10% v/v acetic acid and then soak for 15 min in a 5% solution of acetic acid containing 0.1% glycerol.
3 Lay the gel on a sheet of water-saturated 3MM paper just larger than the gel and cover with a sheet of cling film. Take care to remove all excess water and air bubbles before trimming away the excess cling film with a scalpel blade.
4 Seal the gel into a commercial drier, preferably connected to a high-efficiency oil vacuum pump via two solid CO_2/acetone water traps. A water vacuum pump will do, provided the water pressure is high enough.
5 Turn on the vacuum and heating and dry the gel completely. This may be determined by the change in profile of the gel or when the gel no longer feels cool to the touch, in each case as judged through the rubber sheet of the drier. Do not release the vacuum until the gel is hot.
6 In the dark room, load a metal X-ray cassette with an intensifying screen (if required, see Technical note 2), film and the gel (face down on the film).
7 If an intensifying screen has been used put the cassette at $-70°$, otherwise leave it at room temperature away from direct sunlight, volatile chemicals and any external source of penetrating radiation.
8 Develop the X-ray film according to the manufacturer's instructions. The length of exposure will vary according to the type and amount of radioactivity and should be determined empirically. In some gels, it might be necessary to have both a long and short exposure to gain maximum information; for example, see Fig. 2.6.
9 Blackening of the film in areas corresponding to the protein tracks may be used to infer the presence of radioactive material in the original gel.

Technical notes
1 Direct autoradiography is only possible with the penetrating radiations emanating from ^{131}I, ^{125}I, ^{32}P, etc. Weaker emitters ^{14}C, ^{35}S, ^{3}H, etc. require fluorography; see below.
2 The sensitivity of detection may be increased by the use of:

(a)   Intensifying screens. These are plastic sheets impregnated with heavy metal ion phosphor crystals and are used to trap radiations which pass through the X-ray film. As a consequence, they emit photons and so blacken the X-ray film on the side away from the polyacrylamide gel. In principle, it is possible to use two intensifying screens, one on either side of the film. In practice, however, this can blur the final image because of the greater distance travelled by the radioactive and photon radiations.

(b)   Pre-flashed film. X-ray film is relatively insensitive and therefore single silver atoms may be induced in the silver halide crystals by transient exposure to an electronic flash. The duration of the flash and its intensity (varied by changing the distance between film and electronic flash gun) is critical and should be determined empirically. Set the shortest duration on the flash gun and position the gun at varying distances (increasing in steps of 1 m) from film test strips. Develop the film (and a piece of unflashed original) and use the conditions which just give barely visible fogging.

Exposure of the gel with intensifying screens and pre-flashed film at $-70°$ gives maximal stability both of the nascent image and the sensitised pre-flashed areas.

3   It is convenient to use a mixture of radioactive-purified proteins as molecular weight markers in these gels. Suitable mixtures for different fractionation ranges may either be bought commercially as a ^{14}C-methylated protein mixture (Appendix II) or prepared from an 'in-house' mix of purified proteins treated with ^{14}C-formaldehyde (Appendix II). Intensely coloured 'rainbow markers', which are also radioactive, are available commercially (Appendix II) and offer the dual convenience of visibility during electrophoretic separation and fogging of the X-ray film.

4   Much has been written about the artifacts associated with autoradiography. The two most commonly seen are:

(a)   A homogeneous fogging of the film, often in areas away from contact with the gel. This is due to chemical fogging and probably means that the acetic acid failed to volatilise during drying. Dry the gel with a hot air drier and re-expose to X-ray film.

(b)   Lightning strikes. This is caused by an electrostatic discharge either from your fingers or dampness causing the surfaces of the gel, screen or film to adhere. When you peel the surfaces apart an electrostatic charge is generated. Earth your fingers by touching the bench and make sure the interior of the cassette is warm and dry — especially if it has been exposed at $-70°$ — before you open it.

5   If your cassettes are used communally, it is a wise precaution to line them with plastic benchcote or candy paper. If one becomes contaminated then the liner rather than the cassette can be replaced. Similarly, it is good practice to clean the intensifying screens regularly with an anti-static screen cleaner (Appendix II).

6   As noted in Fig. 2.6, this technique is usually used qualitatively; however, it is relatively simple to quantitate the radioactivity contained in the gel, although there is considerable loss of sensitivity. If you intend to measure the radioactivity, it is helpful to stain the gel, as described in Section 2.10.1, prior to drying the

gel down. This will help you to locate the individual tracks. Remember that quantitation can be carried out after the gel has been exposed to X-ray film, provided that sufficient radioactivity remains.

a   Lay the stained, dried gel on a glass plate and cut it up into its individual lanes using a scalpel blade and straight edge.

b   Cut strips of 1 mm tracing graph paper approximately the same size as the gel tracks.

c   Use spray adhesive to attach a strip of graph paper to each gel track, at right angles to the polypeptide bands.

d   Cut each track into 1 mm strips using a sharp pair of scissors and place each strip in a labelled tube suitable for γ counting.

e   Count in a γ spectrometer and plot a graph of the amount of radioactivity against the distance travelled down the gel.

f   Compare the result with that obtained from the X-ray film.

FLUOROGRAPHY

Weak α and β emitters would be detected very inefficiently by direct autoradiography because of the relatively short distances travelled by these radiations. Instead, a scintillant is incorporated directly into the gel and the energy from the decay of the radioisotope is transferred to the X-ray film as photons of light. In the original method for gel impregnation, the scintillant (usually 2,5-diphenyloxazole, PPO) was dissolved in dimethyl sulphoxide (DMSO), thus causing considerable shrinkage and distortion of the gel. However, aqueous preparations are now commercially available (for example, Enlightening Fluid — New England Nuclear, or Amplify — Amersham International, Appendix II. In both instances available as liquid or spray.) The gel is fixed in an aqueous solution of methanol—acetic acid as above and then soaked in the scintillant solution for 20 min. After drying (without glycerol), the gel is loaded into a metal cassette with X-ray film and exposed at −70°.

2.11   Immuno- or Western blotting

In this technique a sheet of nitrocellulose is placed against the surface of an SDS-PAGE protein fractionation gel and a current applied across the gel (at right angles to its face), thus causing the proteins to move out of the gel and onto the nitrocellulose where they bind firmly by non-covalent forces. Two variants of the basic apparatus are available to accomplish this electrophoretic transfer, the so-called wet and semi-dry blotters. In wet blotters the gel and transfer membrane are immersed in large volumes of buffer whereas semi-dry blotters use only filter paper pads moistened with buffer.

Materials and equipment
Wet blotting apparatus (Appendix II)
Polyacrylamide running buffer, 0.1 M Tris—glycine, pH 8.3, with 500 ml methanol added to 2 litres buffer (Appendix I)

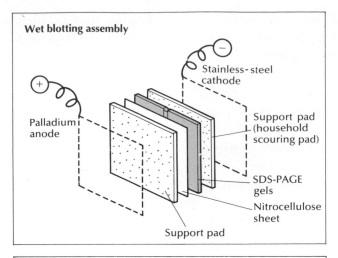

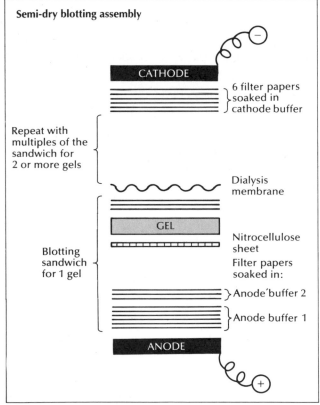

Fig. 2.7 Assembly sequence for sandwich for wet and semi-dry blotting. The precise details of the components will vary with the apparatus used; however, the order of assembly—anode, nitrocellulose sheet, SDS-PAGE gel, cathode — is vital. If reversed by mistake, the carefully separated proteins will be electrophoretically transferred to 5 litres of tank buffer.

The semi-dry blotter not only avoids the use of large volumes of buffer but also can be run as a sandwich of several gel : nitrocellulose sheets interspersed with low molecular weight cut-off dialysis membranes. The dialysis membrane permits the passage of ions but not of proteins.

Nitrocellulose paper (Appendix II)
Whatman No. 1 filter paper (Appendix II)
Scotch-brite pads (Appendix II)

Method

1   Equilibrate the SDS-PAGE gel (containing the fractionated protein) in blotting buffer for 30—60 min.

2 Assemble the blotting sandwich within the blotting cassette taking in order: Scotch-brite pad, nitrocellulose sheet, polyacrylamide gel, and Scotch-brite pad (anode → cathode) (Fig. 2.7). Take care to avoid any air bubbles between the gel and the nitrocellulose.

3 Insert the cassette into the blotting buffer and connect the power supply. The cathode should be on the gel side.

4 Blot for about 3 h at 60 V or overnight at 35 V.

Technical notes

1 Methanol is used in the blotting buffer to prevent the gel swelling.

2 Take great care to ensure that the blotting cassette is assembled in the correct order. Proteins transferred into the filter pads rather than the nitrocellulose will be lost.

3 It is good practice to stain the gel for proteins after blotting over, to ensure that the transfer was complete. Some proteins, for example the relatively insoluble cytoskeletal components, tend to transfer inefficiently and non-quantitatively.

4 Blots may be dried, sealed in a plastic bag and stored at −20° for up to 6 months.

2.11.1 Staining Western blots

Blots may be stained with the usual protein stains but, if it is intended to visualise the polypeptide bands by deposition of enzymically generated colours, 0.02% Ponceau S can be used as a temporary stain. This is usually applied in 3% trichloroacetic acid, which may cause some protein denaturation. The blots are differentiated in running tap water. The stain is completely reversible and removed by washing in tap water.

2.11.2 Blocking protein-binding sites

Before visualisation of protein bands with labelled antibodies it is necessary to block the remaining protein-binding sites on the nitrocellulose. Bovine serum albumin, haemoglobin or skimmed milk powder are frequently used for blocking, sometimes with the addition of 0.05% Tween 20. Tween 20 alone is used by some investigators and has the advantage that, after visualisation with specific antibodies, the whole blot can be stained with protein stains. This provides the double advantage of not only revealing the markers for molecular weight determination but also allowing the visualisation of protein bands which have failed to bind antibody. Unfortunately, Tween alone is not an efficient blocking agent, so when concentrated protein solutions are used, such as serum or ascitic fluid, the background can be unacceptably high.

Materials and equipment

Phosphate-buffered saline, PBS, containing 0.05% Tween 20 and 1% w/v bovine serum albumin, BSA

Plastic box

Method

Place the nitrocellulose blot in the PBS−Tween−BSA and gently rotate on an orbital shaker for about 2 h at room temperature, or overnight in the cold.

2.11.3 Immunostaining nitrocellulose blots

Although proteins separated by SDS-PAGE and blotted onto nitrocellulose have been subjected to harsh denaturing conditions (detergent treatment, boiling, reducing agents and distortion due to adsorption to the highly charged surface of the nitrocellulose membrane) a large proportion of antigenic determinants remain intact and can be revealed by the addition of labelled antibodies. In the past, radiolabelled antibodies or antibodies detected by radiolabelled protein A have been extensively used. Although the technique offers high sensitivity, preparation for autoradiography can be complex and time consuming and carries with it the problems of chronic exposure to low levels of radioactivity. Techniques for the use of enzyme-labelled antibodies have been improved greatly and a range of substrates developed which are not carcinogenic and can be used to deposit a variety of coloured, insoluble products on top of the protein band.

Biotinylated antibodies followed by streptavidin−peroxidase give well-visualised bands with 4-chloro-1-naphthanol as substrate. Carbohydrate determinants maintain their immunogenic properties after SDS-PAGE fractionation and can be detected with biotinylated lectins or antibodies.

Materials

Nitrocellulose blot with immunoglobulin bands

Biotinylated antibody; for example, biotinylated goat anti-human IgG (Appendix II)

Streptavidin−peroxidase (Appendix II)

Phosphate-buffered saline, PBS (Appendix I) containing 0.05% v/v Tween 20 with and without 1% w/v bovine serum albumin, BSA (PBS−Tween−BSA)

4-chloro-1-naphthanol

0.05 M Tris−HCl buffer, pH 7.6 (Appendix I)

Hydrogen peroxide

Method

1   Prepare a dilution of biotinylated antibody in PBS−Tween−BSA; as a guide, high-titred antibodies can be used at a dilution of 1 : 1000. Prepare a sufficient volume of diluted antibody to cover the blot.

2   Immerse the blot in the antibody solution and agitate gently for 2 h on an orbital shaker.

3   Wash the blot thoroughly by immersing in excess PBS−Tween (0.05%); *no* BSA. Mix gently for 10 min on the orbital shaker.

4   Repeat the wash step three more times.

5   Add sufficient streptavidin−peroxidase conjugate (diluted 1 : 1000 in PBS−Tween−BSA) to cover the blot. Mix gently for 1 h on the orbital shaker.

6   Wash the blot by immersing in four changes of PBS—Tween as before.

7   During the final wash prepare the substrate solution by dissolving 6 mg 4-chloro-1-naphthanol in 20 ml methanol and adding it to 100 ml Tris—HCl buffer pH 7.6 plus 12 µl hydrogen peroxide (30 volumes strength).

8   Immerse the washed blot in the substrate solution. Mix gently on the orbital shaker. Bands should develop sufficient colour within a few minutes.

9   Remove the blot and wash with distilled water.

10 Dry the blot and analyse immediately. Although the coloured bands fade with time, the rate of colour loss can be retarded if the blots are kept in the dark.

Technical notes

1   If the antibody is expensive, or the supply limited, a smaller volume of diluted antibody may be applied to the nitrocellulose sheet by means of saturated filter paper. It is essential to achieve good contact between the paper and the nitrocellulose. This may be achieved by sealing the nitrocellulose—filter paper sandwich into a plastic bag or by clamping it between two glass slides.

2   Some of the substrates still in use are known carcinogens; for example, bis diazotized benzidine. *These should only be handled in a fume cupboard.*

3   The colour reaction can be quantitated by scanning densitometry and a permanent record made by photography.

2.11.4   Western blotting with radiolabelled probes

1   Proceed as method above but at step 5 add ^{125}I-streptavidin instead of the enzyme-labelled material. Use about 1×10^6 c.p.m. per track.

2   After washing, dry the blot for 10—20 min between filter papers.

3   Wrap in cling film and insert into an X-ray cassette with autoradiographic film.

4   Leave the autoradiograph to expose at −70° for between 12 h and 1 week depending upon the amount of radioactivity bound. Develop the film according to the manufacturer's instructions.

A typical result is shown in Fig. 2.8.

Technical notes

1   The sensitivity of the detection system may be increased using:

(a) Pre-flashed film. The duration of the flash and its intensity (varied by changing the distance between film and electronic flash gun) is critical and should be determined empirically. Set the shortest duration on the flash gun and position the gun at varying distances (increasing in steps of 1 m) from film test strips. Develop the film and use the conditions which just give barely visible fogging. Exposure of pre-flashed film at −70° gives maximal stability both of the nascent image and the sensitised pre-flashed areas.

(b) Intensifying screens. Screens should be placed on either side of the blot—film sandwich. The screens are impregnated with heavy metal ions coupled to a

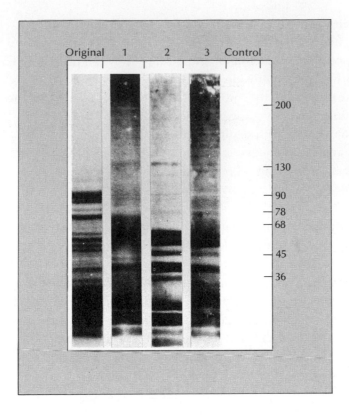

Fig. 2.8 **Immunoblotting with polyclonal sera.** The photograph shows autoradiographs of a detergent-solubilised cell population treated with different antisera. Original: a strip from the nitrocellulose sheet was stained with Coomassie blue to confirm that efficient electrophoretic transfer had taken place. Strips 1–3 and control were treated with different polyclonal antisera or normal rabbit serum, respectively, and the bound antibody detected by ^{125}I-labelled protein A. The migration distance of molecular weight standards was determined by separating a mixture of standard proteins in the original gel and blotting over on to the nitrocellulose sheet prior to Coomassie blue staining. Numbers show molecular weights in kDa.

scintillation system. The efficiency of capture of the emitted radiations is therefore increased and more of them are recorded on the X-ray film because of the photon emissions from the screens. Screens are important for the efficient capture of ^{131}I.

2 The system described above may also be adapted for analysis using ^{125}I-labelled antibodies or unlabelled antibodies detected by ^{125}I-labelled protein A.

2.12 Immunoprecipitation versus immunoblotting

Relatively few studies have been published which have compared these two techniques directly. Immunoblotting is technically more convenient as it does not involve repeated centrifugation and, at least theoretically, might be expected to be more sensitive than immunoprecipitation because it involves antigen presentation on a solid support, thus allowing antibody to bind in a multi-valent, essentially affinity-independent manner. However, in immunoblotting, solubilisation of cell-bound polypeptides relies on harsh denaturing treatment with an ionic detergent with boiling under reducing conditions. Although electrophoretic transfer probably removes most of the detergent and reducing agent, the strong non-covalent forces which bind the polypeptide to the nitrocellulose probably prevent complete renaturation. Thus immunoblotting is likely to favour 'sequence' determinants, whereas immunoprecipitation is likely to permit the detection of both 'sequence' and 'conformational' determinants.

In a direct comparison using polyclonal antisera, both techniques were equally efficient at detecting epitopes on relatively low molecular weight antigens (<50 kDa); however, immunoprecipitation gave more consistent results with epitopes on polypeptides >50 kDa.

2.13   Antibodies in molecular biology

Although the majority of techniques in molecular biology are beyond the scope of this book, some of the contributions of immunology to this important discipline deserve mention.

Foremost of the contributions must be the whole technology for the production and use of monoclonal antibodies. If monoclonal antibodies had not pre-existed, then they would certainly have had to be invented for molecular biology. Similarly, the ability of polyclonal sera to 'view' a polypeptide as a series of discrete epitopes has been crucially important for the detection of incompletely expressed protein sequences fused in the middle of completely unrelated proteins. Antibodies not only provide a means for defining and testing the function of previously unknown protein molecules but also provide an essential tool for the characterisation of the protein via recombinant DNA technology.

2.13.1   Analysis of *in vitro* translation products

The routes from the first definition of an antigen, for example a novel, functionally important cell-surface glycoprotein, to a full determination of its amino acid sequence are now well established. Often the first step in characterisation is to determine its apparent molecular weight by immunoprecipitation (Section 2.9) and SDS-PAGE analysis (Section 2.10). However, several important questions need to be resolved before attempting the full cycle of cloning, expression and sequencing, for example:
(a)   Does the cell really make the antigen or has it been acquired exogenously?
(b)   Is the antigenic determinant protein or carbohydrate based?
(c)   Is the epitope sequence or conformation based? If the latter is the case then it is unlikely that the antibody would react with the unglycosylated, incomplete segment of the original molecule expressed in the middle of a bacterial protein. Immunoprecipitation of *in vitro* translation products from cell-derived mRNA not only definitively resolves these questions but also provides confirmation that the mRNA is acceptable for the preparation of cDNA.

A typical result is shown in Fig. 2.9; mRNA was extracted from the cell expressing the antigen of interest and mixed with ^{35}S-methionine and micrococcal nuclease-treated rabbit reticulocyte lysate (the latter is a rich source of all the molecules to make protein, but devoid of the 'message'). The polypeptides synthesised *in vitro* have been visualised by fluorography after immunoprecipitation and SDS-PAGE analysis. Significantly, the photograph shows discrete polypeptides some of which are in excess of 90 kDa apparent molecular weight, indicating that the mRNA is in

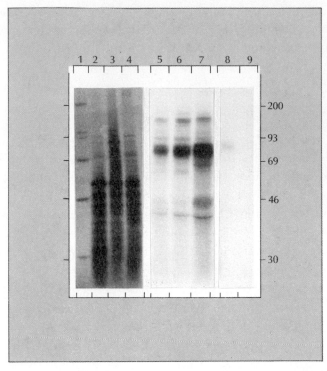

Fig. 2.9 Immunoprecipitation of *in vitro* translation products. Messenger RNA, extracted from three different life-cycle stages of a protozoan parasite, was translated *in vitro* in the presence of ^{35}S methionine. The resulting polypeptides were fractionated on an SDS-PAGE gel, either immediately (tracks 2–4), after inmunoprecipitation with a monoclonal antibody (tracks 5–9) which reacts with a polypeptide in a single life-cycle stage (track 4) or an irrelevant antibody (result not shown). Track 1 contains radioactively labelled molecular weight standards; molecular weight is in thousands and migration position indicated by arrow heads.

Tracks 2–4 show polypeptides in the starting material with molecular weight up to 100 000, indicating good translation. Tracks 5–7 show the effect of increasing the amount of monoclonal antibody added as ascitic fluid. Although the 85 kD band increases in intensity, so does the non-specific binding. Tracks 8 and 9 show the lack of binding of the antibody to the other life-cycle stages (represented in tracks 2 and 3).

good condition. The single, large polypeptide band precipitated by the monoclonal antibody, which is slightly smaller than that synthesised by intact cells (not shown), confirms that the epitope is not carbohydrate dependent, either directly or for its conformation. The techniques for *in vitro* translation are explained in full in Hames and Higgins (1984).

2.13.2 Screening of expression libraries

Antibody can provide a powerful tool by which a mature molecule, for example a cell-surface glycoprotein expressed by a eukaryotic cell, can be related to a set of partial sequences expressed in bacterial fusion proteins. Although the molecular biological background to the manipulations described below is outside the scope of this book, we have used this technique to identify the immunological pitfalls which can result in the unwary investigator cloning a sequence which is unrelated to either the antibody used for screening or the original molecule against which the antibody was generated. The method described was used to screen a cDNA library from a protozoan parasite expressed in the bacteriophage λ gt11. The methods in recombinant DNA technology referred to below are fully described in Glover (1985) or Davis *et al.* (1986).

PREPARATION IN ADVANCE

1   Calculate the titre of the recombinant phage stock and dilute to produce about 300 discrete plaques per plate (adjust the total number per plate according to the size of the plaques).

2   Grow up a stock of the *Escherichia coli* (Y1090) plating cells and mix an aliquot with the appropriate dilution of phage and plate out.

3   Incubate the culture plates at 42° until plaques appear (between 3 and 4 h, but longer if the *E. coli* had been cooled for storage).

4   Transfer the cultures to a 37° incubator, overlay each plate with a sterile, IPTG-impregnated nitrocellulose filter (previously soaked in 10 mM IPTG and dried before use) and incubate overnight to induce fusion protein expression.

5   Before removing the filters, use a syringe loaded with dye and fitted with a large gauge needle to pierce each filter at three places round its periphery to provide orientation marks in the filter and agar. (By this means it will ultimately be possible to match up the black spots on the autoradiograph or coloured spots on the filter with phage plaques on the original culture plate.)

6   Unless you are using a monoclonal antibody produced *in vitro*, it will be necessary to exhaustively absorb all antisera or ascitic fluids to remove the naturally occurring anti-*E. coli* and anti-bacteriophage antibodies. Commercial preparations are now available (Appendix II) which will allow this to be accomplished conveniently, according to the manufacturer's instructions.

Materials and equipment

Nitrocellulose filters bearing replicates of recombinant phage plaques

Antibody, poly- or monoclonal, specifying antigen of interest

10 mM Tris, pH 9.6 containing 150 mM sodium chloride and 0.05% v/v Tween 20 (wash buffer)

Bovine serum albumin, BSA, RIA grade (Appendix II)

3MM paper (Appendix II)

Clear acetate sheets

Pen with water-insoluble ink

Radioactive ink (Appendix II)

Orbital shaker

Bag sealer (Appendix II)

Role of continuous plastic tube

In addition:

Materials for autoradiography (Section 2.11.4) or enzyme labels (Section 2.11.3)

Method

1   Remove the nitrocellulose filters from each plate and immerse them in a large volume of 10 mM Tris, pH 9.6 containing 150 mM sodium chloride and 0.05% v/v Tween 20 (wash buffer). Store the agar plates face down at 4° until immuno-screening is complete.

2   Leave the filters in the wash buffer on the orbital shaker for 10 min at room temperature. Use sufficient buffer to ensure that the filters are moving freely.

3   Transfer the filters to wash buffer containing 3% w/v BSA (RIA grade) and leave rocking for 30 min at room temperature. (The BSA will block the unoccupied protein binding sites on the filters and so prevent non-specific uptake of antibody protein.)

4   Seal the filters into a plastic sac, excluding as much air as possible.

5   Dilute the pre-absorbed antibody (see step 6, Preparation in advance) in wash buffer containing 3% w/v BSA, allowing 5 ml of solution for every 20 filters, and load it into the sac using a syringe and needle. As a guide, dilute the antibody 1:100 or use neat tissue culture supernatant from hybridoma cells.

6   Re-seal the plastic sac and leave it rocking for 1 h at room temperature.

7   Cut open one edge of the sac and recover the antibody solution. So little is consumed during this procedure that it may be stored at −20° for further use.

8   Transfer the filters to a tank of wash buffer and rock gently for 10 min at room temperature. For efficient washing, use sufficient buffer to allow the filters to move freely.

9   Wash twice more under the same conditions.

10 Remove the filters from the final wash, gently blot each one dry on 3MM paper and seal all together into a plastic sac, excluding as much air as possible.

11 Dilute the anti-immunoglobulin antibody or protein A in wash buffer containing 3% BSA. See Technical note 2 for selection of label.

12 Add the labelled second reagent to the plastic sac, using a syringe and needle, and re-seal the sac.

13 After incubating on the rocking platform for 1 h at room temperature, open the sac, recover and store the labelled reagent, and wash the filters three times in wash buffer as in step 8 above.

A   For immunoscreening with enzyme labels:

14 After the final wash, blot each filter dry on 3MM paper, and process with chromogenic substrate to reveal the binding sites of the enzyme-conjugated second reagent, as described in Section 2.11.3.

B   For immunoscreening with radioactive labels:

14 Remove each filter from the final wash solution, blot dry on 3MM paper and mount onto a sheet of card covered with Saran wrap. Finally, cover the filter and card tightly with Saran wrap.

15 Cover each orientation hole on the filters with a small sticky label and mark the position of the hole with radioactive ink (this aids orientation of the autoradiograph when preparing the template for isolation of the phage plaques).

16 Expose to X-ray film using tungsten intensifying screens and process photographically.

17 Prepare a duplicate of the coloured dots on the filter (enzyme labels) or the black dots on the autoradiogaph (radioactive labels) using a clear acetate sheet and a fine pen. Remember to transfer the orientation marks.

18 Mark the regions of the positive plaques on the acetate sheet and use this to guide a pasteur pipette to remove a plug of agar from the corresponding region in the original plate.

The plugs of agar are each dispersed in individual tubes containing a storage buffer. If the original phage plaques were discrete and optimally spaced, each plug should contain one, or a limited number, of types of recombinant phage. It is necessary to repeat the 'screening and picking' process until the phage plaques are uniformly positive on immunoscreening (Fig. 2.10).

You should now have a series of recombinant phages containing segments of the DNA coding for the protein defined by the original antibody.

Technical notes
1 It is necessary to remember that polyclonal sera or ascitic fluids are biological materials and not chemical reagents. The pre-absorption step, to remove the anti-*E. coli* and anti-phage antibodies, must be carried out to completion.
2 Binding of the first antibody can be visualised with an anti-immunoglobulin antibody or protein A, labelled with either a radioactive (Section 2.11.4) or enzyme (Section 2.11.3) label.
3 It is good practice to keep the filters moist during autoradiographic exposure as it is possible to continue the washing procedure, if the radioactive background is

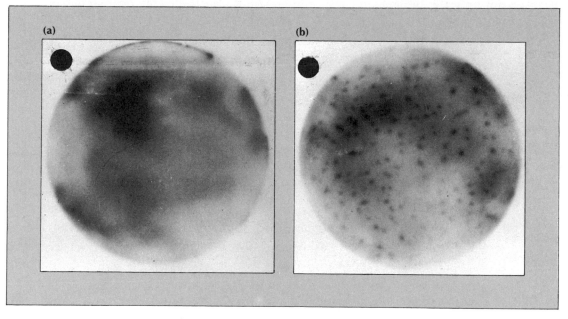

Fig. 2.10 Screening of a λ gt11 expression library with antibodies. A λ gt11 genomic library of the protozoan parasite *Trypanosoma cruzi* was screened with a mixture of antisera from infected patients. (**a**) The first round of screening identified a single-phage colony in this plate (corresponding to the black dot on the photograph of the nitrocellulose filter) producing a fusion protein which contained one or more parasite-derived epitopes. Once the agar plug containing the recombinant phage had been replated onto a fresh culture of *Escherichia coli* (**b**) the proportion of positive colonies increased dramatically.

unacceptably high, or to repeat the immunoscreening, if no signal is detected after 7 days exposure. This is not possible with enzyme labels.

4 All materials and equipment should be sterile and aseptic technique should be used throughout. The screening can take between 7 and 9 days; therefore, even at 4°, microbial contaminants can overgrow and make plaque identification difficult.

2.13.3 From partial sequence to mature protein

The rapid progress seen in the characterisation of important proteins in infectious organisms has been made possible by the application of the techniques of molecular biology, rather than those of protein chemistry. Consequently, there is a frequent need to relate an incomplete, and often unknown, sequence of DNA expressed in a prokaryote to the mature molecule expressed in the eukaryotic cell. The multi-perspective specificity of polyclonal antibodies combined with the discriminatory power of immunoblotting allow this link to be established with relative ease.

Once an unknown sequence has been expressed, for example as a plasmid-derived fusion protein in β-galactosidase, then the whole bacterial lysate may be used to immunise a mouse and so produce an antiserum suitable for immunoblotting (Section 2.11). Again, it is necessary to stress the need for adequate specificity controls when using the antiserum for immunoblotting. It is essential to blot against not only the organism or cell of interest but also the *E. coli* host strain (not infected with the recombinant plasmid). Only then is it possible to be reasonably confident that the mature polypeptide identified on the blot of the SDS-PAGE-fractionated organism really does relate to the fusion protein.

Alternatively, it is possible to adsorb the fusion protein onto nitrocellulose and use it for affinity purification of antibodies from polyclonal sera. This has been particularly useful in clinical situations, where immunisation with fusion protein is not possible.

The technique is, in principle, related to those described above. A small square of nitrocellulose filter is placed in contact with a single clone of recombinant phage growing in *E. coli*, after induction of the fusion protein, the filter is 'blocked' with BSA and pre-eluted with 0.1 M glycine−HCl buffer, pH 2.5 containing 150 mM sodium chloride. Antibody is absorbed from the patient's serum onto the filter, which is then extensively washed and eluted by immersion in a small volume of glycine−HCl buffer. After neutralisation with a few crystals of solid Tris, the affinity-purified antibody can be used for a miniature immunoblot (Section 2.11 and Mini-blotter apparatus, Appendix II). This technique both relates the fusion protein to the mature protein (identified by size in the blot) and establishes its importance to the patient's response to infection.

In some instances it has been possible to relate a DNA sequence of unknown function to a gene product using an antiserum raised against the synthetic oligopeptide inferred from the triplet code. Oligopeptides of <10 amino acids are relatively poor immunogens; however, once their chain length exceeds 10−15 the chances of obtaining an antiserum is high. As expected, this approach tends to favour detection of epitopes in accessible regions of high hydrophilicity and N- or C-terminal regions, even when the resulting antisera are used in immunoblotting.

2.14 Further reading

Barrett AJ and Salvensen G (1986) *Proteinase Inhibitors*. Elsevier, Amsterdam.
Davis LG, Dibner MD and Battey JF (1986). *Basic Methods in Molecular Biology*. Elsevier, Amsterdam.
Glover DM (editor) (1985) *DNA Cloning*, Volumes I and II. IRL Press, Oxford.
Hames BD and Higgins SJ (editors) (1984) *Transcription and Translation*. IRL Press, Oxford.
Oi VT, Glazer AN and Stryer L (1982) Fluorescent phycobiliprotein conjugates for analyses of cells and molecules. *J. Cell Biol.* **93**: 981−986.
Rogers AW (1979) *Techniques of Autoradiography*, 3rd edition. Elsevier, Amsterdam.
Waterlow JC, Garlick PJ and Millward DJ (1978) *Protein Turnover in Mammalian Tissues and in the Whole Body*. Elsevier, Amsterdam.

3 The Lymphocyte: its Role and Function

Having caught measles as a child you became sick. As you obviously survived you are no longer afraid of catching measles, although you may catch chickenpox. The protection afforded by the immune system is specific to those dangerous antigens you have previously experienced and survived! The basic unit of this *specific immune response* is the *lymphocyte*. Throughout this book you will encounter the lymphocyte and its precursors being acted upon and reacting to, not dangerous antigens, such as viruses or bacteria, but to artificial antigens of a much more defined and informative nature. Fortunately lymphocytes react as readily to 'artificial' antigens as 'natural' ones.

Lymphocytes differentiate from precursor cells (derived from the yolk sac, fetal liver and bone marrow at different stages of development) which migrate to the so-called *central lymphoid organs*, i.e. the thymus and the bursa (or its bone marrow equivalent in mammals). When their differentiation is complete lymphocytes migrate to and populate the peripheral lymphoid organs, i.e. blood, spleen, lymph nodes, Peyer's patches, lymphoid appendix, etc. At this stage the animal is usually immunologically mature and able to respond to antigenic challenge.

The mouse has been an invaluable model for the elucidation of the complex interactions which underlie the immune response. However, the steady improvements in *in vitro* technology over the past 5–10 years, combined with the plethora of antibody-based markers for lymphocyte functional subsets, has allowed great advances in the study of the human immune response. However, two insurmountable problems still beset human studies: (a) non-therapeutic experimentation is ethically unacceptable; and (b) most studies are conducted with blood or tonsils as a source of lymphocytes and soluble factors. We know from animal studies that the quality of the immune response can vary greatly with different tissues; it seems likely that the human lymphoid system has the same tissue specific variation.

3.1 Lymphoid organs of the mouse

Figure 1.2 shows the major lymphoid organs of the mouse and their cellular composition. There is a continuous traffic of re-circulating small lymphocytes from the blood into the other peripheral lymphoid organs such as the spleen, lymph nodes, etc. From here the cells enter the other tissues and finally return to the blood via the lymphatic vessels; for example, the thoracic duct. The intact immune response involves great changes in the 'trafficking' pattern of re-circulating antigen-reactive lymphocytes. When specific small lymphocytes are confronted with antigen they will leave this re-circulating pool, congregate at the site of the greatest antigen concentration and migrate to the draining lymph node.

86

The small lymphocyte

Cells from mouse thymus (a central lymphoid organ) and blood (a very important peripheral lymphoid organ) will be stained for morphological examination.

Morphology of thymus and blood leucocytes

BLOOD FILM

Materials and equipment
Mouse or human blood
Microscope slides (cleaned overnight in acetone–ethanol 50 : 50 v/v)
95% methanol in water

Method
1 Grasp the mouse firmly by the nape of the neck using your thumb and forefinger. Hold the mouse's tail between your little and third fingers with its abdomen towards you, use your middle finger to flex its spine slightly so it cannot struggle. This is a general position for immobilising a mouse for intraperitoneal injection or, as here, cutting the tip from its tail with a pair of scissors. Humans are usually more cooperative, in this case a finger prick with a sterile needle will draw sufficient blood.
2 Squeeze out 1 drop of blood and place it at one end of a clean glass slide.
3 Use a second, 'spreader' slide and touch the extreme edge of the drop of blood. Hold this slide at an angle of about 45 degrees.
4 Allow the blood to flow along the edge of the spreader slide and then push it away from the drop to obtain a film of cells (ideally in the shape of a bunsen flame).
5 Wave the slide in the air to dry it rapidly.
6 Fix in 95% methanol for 2 min.

With practice a serviceable, if not perfect, blood film can be produced. It is necessary to vary the size of the drop of blood and the amount taken up on the spreader slide to obtain an optimal distribution of cells.

Smears of single-cell suspensions

The blood plasma is viscous and so protects the cells in whole blood from damage as they are smeared. Smears are more difficult to obtain from single-cell suspensions taken from organs. Although a cytocentrifuge provides an easy answer (Section 3.2.3), it is possible to obtain excellent preparations by simply suspending the cells in neat serum and smearing them as in the previous section.

Materials and equipment
Mouse
Phosphate-buffered saline, PBS (Appendix I)
Fetal bovine serum, FBS
Microscope slides (clean overnight in acetone−ethanol 50 : 50 v/v)
95% methanol in water

Method

1 Kill the mouse by cervical dislocation and remove the thymus into a Petri dish containing PBS or tissue culture medium.
2 Prepare a single-cell suspension as in Section 1.15.
3 Place 1 drop of the cell suspension on a clean slide and smear with a second slide as before (Section 3.2.1).
4 Dry the slide in the air and fix in 95% methanol for 2 min.
5 Wash the slide in running tap water for 30 min to remove the FBS.

3.2.3   ## Cytocentrifuge technique

Materials and equipment
Mouse
Phosphate-buffered saline, PBS (Appendix I)
Fetal bovine serum, FBS
Microscope slides (clean overnight in acetone−ethanol 50 : 50 v/v)
95% methanol in water
Cytocentrifuge (Appendix II)

Method

1 Prepare a single-cell suspension from the mouse thymus as described in Section 1.15. After washing, finally re-suspend in tissue culture medium with 10% FBS.
2 Load cytocentrifuge with glass slides and filter-paper strips.
3 Add 1 drop of cell suspension and 3 drops of tissue culture medium to each carrier block being used.
4 Centrifuge at 300 g for 10 min at room temperature.
5 Unload the glass slides, being careful to keep the slide and filter-paper strip together as you remove them from the carrier.
6 Remove the strip without smearing the cell preparation.
7 Dry the slide in the air and fix in 95% methanol for 2 min.
8 Wash the slides in running tap water for 30 min and then stain as required.

Technical notes

1 The concentration of the cells in the suspension and the volume used should be varied to obtain the required cell density in the smear.
2 Human lymphocytes tend to be more fragile and should be centrifuged at 250 g.

To examine the morphological details of the prepared cells, it is necessary to stain them. Pleasing results can be obtained with May—Grunwald/Giemsa staining.

3.3 May—Grünwald/Giemsa staining

Materials and equipment
Smears of cells, fixed in methanol (Section 3.2.2)
Giemsa buffer (Appendix I)
May—Grünwald stain (Appendix II)
Giemsa stain (Appendix II)
Staining racks and troughs
Neutral mounting medium (DePeX, Appendix II)

Method
1 Immerse the fixed cells in buffer for 5 min.
2 Transfer to May—Grünwald stain (freshly diluted 1:2 with buffer) for 5 min.
3 Rinse the slides in buffer and blot dry.
4 Stain in the Giemsa solution (freshly diluted with buffer) for 15 min.
5 Rinse in the buffer.
6 If the cells are over-stained (too blue) allow them to stand in the buffer.
7 Dry the slides in air and examine them under the microscope. If permanent preparations are required the cells may be mounted in a neutral mounting medium under a coverslip (use DePeX; Canada Balsam, although sold in a neutral form, eventually decolourises the stained cells).

Technical notes
1 These stains are based upon dyes dissolved in methanol which undergo a poly-chromasia upon dilution with water. For this reason stains must be prepared freshly for each staining session.
2 A precipitate forms upon dilution of the stains: this is normal and will not affect the preparation as it is removed during washing of the slides. If you filter the precipitate from the stain you will also remove its staining properties.

EXAMINATION OF CELL SMEARS
During smearing, white cells tend to move differentially to the red cells and so you will find them at the edges and extreme end of the film. Figures 3.1 and 3.2 show the typical morphology of cells encountered in stained blood. Although you should be familiar with their appearance, you will rarely look at stained cells in modern immunology, because, although lymphocytes in the blood are heterogeneous with regard to size and morphology (Fig. 3.1), there is no correlation with their function or antigen specificity.

The stained cells from the thymus are much more homogeneous than those of the blood, the majority have the morphological appearance typical of small lymphocytes (Fig. 3.1a).

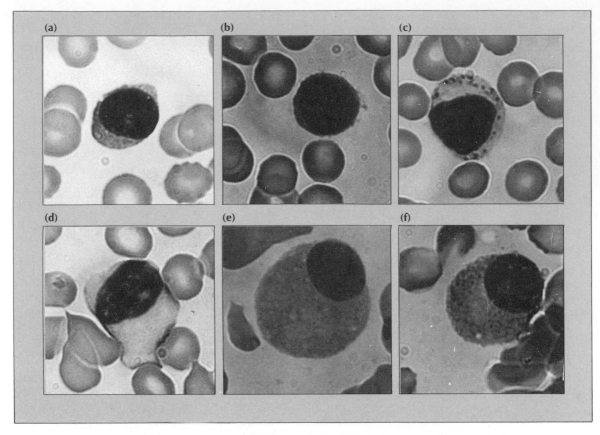

Fig. 3.1 Morphology of lymphoid cells under the light microscope. (a) and (b) show the morphology of typical *small lymphocytes*. The cells have a diameter of about 10 µm and are characterised by a large nucleus : cytoplasm ratio — typical of G_0 or 'resting' cells. In May–Grünwald/Giemsa staining, the cells have a deeply staining nucleus, condensed chromatin and a thin rim of blue cytoplasm.

(c) *Large granular lymphocyte*. Cells with this morphology have been associated with the majority of the NK, LAK and ADCC activity due to peripheral blood mononuclear cells (Sections 4.14 and 4.15). Their azurophilic granules contain perforins, which become integrated into the membrane of target cells during cytotoxic killing. These cells have a characteristic density which facilitates their purification from other lymphoid cells by density gradient centrifugation (Section 1.13).

(d) *Reactive lymphocyte* from a patient with infectious mononucleosis or glandular fever. Viable cell phenotyping (Section 14.1) of this cell would have shown it to be a T lymphocyte, in this case reacting to Epstein–Barr virus infection of B lymphocytes (Section 14.9). The cell has extensive blue cytoplasm and an 'open' chromatin structure, as evidenced by the apparent holes in the nucleus shown in the photograph. T lymphocytes stimulated *in vitro* with an antigen or phytomitogen (Section 4.8) have a similar morphology and the same close 'wrapping' around the exterior of adjacent erythrocytes.

(e) and (f) *Plasma cells* showing the typical characteristics of: large cytoplasm containing an eccentric nucleus with a 'cartwheel' chromatin structure, deep blue cytoplasm rich in RNA and a lucid zone near the nucleus, corresponding to the Golgi apparatus. The cytoplasm is frequently vacuolated, presumably due to intracellular antibodies about to be secreted.

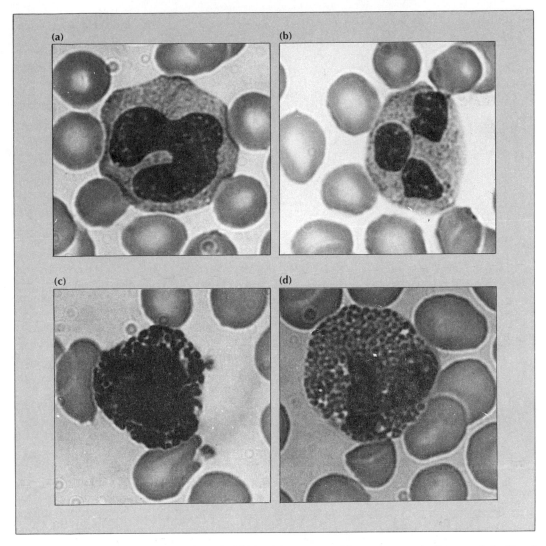

Fig. 3.2 Light microscopy of non-lymphoid blood leucocytes. Monocytes are the largest of the blood leucocytes and, in viable cell preparations, are not easily distinguished from cells of the lymphoid lineage. Granulocytes are classified according to the staining reaction of their granules in response to histological dyes; for example, May−Grünwald/Giemsa staining (Section 3.3).

(a) *Monocytes* have a C-shaped nucleus and grey cytoplasm with a few azurophilic granules on May−Grünwald/Giemsa staining. They are the largest of the blood leucocytes and, on entering the tissues, differentiate into macrophages.

(b) *Neutrophils* are polymorphonuclear cells with neutrophilic cytoplasm. Older cells have a more segmented nucleus and, in general, it is difficult to discern their cytoplasmic granules (except during infection — so-called toxic granulation). These cells account for about 90% of circulating granulocytes — they are about 15 μm in diameter and highly phagocytic.

(c) There are very small numbers of *basophils* in circulation (<1.0% of blood granulocytes). The characteristic deep blue granules obscure the nucleus and contain histamine — very important in type I anaphylactic-type hypersensitivity reactions (Section 5.8.3).

(d) The bi-lobed nucleus shown in the photograph is typical of a human *eosinophil*; the bright red granules makes identification easy. These cells make up about 2−5% of blood leucocytes, but their frequency increases greatly in parasitic infections and allergic reactions. Typically these cells kill invading organisms by secretion of toxic cationic granules (exocytosis) rather than phagocytosis.

Lymphocytes circulate for months, or even years; granulocytes circulate in the blood for about 7 h and thereafter are around in the tissues for only a few days.

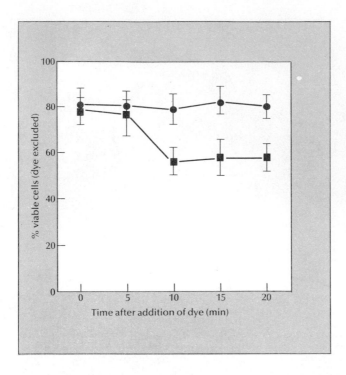

Fig. 3.3 Cell viability in trypan blue and nigrosin dyes. An aliquot of mouse lymph-node cells in phosphate-buffered saline was mixed with an equal volume of 0.2% trypan blue (■) or nigrosin dye (●) and incubated at 37° for 3 min to facilitate dye uptake into dead cells. The suspensions were then returned to 0° (time 0) and the percentage of viable cells determined at the time points shown on the graph.

Although the cell viability decreased rapidly over the first 10 min in trypan blue, it remained at a plateau value of 60% for the next 60 min (full data not shown). The material released from the dead cells bound to the trypan blue and formed a precipitate.

3.4 Viable lymphocyte count

It must be emphasised that at all the following stages in the book, the investigator will be handling living cells. Maximum *in vitro* viability is usually maintained if the cells are kept at 0°, i.e. in melting ice. Guinea-pig lymphocytes, however, are the exception to this rule; they should not be cooled below room temperature.

Cells that are to be used in an experiment must be removed freshly from the animal and the experiment completed, or the cells put into culture or transferred *in vivo* as quickly as possible. In general, living cells will not remain functional if left overnight in a refrigerator.

The plasma membrane of a viable cell does not permit the entry of non-electrolyte dye substances. This phenomenon is used to distinguish dead from living lymphocytes. Many dyes are suitable for this purpose; for example, trypan blue or eosin in dilute, physiological solution. However, we have found that nigrosin has invariably been the least toxic dye for estimation of cell viability (Fig. 3.3).

3.4.1 Chicken thymus and bursa

The chicken has up to nine pairs of thymus lobes running up its neck, alongside the carotid arteries. Unlike the mammalian thymus, which involutes at puberty and is a relatively small and acellular organ thereafter, the chicken thymus increases in cellularity with the onset of each moult. The bursa of Fabricius is found at quite the other end of the bird, it is a large sac-like organ dorsal to the cloaca. Its internal surface is plicated and has a direct connection with the rectum. Cell suspensions from the thymus and bursa provide virtually pure T- and B-lymphocyte populations, respectively.

If you are not familiar with the morphology of viable lymphocytes or the phenotypic differences between T and B cells, then suspensions from these organs provide a good starting point for the techniques described in the next three sections. The cell suspensions should be prepared as in Section 1.15, and the technique for cell-surface immunofluorescence (Section 3.5.1) modified by the use of a rabbit anti-chicken, rather than mouse, immunoglobulin serum.

3.4.2 Dye exclusion test

Materials and equipment
Organs for preparing a lymphocyte suspension
Phosphate-buffered saline, PBS (Appendix I)
Nigrosin dye (Appendix II)
Nylon wool
2 ml syringe barrels
Haemocytometer, improved Neubauer ruling, preferably rhodium plated (Appendix II)

Method
1 Prepare a lymphocyte suspension from each organ to be used (Section 1.14).
2 Loosely pack 1 ml of nylon wool into each syringe barrel, and wash with 5 ml of PBS.
3 Filter each cell suspension through a nylon wool column and wash out with 2 ml of PBS.

Whenever lymphocytes are used for *in vivo* or *in vitro* study they are usually washed by centrifugation to remove any adherent exogenous material. In addition, dead cells are often disrupted during centrifugation and so the percentage cell viability increases during this washing procedure. It is included here merely to concentrate the lymphocytes for further handling.

4 Centrifuge all lymphocyte suspensions at 150 g for 10 min at 4°.
5 Remove the supernatant using a Pasteur pipette connected to a water vacuum pump. Keep the pipette at the meniscus of the buffer at all times to avoid turbulence and cell loss.
6 Re-suspend the cells in 5 ml of PBS.
7 Mix 0.1 ml of each cell suspension with 0.1 ml of 0.2% nigrosin solution and incubate at room temperature for 5 min.
8 Count the number of viable lymphocytes (phase bright, unstained) using a haemocytometer and a phase-contrast microscope.
9 Dead cells may be removed as described in Section 1.16.

Technical notes

1 Prepare a 2% stock solution of nigrosin and dilute with sterile saline for use.
2 If cells are being prepared for sterile work then filtration through nylon wool is not always convenient. It is acceptable to allow the cells to stand at 1 *g* for 10 min and then remove the suspension with a Pasteur pipette.
3 Nylon wool filtration is an essential step if lymphocytes from solid organs are to be used for flow cytometry (Sections 3.9 and 9.11).

3.4.3 Cell counting with a haemocytometer

When counting lymphocyte suspensions it is most convenient to use a × 40 objective lens and to count in the central, triple-ruled area of the haemocytometer (this area is used for red-cell counting in haematology). Count the cells in the large triple-ruled squares (improved Neubauer ruling, Fig. 3.4) until a minimum of 100 unstained (viable) lymphocytes have been counted (see Fig. 3.5).

Calculation of the number of viable cells

$$\text{Number viable lymphocytes ml}^{-1} = \frac{\text{number lymphocytes counted}}{\text{number triple-ruled squares}} \times 25 \times 10^4$$

$$\times \text{ original dilution (if any).}$$

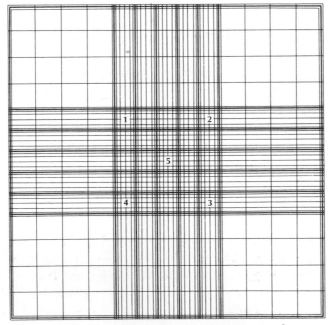

Fig. 3.4 The improved Neubauer ruling haemocytometer. For most applications in experimental immunology, the haemocytometer provides a cost-effect alternative to an electronic particle counter, unless you wish to use it for volume measurements. In principle, the number of cells in small volumes taken at random is counted to pre-determined rules, and this value multiplied up to give an estimate of the total population.

The figure shows the appearance of the central ruled area of the haemocytometer as it would appear under a low-power lens on the light microscope. There are nine squares, each of 1 mm²; as the depth of the counting chamber is 0.1 mm, cells settling into one of these squares have come from a volume of 0.1 mm³.

If dealing with high-density cell populations, use a high-power lens (× 40) and count in the central triple ruled areas (see Fig. 3.5); at low cell density count in one of the four peripheral, single ruled areas. When counting lymphocyte suspensions, it is convenient to use a phase-contrast microscope and so distinguish viable (phase-bright) from dead (phase-dark) cells, as an adjunct to dye exclusion (Section 3.4.2).

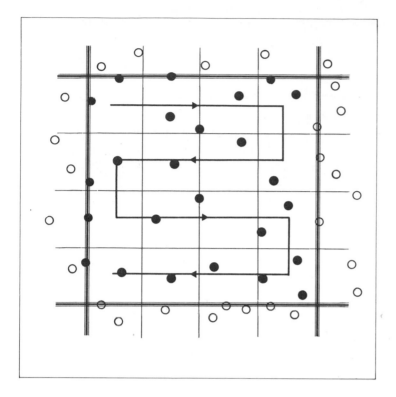

Fig. 3.5 Counting lymphocyte suspensions in a haemocytometer. The figure shows an enlarged view of square 1, in Fig. 3.4. Cells falling across the top and left border lines of a square are considered to be in that square, whereas cells on the bottom and right borders are excluded. The diagram shows 25 cells (filled circles) in an area of 1/25 mm², depth of chamber 0.1 mm. To gain an acceptable degree of accuracy in this technique, you should count cells in the triple-ruled squares in the order shown in Fig. 3.4 until at least 100 cells have been included in the sample.

3.5 Lymphocyte-surface membrane

In a normal animal, the majority of the circulating lymphocytes spend their time apparently doing nothing, they are resting or G_0 cells. As will be seen later, these dormant cells are specifically activated after contact with antigen. Antigen contact occurs as a specific surface event at the plasma membrane and generates a transduction signal which causes nuclear de-repression. The cell enters the cell cycle and divides, it can eventually form a clone of effector and memory cells of the same specificity.

3.5.1 Immunofluorescent staining of lymphocyte membranes

The antisera used in this experiment should be standardised according to the method in Section 2.1.6. Although we have described a method using anti-immunoglobulin antibody to stain B lymphocytes, the method is generally applicable to antisera of any specificity used with any viable cell suspension.

Materials and equipment
Lymphoid organs; for example, from mice (Fig. 1.2)

Tissue culture medium (Appendix I) containing 0.1% w/v bovine serum albumin and 20 mM sodium azide

Nylon wool

2 ml syringe barrels

Haemocytometer

Rabbit anti-mouse immunoglobulin, anti-Ig (Section 1.7.2 or Appendix II)

Fluorescein-conjugated goat, pig or sheep anti-rabbit immunoglobulin, FITC anti-Ig (Section 2.1 or Appendix II)

Mounting medium: 70% glycerol, 30% glycine—saline buffer, pH 8.6 (Appendix I)

Method

1 Prepare a lymphocyte suspension from blood (Section 1.14) or one of the solid lymphoid organs (Section 1.15).

2 Filter cell suspensions from lymphoid organs through nylon wool to remove aggregates.

3 Wash all cells three times in tissue culture medium by centrifugation (150 g for 10 min at 4°).

4 Re-suspend the cells in 10 ml of medium and count the number of lymphocytes per ml using a haemocytometer and phase-contrast microscope (Section 3.4.3).

5 Pipette out 2 aliquots of approximately 10^7 lymphocytes of each cell suspension and centrifuge to obtain a pellet (150 g for 10 min at 4°).

6 Add 0.1 ml of the required dilution of rabbit anti-mouse Ig or normal rabbit serum (NRS) to 1 aliquot of each cell type (antiserum standardised as in Section 2.1.6).

7 Incubate for 30 min on ice.

8 Wash twice by centrifugation (150 g for 10 min at 4°) to remove unbound protein.

9 Add 0.1 ml of the fluorescein-conjugated anti-rabbit Ig (1 mg ml^{-1} total protein) to all cell pellets.

10 Incubate for 30 min on ice.

11 Wash three times by centrifugation (150 g for 10 min at 4°) to remove the unbound conjugate.

12 Re-suspend, add 1 drop of glycerol—glycine mounting medium to the dry cell pellet and mix thoroughly.

13 Put 1 small drop of cell suspension on a microscope slide, add a coverslip and ring with nail varnish.

14 Examine the cell preparations under an incident light UV microscope and identify lymphocytes visible as green rings. (Fig. 3.6b) This is characteristic of cell-surface staining of viable lymphocytes. In addition, note the homogeneously stained dead cells that will inevitably be present (Fig. 3.6d).

15 For each microscope field, count the number of fluorescently stained lymphocytes (green) and then the total viable lymphocytes viewed under phase contrast.

16 Count a total of 200 cells under visible light and calculate the percentage of fluorescing (positive) lymphocytes for each preparation.

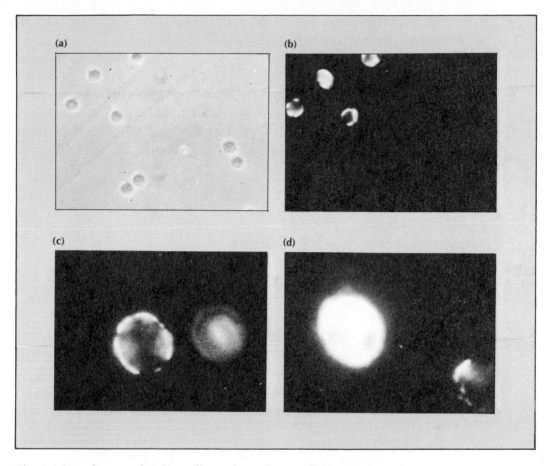

Fig. 3.6 Lymphocytes showing cell membrane immunofluorescence.
(a) Mouse lymph-node lymphocytes viewed under tungsten light.
(b) Same microscope field but viewed under incident UV light. Cells have been stained with a direct conjugate of rhodamine-labelled rabbit anti-mouse light chain. As can be seen, fluorescence is limited to only a proportion of the cells seen in (a).
(c) Lymphocytes stained with rhodamine-conjugated anti-light chain and visualized under UV light. The patchy ring staining is typical of viable lymphocytes. The fluorochrome-conjugated antiserum is unable to cross the cell membrane and so only reacts with surface determinants seen here in optical cross-section. The patching is not inhibited at 4° or in the presence of metabolic inhibitors; for example, sodium azide (20 mM final concentration) and is thought to be due to local cross-linking of membrane determinants.
(d) A dead cell (*top left*) showing bright homogeneous intracytoplasmic fluorescence; such cells should be excluded from all counts of stained (positive) cells.

Technical notes

The technical notes for Section 2.1.6 also apply here.

1 Staining viable cells confines the antibody to the external surface membrane. Staining of internal components can only be accomplished efficiently by cell fixation and membrane permeabilisation (Section 4.4.4).

2 If required, the method may be abbreviated by exposing the cells to each antibody for 10 min on ice, with only slight loss of sensitivity.

3 Precisely the same method may be used to prepare cells for cytofluorimetric analysis (Sections 3.9 and 9.11).

4 Several commercial companies now market an anti-fade fluorescent mounting medium (Appendix II). It is particularly advantageous to use an anti-fade compound for photomicroscopy, and also to remember that the quenched fluorochrome slowly recovers. A cheaper, but slightly less effective anti-fade mountant may be prepared as described below.

Materials

p-phenylenediamine

Phosphate-buffered saline, PBS (Appendix I)

Glycerol

0.5 M carbonate−bicarbonate buffer, pH 9.0 (Appendix I)

Method

1 Dissolve 100 mg *p*-phenylenediamine in 10 ml of PBS in the dark.

2 Add 90 ml of glycerol and mix thoroughly.

3 Adjust to pH 8.0 with the carbonate−bicarbonate buffer.

4 Store the mixture at −20° in the dark.

5 Use as glycerol−glycine mountant, step 12 in method above.

Prepare fresh anti-fade mountant when the stock solution turns brown.

3.5.2 Antigen-binding lymphocytes

We will describe a basic technique by which antigen-binding lymphocytes can be visualised. The applicability of this approach is limited principally by the experimental design to ensure that non-specific binding is avoided. It is, however, difficult in this type of experiment to include a satisfactory specificity control. The approach adopted here is to show that the number of antigen-binding lymphocytes increases after immunisation.

3.5.3 Sheep erythrocyte rosettes

You will perform a rosette inhibition experiment with anti-mouse immunoglobulin at the same time as determining the number of antigen-binding lymphocytes.

PREPARATION IN ADVANCE

1 Immunise a mouse 7 days before the experiment with 10^8 sheep erythrocytes given intraperitoneally.

2 The anti-mouse immunoglobulin and normal rabbit serum must be absorbed

with mouse liver and red blood cells, as well as sheep RBC to be sure they are free of anti-species activity.

Materials and equipment
Sheep erythrocytes, SRBC
Normal and SRBC-immunised mice
Tissue culture medium (Appendix I)
Rabbit anti-mouse immunoglobulin serum, anti-Ig (Section 1.7.2 or Appendix II)
Normal rabbit serum, NRS (Appendix II)
Nylon wool
2 ml syringe barrels
2 ml plastic round-bottomed tubes

Method

1 Kill the mice and prepare single-cell suspension from their spleens (Section 1.15).
2 Remove phagocytic cells (Section 1.17).
3 Wash the cells three times by centrifugation (150 g for 10 min at 4°).
4 Count the number of viable lymphocytes ml^{-1} (Section 3.4) and adjust to 3×10^7 ml^{-1}.
5 Label tubes and add 0.1 ml aliquots of the lymphocyte suspensions as shown in the Protocol.

Protocol

Tube	Lymphocytes from:	Antiserum incubation before rosetting
1	Immune spleen	None
2	Normal spleen	None
3	Immune spleen	Anti-mouse immunoglobulin
4	Immune spleen	NRS

6 Add 0.1 ml of the appropriate sera to tubes 3 and 4. (Use the optimal dilution as determined for immunofluorescence, Section 3.5.1. Alternatively you may wish to do a full titration curve of rosette inhibition.)
7 Incubate tubes 3 and 4 at 4° for 30 min.
8 Add 0.1 ml SRBC suspension (2.4×10^8 SRBC ml^{-1}) to tubes 1 and 2. Mix well.
9 Centrifuge tubes 1 and 2 at 150 g for 10 min at 4°.
10 Add 0.3 ml of 0.5% acridine orange solution to tubes 1 and 2 if UV microscope is available (otherwise use tissue culture medium) and re-suspend the cells on a vertical rotor turning at 8−10 r.p.m. for 5 min. (Alternatively, you may re-suspend the cells using a Pasteur pipette. This, however, reduces the number of rosettes because of the shear forces generated.)
11 Repeat the addition of SRBC, centrifugation and re-suspension for the cells

pretreated with antisera (i.e. tubes 3 and 4). This time, however, add only 0.2 ml of acridine orange solution (or tissue culture medium).

12 Count the number of rosettes in each suspension using a haemocytometer and a microscope. Count at least four samples per tube.

If you are using a microscope with UV light, live cells may be seen at the centre of the rosette by their green fluorescence (dead cells are deep red), thus confirming the cell group as a rosette rather than an aggregate of SRBC. If a UV microscope is not used then 0.1% toluidine blue may be used to visualise nucleated cells. Do not count rosettes with more than one lymphocyte, or clumped red cells without lymphocytes. This is shown in Fig. 3.7.

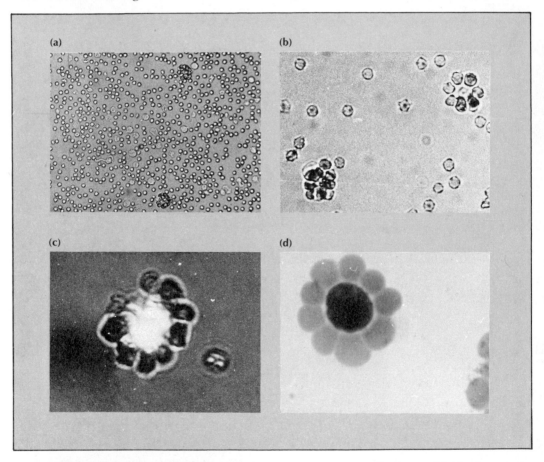

Fig. 3.7 Mouse lymphocytes showing antigen-specific immunocytoadherence with sheep erythrocytes.
(a) Antigen-specific lymphocytes will bind sheep erythrocytes to their surface to form rosettes; two are shown in this field.
(b) At 4° the erythrocytes bind as a single layer.
(c) The nucleus of the lymphocyte at the centre of this rosette has been stained with acridine orange and is visualized under UV and tungsten light.
(d) The morphology of the rosette-forming cell may be seen after Giemsa staining of a cytocentrifuge preparation.
  A rosette may be arbitrarily defined as a single lymphocyte binding five or more erythrocytes. If rosettes are incubated at 37°, in the absence of metabolic inhibition, erythrocyte 'caps' will form in an analogous manner to that shown for anti-immunoglobulin (Fig. 3.14).

Calculation and evaluation of results
1 Calculate the number of rosettes ml^{-1} of suspension and from this the number of rosettes per 10^6 lymphocytes.
2 Compare the number of rosettes per 10^6 lymphocytes from the normal and immune animals (tubes 1 and 2) and calculate the factor of immunisation.
3 You should find that all of the rosettes are blocked by the anti-immunoglobulin serum.

3.5.4 Autoradiographic labelling of lymphocytes

In the previous sections a series of experiments were performed to investigate the surface components of lymphocytes using fluorochrome-labelled antibodies. The sensitivity of this approach can be greatly increased by substituting a radioactive isotope for the fluorochrome. In addition, autoradiography is semi-quantitative, the relative number of grains per cell is dependent upon the number of surface determinants detected. It is therefore possible to estimate the relative distribution of the determinants throughout the cell population and, within the same experiment, the relative concentration and distribution of determinants between two cell populations.

In this way it has been shown that B cells vary widely in the number of available immunoglobulin molecules on their surface (Fig. 3.8) and that T and B cells differ quantitatively in their membrane content of immunoglobulin. The basic autoradiographic method as described below may be used under any situation where a radioactive isotope is introduced into or onto a cell or tissue.

Example: labelling of chicken lymphocytes

Materials and equipment
1-day old chickens
Anti-immunoglobulin antibody, either purified by acid elution (Section 9.6) or an IgG fraction (Section 8.5).
Control, either an irrelevant purified antibody, for example anti-keyhole limpet haemocyanin (anti-KLH), or normal rabbit IgG, NRIgG
Chloramine T
Sodium metabisulphite
Sodium ^{125}I (Appendix II)
Sephadex G-25 (Appendix II)
Glass tubing, internal diameter 6.0 mm
Ilford K5 nuclear emulsion (Appendix II)

Although strictly one should titrate the concentration of antibody used until a plateau value of labelled cells is attained, it has been found in practice that 50 μg of pure anti-immunoglobulin per 10^7 lymphocytes is a vast excess.

Specimen experimental protocol
Anti-immunoglobulin labelling of bursa cells from six 1-day old chicks: *antiserum*; rabbit anti-chicken light chain (anti-LC) purified by acid elution from immunoadsorbent of chicken IgG (Section 9.6), *control serum*; rabbit anti-KLH antibody prepared in a similar manner.

CALCULATION OF INITIAL CONCENTRATION OF REAGENTS FOR PROTEIN IODINATION

Oxidation conditions: use 37×10^6 Bq of ^{125}I per 200 μg of protein in 100 μg ml^{-1} chloramine T (final concentration). The protein concentration must be at or above 5 mg ml^{-1} to avoid excessive denaturation.

Specimen calculation
Rabbit anti-chicken LC and anti-KLH at 20 mg ml^{-1} initial concentration. To label 6 aliquots of bursa cells at 50 μg of antibody per aliquot = 300 μg protein, use 55.5×10^6 Bq ^{125}I. ^{125}I (IMS 30) is supplied at 3.7 GBq ml^{-1}, therefore use 15 μl. To maintain 5 mg ml^{-1} protein concentration calculate permissible volume of chloramine T as follows:

protein used = 15 μl at 20 mg ml^{-1},
maximum permissible oxidation volume = 60 μl at 5 mg ml^{-1}.

Final oxidation mixture
15 μl protein + 15 μl ^{125}I + 20 μl chloramine T (total volume = 50 μl, protein concentration = 6 mg ml^{-1}).
Chloramine T used at 100 μg ml^{-1} final concentration, therefore initial concentration must be 250 μg ml^{-1}, i.e. prepare an initial solution of *25 mg chloramine T in 100 ml PBS*.

Reaction stopped by a twofold excess, by weight, of sodium metabisulphite.

Final mixture
15 ml protein + 15 μl ^{125}I + 20 μl chloramine T + 50 μl sodium metabisulphite. Total volume = 100 μl.
Final concentration of metabisulphite = 200 μg ml^{-1}; initial concentration must be 400 μg ml^{-1}, i.e. prepare an initial solution of *40 mg sodium metabisulphite in 100 ml PBS*.

Method
1 Partially seal the end of two pieces of glass tubing, length 30 cm, internal diameter 0.6 cm, and plug with cotton wool.
2 Pour two columns of Sephadex G-25, height 10 cm.
3 Determine void volume and expanded sample volume of each column using 0.3 ml blue dextran (initial sample volume). Equilibrate columns with PBS (Section 1.5).

4 Pipette out protein for iodination into pointed glass tubes.

5 Add calculated volume of sodium ^{125}I (*carefully*).

6 Add chloramine T and oxidise for 3 min at room temperature.

7 Terminate reaction by addition of sodium metabisulphite.

8 Adjust final volume to 0.3 ml with PBS.

9 Pass the iodination mixture through the Sephadex G-25 column.

10 Monitor the column effluent for the first appearance of radioactivity. (This should be just after the void volume has left the column.)

11 Collect the labelled protein in the expanded sample volume.

The radioactively labelled protein may be stored overnight at 4° before use.

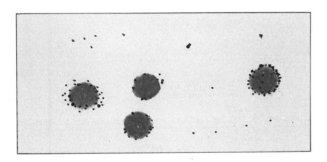

Fig. 3.8 Anti-light-chain labelling of chicken bursa cells.
Cells: 1-day old white leghorn bursa.
Antiserum: ^{125}I-anti-LC antibodies.
Control: ^{125}I-anti-KLH antibodies.

CELL LABELLING

1 Add 50 µg of iodinated protein (either anti-LC or anti-KLH) to aliquots of 10^7 bursal lymphocytes.

2 Incubate at 4° for 30 min.

3 Centrifuge each aliquot of cells through a 2 ml discontinuous gradient of 50% and 100% fetal bovine serum in tissue culture medium (225 *g* for 15 min at 4°).

4 Suck off the supernatant and re-suspend the cells in 1 ml of tissue culture medium.

5 Layer the cells onto a second gradient and centrifuge.

6 Finally re-suspend the cell pellet in a few drops of fetal bovine serum and prepare smears as described in Section 3.2.2 or 3.2.3.

7 Check that the smears are adequate using a phase-contrast microscope, and adjust the cell concentration in the original suspension with fetal bovine serum if required.

8 Prepare at least six smears per cell aliquot, and label the slides for identification.

9 Fix the slides (Section 4.4.4), wash with running tap water for 30 min and finally air dry.

10 Dip the slides in a 1 : 5 solution (v/v) of Ilford K5 nuclear emulsion and dry slides in front of a fan or over silica gel overnight (in a photographic dark room).

11 Leave slides to expose in light-tight containers at 4°. (Do not store near radioactive materials.)

EXPOSURE TIME

1 Under the conditions described, one sample slide should be removed from each group after 4–5 days.

Proportion of labelled cells											
Number of grains	0 5	6 11	12 17	18 23	24 29	30 25	36 41	42 47	48 53	54 59	>60
Anti-LC	0·08	0·15	0·17	0·17	0·10	0·10	0·08	0·06	0·02	0·03	0·04
Anti-KLH	0·95	0·05									
% positive cells	0	11	17	17	10	10	8	6	2	3	4

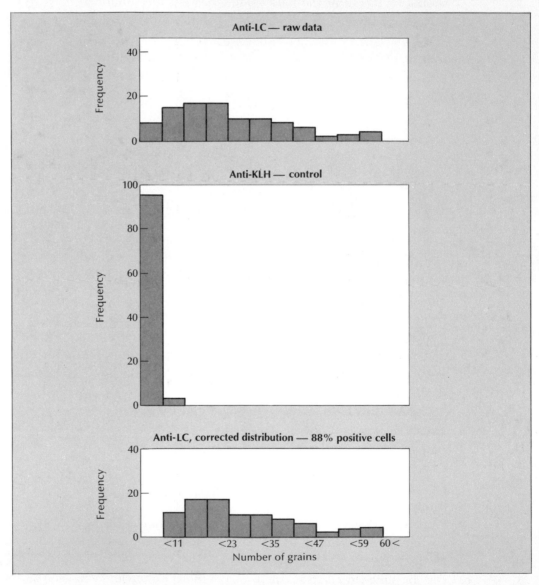

Fig. 3.9 Histograms of grain counts from autoradiographs of ^{125}I-anti-light chain (anti-LC) and anti-keyhole limpet haemocyanin (anti-KLH) labelling of chicken B lymphocytes.

2 Develop, fix and wash the sample autoradiographs and then stain in May−Grünwald/Giemsa (Section 3.3).

3 Examine the slides under oil immersion. If the autoradiographs in the control groups show more than eight to 10 grains per cell, develop all the slides. If, however, the control staining is low, examine the anti-LC treated cells. If the grain counts are clearly above the control values, develop all the slides.

4 Sample the autoradiographs at least every 4 days until satisfactory positive labelling is achieved with a low number of grains on the control cells.

5 At the end of the exposure period (usually 10−14 days under the conditions described), select at least two slides per group for grain counting. Use the following criteria:

(a) The cells must be sufficiently spread so that the grains between two adjacent cells do not overlap.

(b) The cell density must be similar on anti-LC and control slides within each group.

(c) The emulsion over the cells must be free from 'fogging' of any source.

6 Count the number of grains over at least 200 cells per group (Fig. 3.8). Record and rank the grain counts as shown in Fig. 3.9.

7 Calculate the frequency of cells within each ranked group.

CALCULATION OF PERCENTAGE OF POSITIVE CELLS

The proportion of cells showing positive labelling, i.e. grains above those expected by the non-specific binding of labelled protein and for other non-specific reasons, may be calculated by the following equation:

For each grain-count category:

$$C_p = (C_a - C_c) \times \frac{1}{1 - C_c} \, 100$$

where:

C_p = % positively labelled cells,
C_a = proportion cells labelled with antiserum,
C_c = proportion cells labelled with control serum.

Calculate the % positive cells in each category for each group. Plot a graph of cell frequency against grain counts. A specimen result and calculation is shown in Fig. 3.9.

3.6 T- and B-lymphocyte receptors

The terms 'receptor' and 'binding site' are often erroneously considered to be interchangeable. Although a receptor is certainly a binding site, the term imparts some biological significance to the binding event in initiating a positive or negative effect. The cell-surface antigen, mitogen and cytokine receptors undoubtedly deserve this status; however, it remains to be shown whether the so-called Fc and complement receptors deserve this distinction.

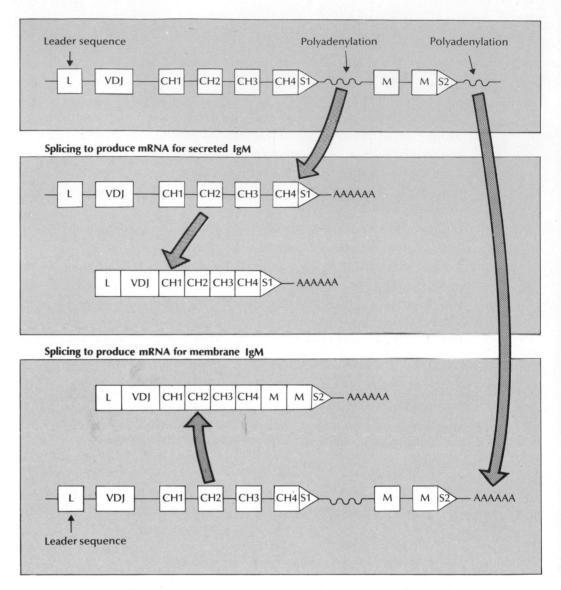

Fig. 3.10 Control of IgM expression. The same genetic information is used to synthesise IgM in two quite different forms: (a) for integration into the lymphocyte-surface membrane as a receptor (Fig. 3.12); and (b) for secretion as an antibody molecule (Fig. 14.1). Control is achieved by polyadenylation at one of two potential sites in the DNA (wavy line in the figure). Poly-A addition at the first site means that transcription does not include the two exons coding for the transmembrane stretches of the molecule, the final stop codon (S2) or the second polyadenylation site. Splicing of the primary transcript results in mRNA which yields the heavy chain of secreted IgM on translation.

Conversely, polyadenylation at the second site allows a primary transcript which includes the two exons coding for the transmembrane sequences and is terminated by the final stop codon. Splicing of the primary transcript removes the first stop codon (S1) and adenylation site to produce an mRNA coding for the heavy chain of an IgM receptor molecule.

The light chain mRNA is the same for either form of IgM.

3.6.1   Range of receptors

Antigen receptors

Both B and T lymphocytes have cell-surface receptors which are able to recognise antigenic determinants (epitopes) by means of their complementary stereo-specificity. Although the chemical nature of the receptors on T and B lymphocytes is profoundly different, both receptor types belong to a highly polymorphic family of molecules with a variable region, which is responsible for antigen binding, held in a relatively constant framework which orientates the receptor in the lymphocyte membrane. In both cases the variability is clonally distributed: all members of a clone have the same type of variable region and antigen-binding specificity.

B lymphocytes have monomeric IgM and IgD molecules integrated into their surface membranes as antigen receptors. Intriguingly, the same base set of information is used for the synthesis of secreted (antibody) and membrane-bound (receptor) IgM. The biophysical problem posed by the same molecule having to function in an hydrophilic (plasma) and hydrophobic (cell membrane) environment is overcome by the addition of an extra sequence of 25 hydrophobic amino acids to the carboxy terminus of the IgM heavy chain destined for membrane integration. The mechanism for this impressively economic use of genetic information is summarised in Fig. 3.10.

Antigen recognition by T lymphocytes is a much more complex affair and requires the interaction of several molecules whose functions have yet to be fully elucidated. In the majority of lymphocytes, the structural diversity required to react to the antigenic universe comes from the variable regions of the α and β polypeptide chains which form the TcR receptor. These chains also have constant regions and are generally considered to share a common evolutionary origin with immunoglobulin. A second molecule, designated CD3, is non-covalently linked to the TcR receptor and consists of at least four invariant polypeptide chains (γ, δ, ε and ζ). The relationship of these chains is shown diagrammatically in Fig. 3.11. Antibodies to CD3 will activate T lymphocytes without regard to clonal specificity, so the molecule is assumed to be associated in some way with transduction of the activation signal.

Whereas B lymphocytes recognise antigen alone, T lymphocytes recognise antigen only when it is combined with self major histocompatibility (MHC) molecules. It is thought that the TcR/CD3 receptors combine, in functional terms, with the CD4 molecules on the surface of helper T lymphocytes or the CD8 molecules on the surface of cytotoxic T lymphocytes to form a complex which recognises antigen in association with class I (cytotoxic T lymphocytes) or class II (helper T lymphocytes) MHC molecules. X-ray crystallographic evidence has revealed an enzyme-like cleft on the outer face of the MHC molecule, thus providing a potential site for the known interaction between MHC molecules and some foreign peptides.

Taken together, the available chemical and biological data suggest that all of these molecules form a single supergene family of recognition molecules (Fig. 3.12).

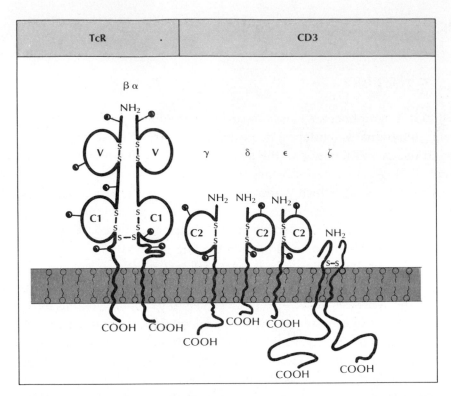

Fig. 3.11 T-lymphocyte receptor for antigen. The T-lymphocyte receptor is a complex of at least three main components: the polymorphic TcR chains determining antigen specificity, combined with the CD3 complex and, in helper T lymphocytes, the CD4 molecule or, in suppressor / cytotoxic lymphocytes, the CD8 molecule. The molecular features of the main arrays are shown in the figure.

In the majority of lymphocytes, the TcR component is composed of an α- and β-glycoprotein heterodimer, which determines antigenic specificity. However, in a small proportion of cells (0.5–10% of human peripheral blood T lymphocytes and 0.2–0.9% thymocytes) a γδ dimer is expressed. The precise significance of this substitution is unknown; however, a high proportion of T lymphocytes in the skin, gut and rheumatoid joints use the γδ combination of polymorphic chains.

The CD3 component is an array of invariant polypeptide chains, termed γ, δ, ε and ζ. These integral membrane proteins are thought to be associated with signal transduction after activation of the TcR by antigen. The observation that serine or tyrosine residues on the CD3 chains become phosphorylated after lymphocyte stimulation, is in accord with this hypothesis.

Intriguingly, the TcR/CD3 complex is pre-formed in the endoplasmic reticulum prior to glycosylation in the Golgi complex and insertion into the cell membrane.

Fc and complement receptors (binding sites)

Many cells, for example mast cells, monocytes, neutrophils, lymphocytes, platelets and placental syncytiotrophoblasts, carry receptors for the Fc region of immunoglobulin molecules. Although there is a weak, easily reversible binding of native (monomeric) IgG to such cells, the strength of binding is greater with IgG antibody complexed either with antigen (Section 3.6.2) or aggregated by heat. This is in direct contrast to the high affinity shown by mast-cell Fc receptors for monomeric IgE (affinity constant around 10^9–10^{10} M^{-1}).

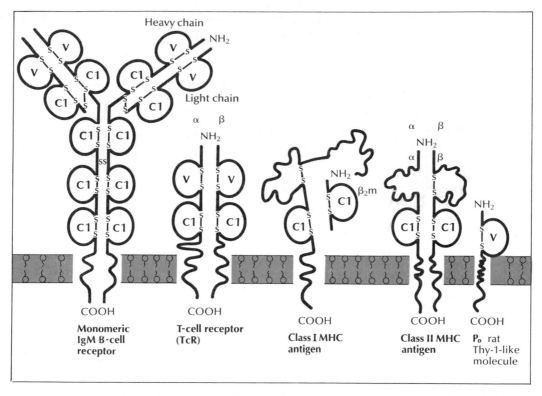

Fig. 3.12 Molecules in the immunoglobulin supergene family. The figure shows the folded polypeptide chains of the members of the immunoglobulin supergene family with a known immune function. Each of the constant (C) or variable (V) region loops is stabilised by an intrachain disulphide bond, and in the case of secreted and receptor (shown here) IgM the heavy (H) and light (L) chains are held together by interchain disulphide bonds in addition to non-covalent interactions.

The different molecules depicted here each represent multi-gene families, for example the heavy and light chains of immunoglobulin, and are thought to have diverged from a single primordial molecule by gene duplication and mutation. It is obvious from the figure that the loop or domain is a repeating feature and suggests that the primordial molecule might have been similar in structure to the single-copy, but variable, gene encoding the Thy-1 molecule found on the surface of mouse T lymphocytes (Fig. 3.15). Although the structural homology between the different molecular families in this series is high, they have relatively low sequence homology and, on present evidence, serve different functions.

Similar sequences have been grouped into three categories called V-SET, C1-SET and C2-SET. The first set includes the antigen-specific receptor V-domains and other sequences likely to have a similar fold. The C1-SET is composed largely of receptor-constant domains and major histocompatibility complex (MHC) antigen domains. C1 is defined by similarities in conserved sequences which serve to distinguish it from C2. Both C1 and C2 sequences are likely to fold as for immunoglobulin constant region domains.

It is also possible to demonstrate a site for the binding of the activation products of C3 (presumably *in vivo* in the form of antigen−antibody−complement complexes) to many cells, including B lymphocytes.

In many cases the function of the Fc or C3 receptors is clear, for example, both types of receptor are involved in promoting the phagocytic activity of macrophages, and the transplacental passage of IgG via receptors on placental syncytiotrophoblasts is well understood. However, the physiological significance of such receptors on T and B lymphocytes remains to be determined.

3.6.2 ## Detection of Fc receptors on lymphocytes

Materials
Mice
Sheep erythrocytes, SRBC (Appendix II)
Anti-SRBC serum, mouse or rabbit (Section 6.14.1)
Saline (Appendix I)
Tissue culture medium (Appendix I)
Tris−ammonium chloride (Appendix I)

Method
1   Wash SRBC three times in saline by centrifugation (300 *g* for 5 min).
2   Re-suspend pellet to 2×10^8 cells ml^{-1} (approximately 1% v/v) in tissue culture medium.
3   Incubate aliquots of the erythrocytes with the antiserum dilutions in a total volume of 0.5 ml (shown in the Protocol) for 30 min at 37°.

Protocol

	Tube number			
	1	2	3	4
SRBC (2×10^8 ml^{-1})	0.5 ml ————————————————→			
Final antiserum dilution	1:5	1:10	1:20	1:40

4   Wash each aliquot of SRBC three times in tissue culture medium by centrifugation and re-suspend to 1 ml.
5   Take a sample from each aliquot of SRBC and examine under a microscope. Discard all aliquots showing visible agglutination.
6   Prepare cell suspensions from thymus, lymph nodes and spleen (Section 1.15) and wash three times in tissue culture medium by centrifugation (150 *g* for 10 min at 4°).
7   Count lymphocytes and adjust to 5×10^6 cells ml^{-1} (Section 3.4.3).
8   Mix 0.1 ml of each lymphocyte suspension with 0.2 ml of sensitised SRBC. Use SRBC suspension with the lowest antiserum dilution not giving agglutination.
9   Incubate at room temperature for 60−90 min.
10   Add acridine orange or toluidine blue dye (Section 3.5.3).
11   Determine the number of rosettes ml^{-1} as in Section 3.5.3.
12   Count the number of viable lymphocytes ml^{-1}.
13   Calculate the percentage of lymphocytes forming Fc rosettes.

The appearance of typical rosettes is shown in Fig. 3.13.

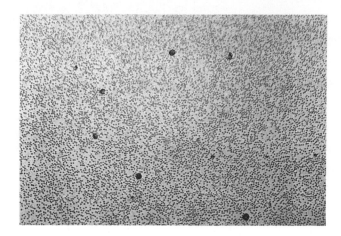

Fig. 3.13 Fc receptors on lymphocytes detected by sheep erythrocyte—antibody complexes. The Fc of the antibody—erythrocyte complex binds to the Fc-binding site on the lymphocyte forming a rosette which can be seen easily, even at low magnification. The majority of the Fc-binding lymphocytes are B cells, although recent evidence indicates that 3% of small T lymphocytes and 40% of antigen-activated T cells have Fc-binding sites that can be detected by this technique.

3.7 Mobility of the lymphocyte-surface membrane

Current models of eukaryotic cell membranes view the surface antigens of cells as though they were in a viscous, (virtually) two-dimensional solution in the phospholipid bilayer. Consequently, they move relatively freely and at random in the plane of the membrane but, because the majority of transmembrane molecules have polar outer and apolar inner regions, never change their position by a 'flip flop' re-orientation. Treatment of eukaryotic cells with bi- or multi-functional cross-linking agents, such as antibody or antigen, causes a dramatic but selective change in the distribution of surface antigens (as demonstrated in Section 3.7.1). There is rapid, local micro-precipitation to form surface patches (as viewed using fluorescent probes), this process is energy independent and temperature insensitive. Thereafter, the patches slowly coalesce to form a 'cap' which is then either internalised or 'shed' into the surrounding medium. This latter response is probably brought about by a re-distribution of the cytoskeletal components of the cells and as a consequence is energy dependent (metabolic poisons, such as sodium azide inhibit 'capping' reversibly) and greatly retarded by cooling to near 0°.

Significantly, capping of one type of two unrelated surface antigens re-distributes or removes one but leaves the other unaffected. This property may be used to investigate the nature of the interaction between cell-surface molecules. Evidence of co-capping of two distinct molecules in the presence of cross-linking agent reacting with only one of them, is sufficient to demonstrate even weak chemical interactions. This technique was used to provide the first evidence of an interaction between the TcR and CD3 surface molecules of T lymphocytes. An interaction too weak to be demonstrated initially by classical detergent extraction and immunoprecipitation.

3.7.1 Capping of lymphocyte receptors

Materials and equipment
Mouse-spleen or lymph-node suspension on ice

Tissue culture medium with and without sodium azide, 20 mM, final concentration
 (Appendix I)
Rabbit anti-mouse immunoglobulin serum (Section 1.7.2).
Fluorescein-conjugated goat or sheep anti-rabbit immunoglobulin (Sections 2.1 or
 Appendix II).

Method

1 Prepare a cell suspension from spleen or lymph node (Section 1.15), using tissue
   culture medium *without* sodium azide.
2 Wash the suspension three times by centrifugation (150 g for 10 min at 4°).
3 Count the viable lymphocytes and dispense aliquots of 10^7 cells into each tube
   shown in the Protocol. Centrifuge (150 g for 10 min at 4°) to obtain a cell pellet.

Protocol

		Incubation		
Tube number	Antiserum added	Temperature	Time (min)	Medium
1	Anti-mouse Ig	4°	30	With azide
2	NRS control	4°	30	With azide
3	Anti-mouse Ig	37°	5	Without azide
4	Anti-mouse Ig	37°	10	Without azide
5	Anti-mouse Ig	37°	15	Without azide
6	Anti-mouse Ig	37°	20	Without azide
7	Anti-mouse Ig	37°	30	Without azide
8	Anti-mouse Ig	37°	60	Without azide

4 Add 0.1 ml of anti-mouse Ig or normal rabbit serum to tubes 1 and 2. (The
   antiserum must be diluted with medium containing sodium azide, 20 mM final
   concentration. The sera should have been standardised for immunofluorescent
   staining, Section 2.1.6.)
5 Incubate tubes 1 and 2 on ice for 30 min.
6 Add the same dilution of anti-mouse Ig to tubes 3−8; however, this time dilute
   the antiserum with medium *without* sodium azide.
7 Incubate tubes 3−8 in a water bath or incubator at 37°.
8 Remove tubes from the 37° incubator at the intervals shown in the Protocol and
   fill them with medium containing sodium azide, 20 mM, and stand on ice.
9 At the end of the incubation period for tubes 1 and 2, fill these with medium
   containing azide and store on ice.
10 At the end of the total incubation period (60 min), wash all cell suspensions
   (tubes 1−8) twice by centrifugation (150 g for 10 min at 4°).
11 Incubate all cell aliquots with 0.1 ml of goat or sheep anti-rabbit Ig conjugate
   (1 mg ml^{-1} final dilution) for 30 min at 4°. (Again the diluted conjugate must
   contain sodium azide.)
12 Wash cells three times by centrifugation (150 g for 10 min at 4°).
13 Re-suspend the cell pellet in glycerol/glycine−saline mounting medium and

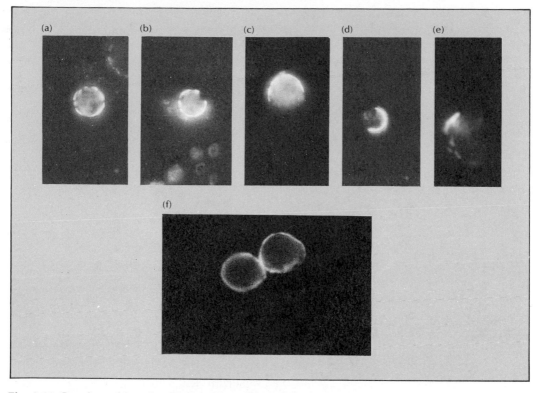

Fig. 3.14 Capping of lymphocyte receptors. If lymphocytes are treated with divalent anti-immunoglobulin antibodies the surface immunoglobulin determinants are cross-linked to form aggregates visible as a patchy ring of surface fluorescence (**a**).

At 37° and in the absence of metabolic inhibitors these patches coalesce (**a**–**d**) to form a 'polar cap' (**e**) which within 30 min is usually pinocytosed or shed into the medium. (Photograph (**e**) is at twice the magnification of the others.)

Monovalent Fab anti-immunoglobulin antibodies are not able to cross-link the determinants and so ring staining is obtained (**f**), even at 37°. Pinocytosis still occurs on a limited scale even though patch and cap formation is not induced. Surprisingly, ring staining is obtained when mouse T cells are stained with directly conjugated anti-Thy-1 serum (Section 3.8.3) presumably because of the low density of Thy-1 determinants.

observe the fluorescing lymphocytes, preferably with an incident light UV microscope.

Observations

Tube 1. Here you should see the normal 'broken ring' immunofluorescence (Fig. 3.14a) already seen for mouse lymphocytes (Fig. 3.6c).

Tube 2. This is the control and should show no staining. If not, proceed as in Section 2.1.7.

Tubes 3–8. You should observe staining as shown in Fig. 3.14, photographs (a) to (e) with a progressive clustering of the fluorescence to a polar 'cap'. With some anti-Ig sera this cap is then endocytosed and appears as pin-points of fluorescence within the cell. With other antisera, which do not induce endocytosis, the stained membrane components are shed into the medium at 37° in the absence of respiratory inhibitors (e.g. sodium azide).

14 Determine the percentage of cells in each suspension showing: (a) broken ring; and (b) capped staining. If your antiserum induces endocytosis, determine the percentage of cells containing ingested fluorochrome.

15 Plot a graph against time for each set of data.

3.7.2 # Differential mobility of membrane components

This experiment requires techniques and antisera found later in the book. We include it here simply as it is an extremely useful research tool.

Capping of unrelated membrane components

In Section 3.7.1 you observed that surface components of the membranes of nucleated cells could be made to change their distribution by the use of bi-functional cross-linking agents; in the experiment described the cross-linking agent was an anti-immunoglobulin molecule. We now wish to show that this re-distribution of surface components is specific to the cross-linking agent used. In other words, in the experiment described an anti-Ig antiserum will cause Ig receptors to cap but will leave other, unrelated components undisturbed.

Materials and equipment
Mouse lymph-node or spleen lymphocytes
Tissue culture medium with and without 20 mM sodium azide
Directly conjugated rabbit anti-mouse Ig (fluorescein)
Directly conjugated anti-MHC monoclonal antibody (labelled with rhodamine or phycoerythrin, Appendix II)
UV microscope, capable of dual excitation — to allow the use of the direct conjugates this should have incident UV illumination (it is complex and soul-destroying to perform this experiment by indirect immunofluorescence)

INITIAL PREPARATION OF ANTISERA
We are going to stain the same cell with both antisera; it is therefore essential to ensure that the antisera do not cross-react.

1 Prepare a suspension of mouse thymus cells in medium.
2 Wash three times by centrifugation (150 g for 10 min at 4°).
3 Add an equal volume of rabbit anti-mouse Ig to the dry cell pellet.
4 Mix at 4° overnight, then spin off the cells at 300 g for 20 min at 4° and store the antiserum at −20°.
5 Prepare the γ-globulin fraction of mouse serum using 40% saturated ammonium sulphate (Section 1.3.2) and insolubilise with glutaraldehyde (Section 2.1.8).

6 Mix an equal volume of insolubilised mouse immunoglobulin with the rabbit anti-mouse lymphocyte serum. Mix overnight at 4° or at 37° for 3 h.

7 Spin off the antiserum (500 g for 20 min at 4°) and store at −20°.

We are using a vast excess of immunoadsorbent to ensure complete absorption.

Method

1 Incubate 10^7 lymphocytes with fluorescein-conjugated anti-mouse Ig serum at a suitable dilution (Section 2.1.6) for 30 min at 37°. The medium must not contain azide.

2 Spin the cells down in medium containing sodium azide, final concentration 20 mM (150 g for 10 min at 4°) and incubate with rhodamine or phycoerythrin-conjugated anti-mouse MHC antibody (the antibody should have been standardised for immunofluorescent staining, Section 2.1.6) for 30 min at 4° in the presence of 20 mM sodium azide.

3 Wash the cells by centrifugation and prepare them for examination under the UV microscope (Section 3.5.1).

Observations

Using sequential UV excitation for fluorescein and rhodamine or phycoerythrin dyes, you should see cells with green caps and red bodies, showing that the re-distribution has affected the Ig molecules alone. Here only one antiserum was used under 'capping' conditions. We suggest you repeat the experiment using the antisera as a mixture under 'capping' conditions and observe the localisation of the two caps, one relative to the other.

The basic ability to selectively remove cell-surface components as defined by bi- or multi-functional cross-linking agents has very wide applicability. One could, for example, investigate whether two cell-surface components are distinct by causing one or the other to cap; co-capping would then indicate a close association between the two components. In addition, one can overcome the problem of potential steric hindrance between two surface components by simply capping one away.

3.8 Antibodies to cell-surface antigens

In addition to monoclonal antibodies, polyclonal antisera against polymorphic cell-surface antigens may be produced reproducibly by immunisation between congenic strains of animals (almost invariably mice, Section 1.19.1). Because the two strains of animals are identical except for the locus carrying the two allelic genes, only the antigens of interest (alloantigens) will be recognised as foreign and elicit an antibody response.

Hybridoma-produced antibodies are commercially available to many alloantigens, including H-2 and Thy-1 gene products (Appendix II).

3.8.1 Anti-lymphocyte serum

Anti-lymphocyte sera (ALS) have been used to suppress the cells mediating the immune response in both humans and animals. Anti-lymphocyte sera are potentially more specific immunosuppressive agents than, for example, X-irradiation or cyto-toxic drugs which also suppress haemopoietic function. For use *in vivo* the hetero-antiserum is fractionated to obtain γ-globulin or IgG to reduce the amount of foreign protein injected into the recipient. Additionally, the antiserum is ultracentrifuged to remove soluble aggregates and so reduce its immunogenicity to a level where it might become tolerogenic.

Materials
Mice, preferably inbred, 4–6 weeks of age
Rabbits

Method
1 Remove thymuses from mice and prepare a single-cell suspension.
2 Inject 10^9 viable lymphocytes into the marginal ear vein of the rabbit.
3 Two weeks later repeat the injection; however, the rabbit must first receive an anti-anaphylactic agent; for example, 25 mg promethazine hydrochloride given intravenously.
4 Two weeks later exsanguinate the rabbit by cardiac puncture.
5 Separate the serum, inactivate the complement components at 56° for 30 min and store at −20°.

3.8.2 Mode of action of ALS *in vivo*

Anti-lymphocyte sera are able to kill both T and B cells in *in vivo* assays; surprisingly, however, there is a marked T-cell specificity when used *in vivo*. Hence, in mice, the system most extensively studied, T-dependent areas of the spleen and lymph nodes are markedly depleted, and only T-dependent, but not T-independent, humoral responses are suppressed after ALS treatment. Accordingly, adult thymectomy accompanied by ALS treatment is as effective at suppressing the T-cell pool as neonatal thymectomy.

It is known that ALS do not penetrate lymphoid tissues appreciably and so only cells in the re-circulating pool, mainly T cells, are susceptible to ALS killing. Although ALS can kill lymphoid cells with the aid of complement, it is likely that immune adherence and opsonisation followed by phagocytosis by the reticuloendothelial system is the main mechanism by which immunosuppression is effected.

3.8.3 Polyclonal antisera to lymphocyte-surface antigens

H-2 congenic mice can be cross-immunised to produce antisera which can be useful strain-specific reagents for cell and animal strain typing. In addition, several useful

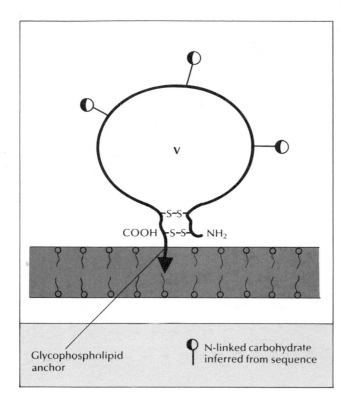

Fig. 3.15 Thy-1 molecule — a primordial member of the immunoglobulin supergene family. The Thy-1 antigen is expressed in large amounts on T lymphocytes (both peripheral blood T cells and thymocytes), neural tissue and fibrobasts. It is a 25 kDa glycoprotein bound to the cell membrane through a phosphoinositol-containing, membrane-binding domain. Although its usefulness as a murine T-lymphocyte marker is beyond doubt, its function is unknown. It is thought to be a modern example of one of the primitive molecular ancestors of the immunoglobulin supergene family (Fig. 3.12) and has interesting similarities to a glycoprotein from squid neural tissue.

Although it is common practice to draw carbohydrate moieties as small sticks, in an accurate space-filling model, the sugar residues would occupy over 90% of the molecular volume.

alloantigens have been recognised on mouse lymphocytes and plasma cells. These antigens are strain-specific differentiation antigens and occur on subpopulations of cells; for example, the Thy-1 antigen (Fig. 3.15) which occurs predominantly on thymocytes and T lymphocytes. Thy-1 occurs as two alleles: (a) gene Thy-1[a], gene product Thy-1.1 on T cells of AKR, RF and several substrains; (b) gene Thy-1[b], gene product Thy-1.2 on T cells of most other inbred and outbred strains. Antisera may be raised to these antigens by cross-immunising congenic mice using cells which carry the antigen of interest. We will describe a technique for the production of an anti-Thy-1 polyclonal serum — a precisely similar approach may be taken for the production and validation of other polyclonal alloantisera; for example, anti-H-2.

Materials
AKR and C3H or CBA mice; alternatively use AKR/J and AKR/Cum mice — these are congenic strains differing only at the Thy-1 locus

Method
1 Prepare a thymocyte suspension from AKR donors (Section 1.15).
2 Inject 3×10^7 thymocytes intraperitoneally into each C3H or CBA recipient weekly for 10 weeks.
3 Take a sample bleed from the tail of immunised mice on week 11, pool serum and test by cytotoxicity (Section 7.5).

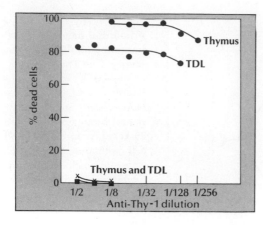

Fig. 3.16 Complement-mediated cytotoxicity with anti-Thy-1 serum.
●———● Anti-Thy-1 plus complement.
×———× Normal AKR serum plus complement.
■———■ Anti-Thy-1 serum alone.
Percentage immunoglobulin positive B lymphocytes by immunofluorescence: thymus 0.3% thoracic-duct lymphocytes 18.9%.

A specimen titration curve is given in Fig. 3.16. Exsanguinate the mice when a high-titre antiserum has been obtained.

Technical note

As the mice (AKR,C3H and CBA) are histocompatible at the MHC, no anti-H-2 antibodies are produced by this immunisation procedure. Several other contaminating antibodies have been identified, however, such as anti-thymocyte autoantibody and anti-immunoglobulin allotype antibody. In the assay systems described in this book, these contaminating antibodies are not detected and so the anti-Thy-1 serum may be used specifically to detect, kill or inhibit T cells.

3.9 Analytical continuous-flow cytofluorimetry

The technique of analytical continuous-flow cytofluorimetry is analogous to the visual assessment of the intensity of fluorescence that is sometimes made while

Fig. 3.17 (*Facing page*) **The continuous-flow cytofluorimeter**. Cells, in dilute suspension, are injected into the centre of a plastic nozzle through which a stream of sheath fluid flows continuously. As the cell and sheath buffer inlets are at different pressures, the concentric buffer streams emerging from the nozzle run at different rates and therefore do not mix; the cells are thus constrained at the centre of the carrier stream. Under stable conditions, each cell should follow virtually the same path.

Laser light, usually from an argon ion laser, is passed through a set of shaping lenses to produce a beam with an elliptical cross-section, which is aimed at the buffer stream falling to waste. The buffer stream acts as a vertical cylindrical lens and disperses a small proportion of the laser light in the same horizontal plane as the beam. However, the majority of the light continues forward through the buffer stream and is absorbed harmlessly by the cylindrical beam dump. The optical system is aligned so that, provided the laser beam does not hit a cell, no light signal is recorded by the instrument; the horizontally dispersed light is absorbed by obscuration bars placed across the front face of the collecting lenses in the forward angle and at 90 degrees to the incident beam.

Any cell interacting with the laser beam acts as a spherical lens and disperses the light in all directions out of the horizontal plane (shown in the inset). Light is collected by detector systems placed in the direction of travel of the beam (forward-angle light scatter) and at right angles to the direction of travel (90-degree light scatter). It the cell is labelled with one or more fluorochromes, the emitted light, which is shifted to a longer wavelength, is resolved from the original exciting

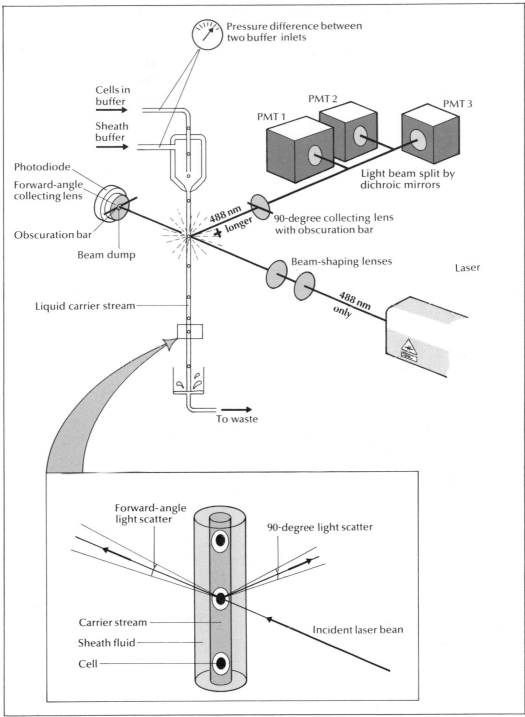

wavelength of the laser (for example, 488 nm for the laser and fluorochrome combinations most frequently used) by a combination of dichroic mirrors and long- and short-pass filters which direct the light to a series of photomultiplier tubes PMT2 and PMT3 in the figure. PMT1 is being used in this case for the detection of the 90-degree light scatter signal. The integral of the electrical impulse thus generated is digitised and stored or analysed in a computer.

Although the laser beam can be of sufficient intensity to burn a hole in a piece of card, the high thermal capacity of water protects the cells from harm. Viable cells can be sorted using this instrument, as described in Section 9.11.

counting cells stained with a fluorescein-conjugated antibody under a UV microscope (Section 3.5.1). However, as this technique allows accurate quantitation of fluorescence for each cell, determines the distribution of fluorescent intensities of the sample population (measurements on an average of 10 000 cells per sample can be made in a few minutes) and can be used to sort and select the cells individually (Section 9.11), it may be appreciated that the analogy is a very loose one. Even so, the microscope is a very useful tool in the flow cytometer room. Visual inspection of cells, particularly under new experimental conditions, can avoid operation of the flow cytometer in its 'garbage in, garbage out' mode.

The basic components of a flow cytometer are shown in Fig. 3.17. Cells are individually interrogated by the laser beam and the scattered or emitted light analysed in the forward angle and at 90° to the incident beam.

FORWARD-ANGLE LIGHT SCATTER, FALS

The amount of light scatter in the forward angle is proportional to the volume of a spherical cell (Fig. 3.18). This can be a very useful parameter at several stages in this technique:

(a) It is a very strong signal and may be detected by a photodiode — it tends to be a very 'robust' parameter for the initial 'setting up' of the instrument.

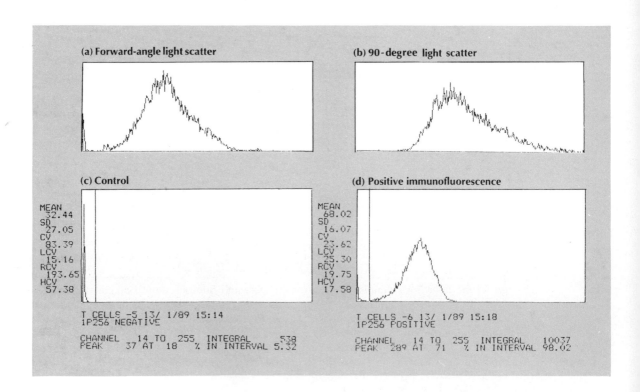

(b)   Viable cells tend to produce a larger degree of low-angle light scatter than dead cells — this attribute may be used to distinguish live from dead cells.

(c)   All cells, whether fluorescently labelled or not, must have a size. Counts based on this parameter are therefore used to set the sample size, usually 10 000 cells (events) per sample.

NINETY-DEGREE LIGHT SCATTER, 90°LS

The degree of light scattered out of the horizontal plane, measured at 90° to the

Fig. 3.18 (*Facing page*) **Flow cytometry parameters**. The data in the figure were derived from the analysis of the T-cell line CEM using a Coulter EPICS V cytofluorimeter, in each case analysing 10 000 events. Forward-angle light scatter, 90-degree light scatter and fluorescent data are plotted as frequency histograms using an ascending logarithmic horizontal scale divided into 256 channels.

(**a**) *Forward angle light scatter — FALS*. The intensity of the FALS signal is directly proportional to the volume of the cell being measured. The data have a clear bimodal distribution; a minor population of particles with a very low FALS signal (extreme left of distribution) probably due to cell debris and inorganic particles (described in flow cytometry jargon by a variety of epithets of Anglo-Saxon derivation) and a major population with a peak value just mid-way along the axis — these are the viable CEM cells. Although the standard polystyrene beads used to set up the instrument would have given a FALS distribution with a very low coefficient of variation, living cells — even from a cloned cell line — show marked variation in cell size. It is possible to examine a proportion of the above population only by setting an electronic 'gate'. In this instance the lower gate would be set to the right of the minor population, and the upper gate to the extreme right of major population. It is then possible to confine the measurement of a second parameter purely to those cells falling within the pre-set FALS values — they are 'gated in'.

(**b**) *90-degree light scatter — 90°LS*. This signal is proportional to the volume of the cell, but is also affected by other parameters such as granularity, surface topography, etc. Although in this instance, where we are using a tumour-cell line with a homogeneous cytoplasm, this parameter yields little additional information over FALS alone, its true value may be appreciated with reference to Fig. 3.21a and b.

Histograms (**c**) and (**d**) show the *relative fluorescent intensity* of cell populations stained with a directly conjugated irrelevant monoclonal antibody (histogram (**c**)) or a pan-T monoclonal antibody (histogram (**d**)). In each case, we are examining the fluorescence associated with the FALS 'gated-in' population alone.

(**c**) The majority of the signals given by the cells in this population could not be detected above the electronic 'noise' of the instrument. In order to set the fluorescent intensity limits for this negative control, it is convenient to set the lower cursor (depicted as vertical line) to a channel number which excludes (to the left) about 95% of the population — in the example shown, 5.3% of the cells fall in the interval between channels 14—255 (to the right of the cursor).

(**d**) This population of cells has been analysed with the same instrument settings as in (**c**), and 98% of the 10 000 cells analysed gave a fluorescent signal falling in the channel interval defined in (**c**). They are the specifically stained population. The computing software used on this instrument can use much more precise definitions of the positive and negative populations and carry out a 'channel-by-channel' analysis to obtain full information from the data.

In examples (**c**) and (**d**) we have used electronic cursors to define the fluorescent population only for analysis and integration. It is possible, however, to define a 'gated-in' population, either alone or with reference to the FALS gates already set from histogram (**a**). One may then examine a third parameter in relation to cells of a certain size (perhaps lymphocytes rather than platelets) and with a certain fluorescent attribute (for example, pan-T-positive lymphocytes in a population of peripheral blood mononuclear cells). The ability to measure using correlated parameters on a *per cell basis* provides these instruments with exquisite analytical and preparative (Section 9.11) capabilities.

incident beam, is also proportional to cell volume (Fig. 3.18). However, this parameter is also affected by cell-surface topography (for example, the number of surface villi or blebs), nucleus : cytoplasm ratio and the homogeneity of the cell's cytoplasm (for example, the size, number and optical properties of intracellular granules), etc. If a lymphocyte and a neutrophil had the same volume they would give a similar FALS signal but a different 90° light-scatter signal (cf. Fig. 3.21b).

QUANTITATION OF FLUORESCENCE

Although the number of fluorescein molecules attached to a single stained cell is low, the intensity of the laser irradiation and the sensitivity of detection is sufficient to permit the measurement and discrimination of the emissions from up to three different fluorochromes, provided the instrument has an appropriately equipped optical bench.

Reagent and sample preparation are precisely the same as described for microscope-based immunofluorescent techniques (Sections 2.1 and 3.5); however, the result is quantitative and derived from a larger sample (10000 cells [Fig. 3.18] compared to 200).

The introduction of phycoerythrin as a second fluorochrome, for use with fluorescein, has greatly simplified and extended the applications of this technique. The two dyes can be excited by the 488 nm line of a single argon-ion laser (Fig. 3.19) and easily resolved into two signals of comparable strength by a combination of dichroic mirrors and absorbance filters (Fig. 3.20).

MULTI-PARAMETER ANALYSIS

Each of the parameters described above (and several more not described) may be used interactively, to permit analyses of great precision and sophistication. One such

Fluorochrome	Maximum excitation (nm)	Peak emission (nm)	
Fluorescein isothiocyanate	495	525	Argon laser 488 nm
Phycoerythrin	475–560	576	
Texas red	596	615	Krypton laser 568 nm
Tetrarhodamine isothiocyanate	554	573	

Fig. 3.19 **Excitation and emission maxima of commonly used fluorochromes.** Note that in each case the emitted light is always shifted to a longer wavelength than that used for excitation. Although neither the argon nor krypton lasers have spectral lines which coincide precisely with the excitation maximum of the dyes used both the excitation and emission spectra are sufficiently broad to permit useful energy capture and light emission. The stability and ease of operation of these instruments is greatly enhanced when using only a single laser (they also cost less); consequently, the combination of fluorescein with phycoerythrin (Section 2.1) is virtually ideal for immunological investigations.

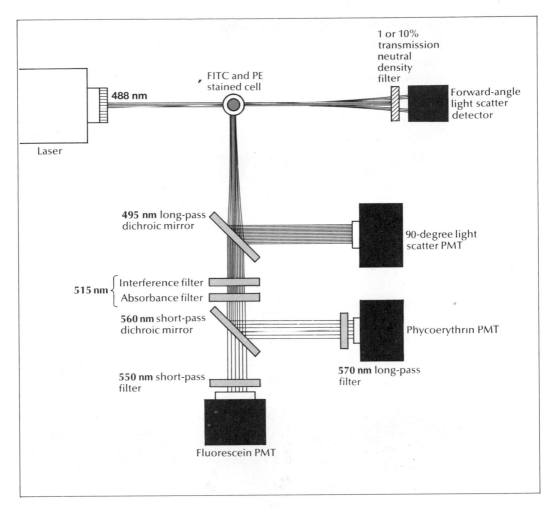

Fig. 3.20 Lens and mirror combinations used to resolve the signals emitted by stained cells. Laser light is monochromatic, stable and very powerful. Thus even subtle shifts of wavelength and minor changes of direction caused by refraction through a single cell can be detected by judicious selection of filters and dichroic mirrors. In principle, light near the original exciting wavelength is used to measure forward-angle light scatter (FALS) (using a photodiode placed in the forward angle) and 90-degrees light scatter (90°LS) (a weaker signal so it is detected using a photomultiplier). Thereafter, light of the exciting wavelength is stripped off using a pair of 515 nm filters which pass only longer (emitted) wavelengths. The dichroic mirror placed at an angle of 45 degrees to the light beam, and after the stripping filters, directs long wavelength light to the photomultiplier set to detect red light (phycoerythrin PMT), shorter wavelengths are not interrupted in their passage to the photomultiplier set to detect green light (fluorescein PMT). As the mirror does not split the wavelengths perfectly, it is 'backed-up' by long- and short-pass absorbance filters, as shown in the diagram. The final traces of 'breakthrough' between the red and green channels can be removed by electronic processing of the photomultiplier signals.

application is described in Fig. 3.21 where the aberrant expression of a T-cell marker is demonstrated on a single clone of B lymphocytes, analysed in the presence of whole blood. The example stopped at analysis; however, the full power of the technique can be appreciated when one realises that exactly the same approach could have been used to physically isolate viable cells from this clone for further investigation and experimentation (Section 9.11).

We have concentrated on a detailed consideration of the utility of this technique, and the interpretation of the data that can be obtained; rather than the instruments themselves. If you buy a flow cytometer, the instrument-based training takes about 5 days.

3.10 Summary and conclusions

The lymphocyte is a cell destined for great things after contact with antigen. Before antigenic stimulation most lymphocytes are dormant. They have, however, an array of surface receptors which in the case of B lymphocytes are modified immunoglobulin molecules of the same antigenic specificity and overall structure as the antibody ultimately secreted by the plasma cell. In contrast, the T-lymphocyte receptor for antigen seems extravagant in its complexity; antigen diversity is probably invested primarily in the TcR receptor, but this is then 'fine tuned' by interaction with the invariant CD3, CD4, CD8 and MIIC molecules.

The receptor molecules do not have a fixed distribution in the cell membrane but

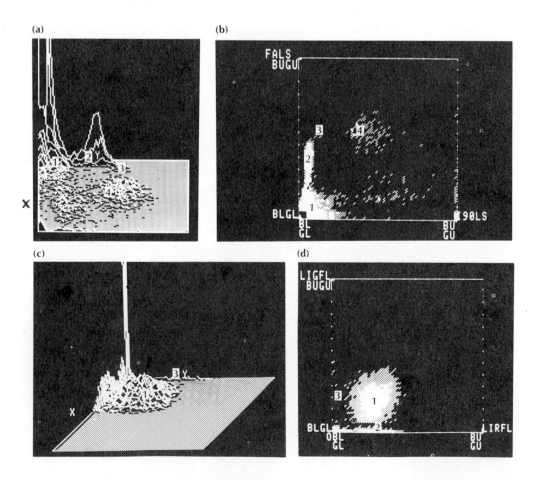

can be drawn together by cross-linking agents; for example, anti-Ig in the case of B lymphocytes. However, such blocked receptors are removed from the cell surface either by endocytosis or shedding. This may be a physiological process, probably occurring after antigenic contact, to allow the cell to re-synthesise new receptors.

Our understanding of the processes of intercellular signalling, activation and differentiation has developed enormously over the past 5 years. Even so, it is clear that much still remains to be discovered, particularly with regard to the intriguing complexities of the T-cell receptor.

Fig. 3.21 (*Facing page*) **Multi-parameter cytofluorimetry**. Figures (a) and (b) show an isometric (three-dimensional) and planar (two-dimensional) projection of the same data. Whole blood was stained with fluorescein- and phycoerythrin-conjugated antibodies, the erythrocytes lysed by osmotic shock and the resulting cell suspension washed by centrifugation, prior to analysis on a Coulter Electronics cytofluorimeter (EPICS V).

(a) In this histogram, forward-angle light scatter (FALS) is plotted along the y (rear) axis; 90-degree light scatter (90°LS) along the x (left) axis and frequency on the z (vertical axis). Although the relative numbers of cells in the different populations may be easily appreciated from this type of display, the nature of the populations (in terms of the parameters being measured) is more easily appreciated from a planar view, as in (b).

(b) An approximation to the relative abundance of the different populations is achieved in the two-dimensional display by different pixel densities, representing three selected 'levels' in the frequency data. The four populations of cells marked in the figure have the following characteristics and identity:

1 Low FALS and 90°LS — red-cell ghosts and platelets.
2 Medium FALS and low 90°LS — lymphocytes.
3 High FALS and low 90°LS (also low abundance) — monocytes.
4 High FALS and high 90°LS — granulocytes.

Electronic gates were set about the 'lymphocyte' population which was then analysed for the presence of a T- and B-lymphocyte marker. Even though other cells were present, both stained and unstained, they are now 'gated out' from further analysis.

Histograms (c) and (d) show three- and two-dimensional plots of fluorescent emissions of the cells examined in (a) and (b).

(c) It is possible to discern three distinct populations, one massive population in the centre of the distribution (1), and more minor populations on the x (2) and y (3) axes. The x axis corresponds to the red fluorescence associated with an antibody against a T-cell marker; whereas the y axis corresponds to the green fluorescence associated with an antibody against a B-cell marker. The three cell populations (more easily seen in (d)) have the following characteristics and identities:

1 High red and high green fluorescence — this is a population of B lymphocytes (see below) expressing a T-cell marker.
2 High red, low green — this is the staining pattern of the normal blood T-lymphocyte population.
3 Low red, high green — this is the staining pattern of the normal B-lymphocyte population in the blood, however, in this patient it is a very minor population.

These cells are derived from a patient with B-cell chronic lymphocytic leukaemia and so contain a monoclonally expanded population of aberrant B lymphocytes (Section 14.2). The residual normal B lymphocytes (on the y axis in (c)) have been virtually replaced by leukaemic cells, whereas the T-lymphocyte population is virtually unchanged. This type of qualitative and quantitative analysis can provide crucial data for haematological diagnosis of disease.

3.11
Further reading

Butler EB and Stanbridge CM (1986) *Cytology of Body Cavity Fluids*. Chapman and Hall, London.

Henry K and Farrer-Brown G (1981) *Colour Atlas of Thymus and Lymph Node Histology with Ultra-structure*. Wolfe Publishing, London.

Janossy G and Amlot PL (editors) (1986) *Lymphocytes in Health and Disease*. MTP Press, Lancaster.

Shapiro HM (1988) *Practical Flow Cytometry*, 2nd edition. Alan R Liss, New York.

4   Lymphocytes and Effector Cells

Immunological protection

To all external appearances the majority of small lymphocytes are undoubtedly uninteresting cells to the average immunologist who likes to observe spectacular dynamic change. The sheer diversity of their antigenic reactivity probably guarantees that many small lymphocytes never meet their specific antigen and so are never called upon to express their pre-ordained effector function. They simply spend their lives slowly turning over and divide only rarely.

Under the influence of antigen, however, the lymphocyte changes dramatically. Concurrent with the easily observable morphological changes, the lymphocyte nucleus becomes de-repressed, the cell enters the cell cycle and begins to divide to produce daughter cells all of the **same antigenic specificity**. Each stimulated cell can form a **clone** of effector cells each reacting with the same antigen. However, lymphocyte proliferation is asymmetric: very soon after antigen contact some of the proliferating cells revert to quiescent small lymphocytes known as **memory cells**. It is not known how this asymmetry is controlled or directed.

Eventually as the immune response declines, the effector cells are no longer active and are totally replaced by clones of small lymphocyte memory cells. Within a clone all of the cells have the same antigenic specificity as the original single lymphocyte. Memory cells loose their virgin status through contact with antigen and, in the case of B lymphocytes, are known to produce a changed effector function (a different class of immunoglobulin with the same antigen-binding specificity) upon second contact with the same antigen (Fig. 4.1).

This increase in number of initiator cells and the change in the quality of their effector function (for example, an IgM to IgG switch in the case of some B-lymphocyte subpopulations) is sufficient to explain all the characteristics of the memory or **anamnestic** response seen upon a second contact with the same antigen. Accordingly, as discussed in the previous chapter, when one has measles and recovers, there is an increase in the size of measles-specific lymphocyte clones — usually sufficient to ensure that the measles virus becomes only minimally established upon subsequent contact, and is unable to replicate to the numbers required to cause disease or to permit onward transmission.

The immunity thus gained is specific to the same or closely related antigens, i.e. cross-reacting viruses or antigens, and is protective (cf. autoimmunity [Sections 5.8.1 and 14.4.2] — a bad thing?). The reader will realise, without requiring to do the experiment, that this is the basis of vaccination. The subject is given a controlled exposure to a killed or avirulent strain of the pathogen to stimulate the immune system and prepare it to confront the virulent organism. It is important to realise the conceptual difference between infection and disease in this context. Protection may prevent disease but not necessarily by preventing infection. It has become apparent from epidemiological studies that subclinical infection after effective vaccination often consolidates immunity. Widespread application of the commonly used vaccines, which were previously thought to be totally effective, has now reduced the rate of natural infection and immune consolidation. Consequently, vaccine efficacy appears (artifactually) to be declining — they were probably never totally effective!

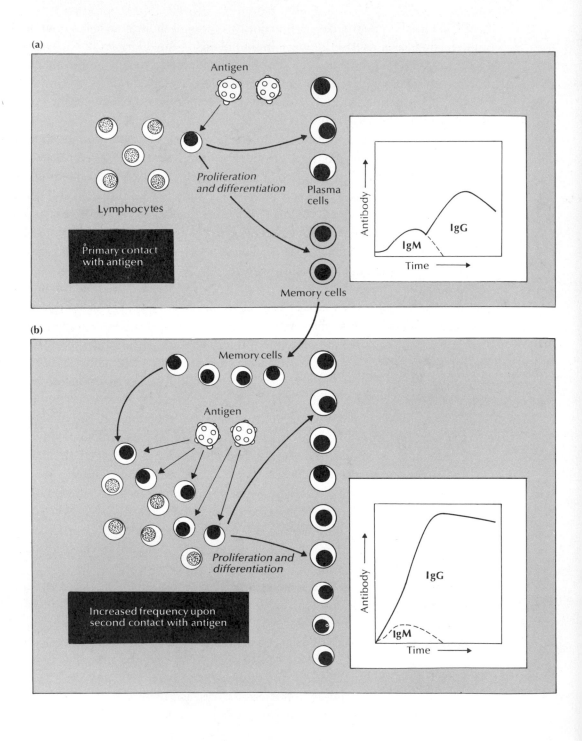

Antigen-specific effector cells

It is convenient to use the basic division of lymphocytes into the thymus- and bursa (bone marrow)-dependent subpopulations when examining their effector functions. B cells normally transform to **plasma cells** after antigenic stimulation. Plasma cells produce antibody for secretion at the rate of $1-3\times10^3$ molecules sec^{-1}. T lymphocytes become **blast cells** after antigenic stimulation and do not produce antibody for secretion. The specific effector function of these cells, for example the killing of foreign cells, is brought about by direct cell contact or is via mediator molecules that, unlike immunoglobulin, show no antigen specificity. It should be noted that the properties demonstrated for T blasts and effector cells have been shown to have *in vivo* importance in only a few instances. Accordingly, we have a better understanding of the role of B lymphocytes *in vivo*.

The intact immune response is never limited to one cell type. The Mantoux reaction to purified protein derivative (PPD) of *Mycobacterium tuberculosis* is often cited as the classical example of cell-mediated immunity yet it involves a variety of cell types, some of which are not even of lymphoid lineage, which change in relative importance and numbers as the reaction progresses. Early in the development of a Mantoux reaction (for example at 24 h) a biopsy would reveal a cellular infiltrate virtually identical to that recruited to an immediate-type hypersensitivity reaction.

Many basic experiments are still required to understand the nature of the molecules mediating cell—cell interactions and how these interactions are controlled and directed in the complex milieu of the intact immune system. A return to *in vivo* immunology, with defined and more effective tools for immune manipulation, is an important current goal.

Fig. 4.1 (*Facing page*) **Cellular and molecular kinetics of the humoral immune response**.
(a) In the initial population of virgin lymphocytes, the specific antigen-reactive clone (represented here by a single cell with filled nucleus; but *in vivo* each clone could have an estimated 100—10 000 members) is relatively rare and requires considerable multiplication to generate a detectable antibody response. Proliferation and differentiation is antigen driven, and except for a relatively few rapidly catabolised antigens, is accompanied by a rapid maturation of antibody class from IgM to IgG even upon first contact with antigen.
    Plasma cells are terminally differentiated and so they die once antibody production has ceased. However, the effects of immunisation are not lost. The asymmetry of the proliferation and differentiation pathway ensures that a clonally expanded pool of small memory lymphocytes remain. These cells are already committed to IgG, rather than IgM, production.
(b) Upon second contact with the same antigen, there are more antigen-specific cells available to respond, so antibody production is detectable without any lag, plasma concentrations rise rapidly to a higher peak than detected previously and the majority of antibodies are of the IgG isotype. An IgM response can often be detected second time around; however, it shows no adaptation.
    The change in cellular and molecular kinetics between the primary and secondary immune response can be explained completely by this increase in the frequency of antigen-reactive cells. Although lymphocytes can change immunoglobulin isotype in response to antigen stimulation, their rate of antibody production does not vary.
    Of course, this adaptive response is expressed only upon second contact with the same or a closely related antigen. Challenging an immunised animal with an unrelated antigen will result in a primary response.

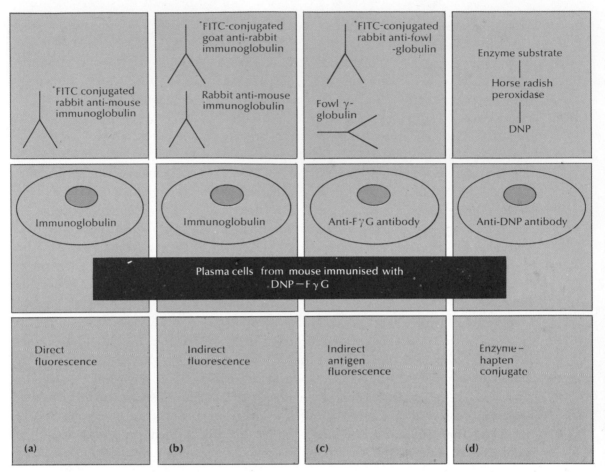

Fig. 4.2 Assays for the demonstration of immunoglobulin and antibody synthesis in plasma cells.
The cells used in these assays (Section 4.4) are prepared from the spleen of an immunised mouse.
Although the majority of plasma cells will have been elicited in response to the immunising
antigen, there is always a background of antibody production against altered-'self', environmental
and food antigens, gut bacteria, subclinical infections, etc. Consequently the total number of
immunoglobulin-synthesising cells detected by the techniques (a) and (b)above should be greater
than the number detected by antigen probes (c) and (d).

Immunoglobulin is a chemical term applied to those glycoprotein molecules with a characteristic
structure of light and heavy polypeptide chains with variable and constant-region repeating
domains. If we use a functional probe — antigen — the reacting immunoglobulins can be further
identified with regard to their ability to act as antibody. All immunoglobulins are undoubtedly
antibodies, but we frequently do not know their relevant antigens.

The techniques summarised above differ in their relative sensitivities; indirect immunofluorescence is more sensitive, and technically often more convenient, than direct immunofluorescence. Enzymic detection is potentially the most sensitive of all the techniques shown above
and offers the added convenience that it can be visualised without a special microscope or
darked room.

4.3   Effector B cells

Most of the assays described in this section are carried out on plasma cells *in vitro* or
their soluble products, i.e. immunoglobulin. In some of the assays, their soluble

products are detected by means of a functional probe (antigen) and so we are able to delimit that subset of immunoglobulin-synthesising plasma cells that are producing a relevant, antigen-reactive antibody. The approaches are summarised in Fig. 4.2.

4.4 Plasma cells and antibody production

PREPARATION IN ADVANCE
Prime mice 7—8 days before the experiment with 400 μg of alum-precipitated DNP—FγG (dinitrophenyl—fowl γ-globulin; Section 1.8) plus *Bordetella pertussis* (Section 1.9.2).

4.4.1 Demonstration of plasma cells

This can be done either on spleen sections or with single-cell suspensions smeared on microscope slides.

Frozen sections

Materials and equipment
Immune mouse (immunised; for example, as above)
Acetone
Solid carbon dioxide (dry ice, see Appendix II)
OTC compound, Tissue Tek II (Appendix II)
Freezing microtome

Method
1   Add small pieces of solid CO_2 to acetone in an insulated metal container until bubbling stops.
2   Kill the mouse, remove the spleen and chop it transversely into about five pieces.
3   Drop the spleen fragments into the freezing mixture.
4   Mount one of the fragments on a microtome chuck using OTC compound and cut 5 μm sections. These must be air dried and can then be stored at $-70°$ for up to 3 months.

Isolated cells

Materials and equipment
Immune mouse (as above)
Tissue culture medium at 4° (Appendix I)
Fetal bovine serum, FBS (Appendix II)
Cytocentrifuge (Appendix II)

Method

1 Kill the mouse, remove the spleen and prepare a single-cell suspension in tissue culture medium (Section 1.15).

2 Allow the aggregates to settle for 10 min at 1 g. Do not filter the cells through nylon wool because you are going to look at large cells which are easily damaged and trapped in nylon wool.

3 Wash the cells twice with medium by centrifugation (150 g for 10 min at 4°).

4 Count the cells and adjust to 2×10^7 ml^{-1}.

5 Add an equal volume of FBS to the cell suspension.

6 Prepare cell smears on a cytocentrifuge (Section 3.2.3). Spin at 100–150 g for 20 min. It will be necessary to vary the number of drops of cell suspension used to obtain a good smear; however, the total volume of liquid should be maintained at 4 drops per well.

7 Dry the smears thoroughly and fix in 95% methanol.

It is possible to prepare these smears as described for small lymphocytes in Section 3.2.2, but the plasma cells are large and fragile, so you must not use a 'spreader' slide. Simply shake the slide to spread out the drop and air dry before methanol fixation.

4.4.2

Staining of sections or cytosmears for antibody-producing cells

We will demonstrate that there are antibody-producing cells present, and that many of them are specific for antigenic determinants on the immunising antigen, either carrier (FγG) or hapten (DNP).

Materials

Frozen section or smears from immunised mice

Fluorescein isothiocyanate (FITC)-conjugated rabbit anti-mouse immunoglobulin
    (Section 2.1 or Appendix II)

Guinea-pig or pig-liver powder (Section 4.4.6 or Appendix II)

Phosphate-buffered saline, PBS (Appendix I)

There is a serious problem of non-specific adsorption of conjugated antisera to fixed material, in contrast to the very low background associated with viable cell immuno-fluorescence. You should use antisera with a low substitution ratio (Section 2.1.2) and in addition absorb the antiserum with liver powder (Section 4.4.6) as follows:

Method

1 Dilute the antiserum 1 : 5 with PBS and absorb 1 ml with 100 mg of pig-liver powder (use pro rata).

2 Mix for 30 min at 4° and spin off the liver powder (500 g for 20 min at 4°).

This absorption must be done at the beginning of each staining session.

4.4.3   Detection of intracellular immunoglobulin

1   Dilute 2 aliquots of the absorbed antiserum to a final dilution of 1:10, 1:20 and 1:40 with PBS.

2   Apply 1 drop of each FITC-conjugate dilution to separate spleen sections or cytosmears.

3   Incubate for 20 min at room temperature.

4   Wash off the excess antiserum. This can be done by putting the slides in a tray (face up!) and flooding them with PBS. Washing can be made more effective by placing the tray over a magnetic stirring platform with the mixing bar at the extreme end of the tray from the slides. Mix slowly for 5 min.

5   Change the PBS and mix for a further 5 min.

6   Add 1 drop of mounting medium (Section 3.5.1 Technical notes) and add a coverslip. Ring with nail varnish.

7   Examine the slides under a UV microscope.

Plasma cells should be easily visualised as shown in Fig. 4.3.

Technical notes

1   You may see a high background reaction when staining spleen sections for immunoglobulin because of secreted antibody entrapment. This should not be a problem with cytosmears.

2   Slides of tissue sections may be stored at −20° for several weeks after drying. Remove from the deep freeze and dry before use.

3   The antigen detected above (immunoglobulin) is relatively insensitive to drying-induced denaturation. For long-term storage, cells may be fixed after smearing (Section 4.4.4).

4   Sometimes antigen reactivity can be lost if cells are allowed to dry out before or

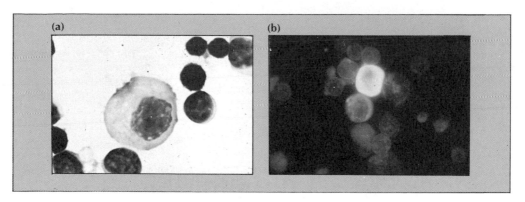

Fig. 4.3 Plasma cells.
(a) May−Grünwald/Giemsa staining of a cytocentrifuge preparation, viewed under transmitted light.
(b) Plasma cell stained with fluorescein-conjugated anti-mouse IgG and visualised under a UV microscope. The single stained plasma cell is seen slightly above centre.

after fixation (Fig. 4.4a and b). In this case, apply a concentrated suspension of cells to a slide pre-treated with 1% w/v solution of poly-L-lysine (to aid adhesion), allow them to settle at room temperature in a humid chamber for 5−10 min and then add an aqueous fixative (Section 4.4.4).

5 An essentially similar technique can be used for staining paraffin-embedded tissue sections with monoclonal antibodies, thus gaining additional information from the better preservation of histological structure (Section 12.13.1).

We have described a direct immunofluorescence technique here as this usually gives sufficient sensitivity to detect the relatively large amount of immunoglobulin in the average plasma cell. It is often more convenient, and sometimes essential, to use an indirect staining technique if the antigen to be detected is scarce or if it was poorly immunogenic when the detecting antiserum was raised. In the indirect technique the

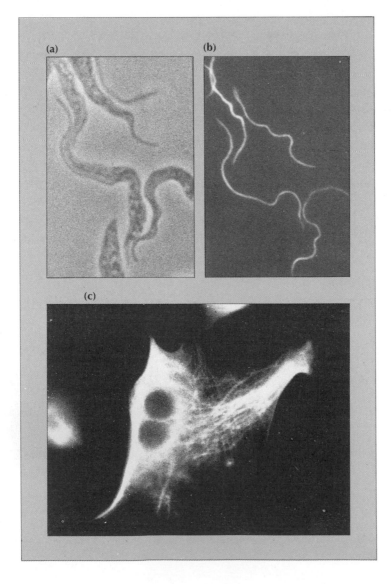

Fig. 4.4 Immunofluorescent staining of cells for intracytoplasmic epitopes. Photographs (a) and (b) show the flagellate *Trypanosoma cruzi* stained with a monoclonal antibody against an epitope in the paraxial rod (a structure associated with the flagellum), viewed under: (a) transmitted light; and (b) UV light. The staining reaction was completely lost if the preparation was allowed to dry out after fixation.

Photograph (c) shows a Swiss 3T3 cell treated with the detergent Triton X−100 to remove the majority of the cell cytoplasm prior to staining with with an anti-microtubule monoclonal antibody.

first antibody, in this case rabbit anti-mouse immunoglobulin, is unconjugated. Its binding is visualised by a second antibody; for example, FITC-conjugated goat anti-rabbit immunoglobulin (as illustrated in Fig. 4.3). The indirect technique gives a significant gain in sensitivity (up to eight second antibodies may bind for each first antibody), with only a marginal increase in the background of non-specific fluorescence, and can offer the convenience of having to prepare only a single conjugate of an antiserum from a large animal rather than a series of direct conjugates; for example, an FITC-conjugated IgG fraction of goat or sheep anti-rabbit immunoglobulin may be used to visualise a range of rabbit antisera to different antigens. However, the indirect technique takes more time and can be cumbersome if used for the simultaneous detection of different antigenic determinants in two-colour immunofluorescence. If you use indirect immunofluorescence to stain tissue sections, only the fluorescent conjugate need be absorbed with liver powder.

4.4.4   Cell fixation and permeabilisation

With the advent of monoclonal antibodies, a careful control of the procedures for cell fixation and permeabilisation by removal of some or all of the membrane lipid has become more critical. In the past a fixative might ruin the majority of epitopes recognised by a polyclonal antiserum; however, sufficient might remain to allow a visible antigen−antibody interaction still to take place. Monoclonal antibody binding is essentially an 'all or nothing' event; if the epitope is ruined no binding can take place.

For general use, we favour fixation with 4% paraformaldehyde in 0.1 M phosphate buffer, pH 7.4 for 20 min at room temperature followed by treatment with an organic solvent (methanol, acetone, etc.), as a way of optimising structure preservation and permitting good permeabilisation for antibody penetration for most mammalian cell types. The serological reactivity of surface H-2, immunoglobulin-receptor molecules and Thy-1 antigens is retained after fixation if the buffered paraformaldehyde solution is supplemented with paraperiodic acid (9 mg ml^{-1}) and 0.1 M L-lysine. Some antigenic determinants are destroyed by this procedure; in this case we recommend fixation directly in acetone for 5 min at −20°.

Effective permeabilisation can also be achieved by treating cells with a detergent solution (1% v/v Triton X-100 or Nonidet P-40) after formaldehyde fixation. Highly insoluble cellular proteins, such as those found in the cytoskeleton, may be prepared for immunofluorescent staining by detergent treatment without fixation (Fig. 4.4c).

In general, time spent in optimising fixation, permeabilisation and staining techniques for each individual monoclonal antibody will usually yield dividends in the quality of the final result.

4.4.5   Detection of specific antibody using fluorescent probes

To demonstrate the antigen-binding specificity of intracellular antibody it is necessary to incubate spleen sections or cell preparations with fluorescein-conjugated FγG or unconjugated FγG visualised by FITC-conjugated rabbit anti-FγG antibody. We have described the indirect technique which is more sensitive.

Materials
In addition to Section 4.4.2:
Fowl γ-globulin, FγG (Section 1.3.1)
Fluorescein-conjugated anti-FγG (Section 2.1)

Method
Again you should absorb the fluorescent conjugate with liver powder (Section 4.4.6) and, in addition, absorb or ultracentrifuge the FγG as this is also 'sticky'.

1 Dilute FγG to 1 mg ml^{-1} and put 1 drop onto each of three sections or cytosmears of FγG-immune spleen.
2 Incubate for 20 min at room temperature.
3 Wash away the unbound antigen with PBS (Section 4.4.3).
4 Add 1 drop of 1:5, 1:10, 1:20 fluorescein-conjugated anti-FγG to each slide, respectively, and incubate for 20 min at room temperature.
5 Wash away the excess conjugate, blot dry and mount (Section 3.5.1).
6 Examine the preparations under a UV microscope.

Technical note
It is important to ensure that the FITC-conjugated rabbit anti-FγG does not cross-react with mouse immunoglobulin, i.e. it does not bind directly to the contents of the murine plasma cells. If it does, absorb with glutaraldehyde insolubilised mouse γ-globulin (Section 2.1.8).

4.4.6   Preparation of pig-liver powder

Materials and equipment
Pig liver
0.14 M saline
Acetone
Waring blender

Method
1 Remove blood from the isolated liver by an intravenous infusion of saline.
2 Chop liver into pieces and homogenise with 4 volumes of saline using a Waring blender.
3 Concentrate and wash in saline by centrifugation (600 g for 45 min at 4°).
4 Remove large aggregates by filtering through a pad of glass wool or muslin.
5 Centrifuge filter effluent at 600 g for 45 min at 4° and re-suspend pellet in acetone.
6 Filter through a Buchner funnel and wash filtrate with acetone until the preparation is white on drying.
7 Grind up into a powder and store at 4° under desiccation.

4.4.7 Detection of plasma cells with hapten−enzyme conjugates

This technique is similar in principle to that used for anti-carrier antibodies (Section 4.4.5). However, in this instance the detection molecule (enzyme) is much bigger than the antigen (the hapten, DNP).

PREPARATION IN ADVANCE

This method works equally well using horse radish peroxidase (HRP) or alkaline phosphatase (AP). Conjugate the enzymes with DNP according to the method in Section 1.6.1. Although AP may be conjugated at room temperature (optimum substitution ratio DNP_{10-15} AP), HRP should be conjugated at 4° to slow the rate of reaction and so obtain the necessary low substitution ratio (optimum DNP_{1-2} HRP). Enzyme activity is lost if HRP is over-substituted, probably because of the addition of DNP groups into the catalytic site.

Technical note

Determine the 280 and 360 nm absorbance values before conjugation as HRP has significant absorbance up to 403 nm. It is necessary to subtract the initial absorbance reading at 360 nm from that obtained after conjugation, to calculate the true degree of dinitrophenylation.

Materials and equipment

Cryostat sections (or cytosmears) from immunised mouse (Section 4.4.1)
Acetone
Methanol
Hydrogen peroxide
Hapten−enzyme conjugate; for example, dinitrophenyl−horse radish peroxidase, DNP−HRP
Diaminobenzidine, DAB (Appendix II). *Take care — this is a carcinogen*
Phosphate-buffered saline, PBS (Appendix I)
Bovine serum albumin, BSA

Method

1 Air dry the cryostat sections and fix for 30 min in acetone containing 0.2% v/v hydrogen peroxide at room temperature, to inactivate any endogenous peroxidase.

2 Rinse three times in PBS and wipe the slide around the section.

3 Overlay with DNP−HRP diluted to 0.5 mg ml^{-1} in PBS containing 0.1% w/v BSA. Leave for 30 min at room temperature in a humid atmosphere.

4 Wash in PBS, as in Section 4.4.3, and finally wipe the slide around the section.

5 Prepare the DAB substrate by adding 4 µl hydrogen peroxide to 10 ml PBS containing 6 mg DAB; filter and use immediately.

6 Add a few drops of DAB solution to each section and allow the colour reaction to develop for 20 min at room temperature in a humid chamber.

7 Wash carefully under tap water and counterstain; for example, with Harris haematoxylin (Section 12.13.1).

8 If permanent mounts are required, the sections may be dehydrated through graded alcohols, treated with xylene and mounted in DePeX.

9 Observe the sections under bright field illumination; cell nuclei should be blue while plasma cells containing anti-DNP antibody should have blue cytoplasm.

4.5 Enumeration of antibody-secreting cells *in vitro*

Many of the values given later in this chapter, especially for cell numbers and expected responses, can only be taken as a guide. Biological materials do not behave in an exactly similar manner between laboratories and so each system must be standardised for research purposes.

We have shown in the previous section that plasma cells synthesise intracytoplasmic antibody. It is possible to show that these cells synthesise antibody for secretion and this can be used to quantitate the number of antibody-producing cells in an organ. The basic assay which we will describe was developed by Jerne and Nordin to detect cells producing antibody against erythrocyte antigens. Spleen cells from immune mice are incubated in an agar gel with the immunising erythrocytes. After the addition of complement, the erythrocytes in the locality of the plasma cells are lysed, producing macroscopic holes or plaques in the erythrocyte suspension. This relatively simple and robust assay has undergone several modifications to improve its convenience and application range.

4.5.1 Enumeration of total plasma cells by reverse plaque assay

This assay is particularly useful for the enumeration of total immunoglobulin-secreting cells. Secreted immunoglobulin is captured by protein A coated onto indicator erythrocytes (see Section 9.1 for species specificity of immunoglobulin adsorption by protein A), which are then lysed by the addition of a developing anti-immunoglobulin serum plus complement.

PREPARATION IN ADVANCE—COATING OF SHEEP ERYTHROCYTES WITH PROTEIN A

Materials and equipment
Sheep erythrocytes, SRBC, in Alsever's solution (Appendix II)
0.14 M sodium chloride in distilled water (saline)
Protein A (Appendix II) (2 mg ml^{-1} in saline)
Chromic chloride (0.1 mg ml^{-1} in saline)
Phosphate-buffered saline, PBS (Appendix I)

Method
1 Wash SRBC six times by centrifugation (300 g for 10 min at room temperature).
2 Add 1 ml of protein A solution (2 mg ml^{-1} initial concentration) to 1 ml of packed erythrocytes.

3 Add 6 ml of chromic chloride solution (0.1 mg ml^{-1}) dropwise. After mixing add 10 ml saline and incubate overnight at 4°.

4 Wash the erythrocytes three times by centrifugation (300 g for 10 min at room temperature) and re-suspend to 10% v/v in PBS.

Coated erythrocytes may be used for up to 2 weeks.

ASSAY

Materials and equipment
Cell suspension for assay; for example, spleen from immunised mouse
Protein A-coated erythrocytes (prepared as above)
Phosphate-buffered saline, PBS (Appendix I)
Agarose, 1.8% w/v in distilled water
Tissue culture medium, three times concentrated (Appendix I)
Bovine serum albumin, BSA, 7% w/v in PBS
Anti-mouse immunoglobulin, developing serum
Guinea-pig serum, as complement source (Appendix II)
Plastic Petri dishes, 50 mm

Method
1 Mix 14 ml agarose solution with 5.5 ml of tissue culture medium, which has been concentrated three times, and add 1.5 ml of BSA solution.

2 Dispense 0.7 ml volumes of agarose mixture into glass test tubes in a water bath at 45°.

3 For each assay dish: add 0.2 ml of lymphoid cell suspension, 0.1 ml of anti-immunoglobulin serum and 0.05 ml of protein A-coated sheep erythrocytes to each tube containing 0.7 ml agarose mixture. Mix thoroughly and pour into a plastic Petri dish. Swirl the dish to ensure an even covering of agarose−cell suspension.

4 Incubate for 1−1.5 h in a humid 37° incubator gassed with 5% CO_2 in air.

5 Add 1 ml of diluted guinea-pig serum, as a complement source (the dilution must be pre-determined empirically) and continue incubation at 37° until haemolytic plaques are visible (within 30−60 min).

6 Count the number of haemolytic plaques and calculate the number of antibody-secreting cells in the original cell suspension.

Technical notes
1 The optimal dilution of anti-immunoglobulin serum and complement source must be determined as in Section 4.5.2.

2 Illuminate the assay dish with light at a low angle of incidence to aid visualisation of the plaques. They will appear as uniform dark holes in a light, birefringent layer of erythrocytes.

3 The cell suspension for assay should be used at a concentration to give not more than 100−200 plaques per assay dish.

4.5.2 Enumeration of antigen-specific plasma cells

By analogy with the method used for detecting antigen-specific, antibody-synthesising plasma cells in tissue sections (Section 4.4.2), the Jerne haemolytic plaque-forming cell technique uses the original immunogen, sheep erythrocytes (SRBC), in an antibody−antigen binding reaction to detect antibody-secreting plasma cells. In this case, the addition of complement results in the formation of a lytic halo associated only with SRBC antigen-secreting plasma cells.

PREPARATION IN ADVANCE

1 Immunise two mice with 2×10^8 SRBC given intraperitoneally 5 days before the experiment.
2 Agar underlay. Make up 1.4% Difco Bacto Agar in Hank's saline (Appendices II and I, respectively). Melt the agar in a microwave oven and then directly over a bunsen flame to get rid of all of the lumps. Take care to swirl the agar gently to avoid charring. Add enough of the agar solution to a 5 cm plastic Petri dish to just cover its base. An underlay is used to ensure that the base of the assay dish is reasonably flat, so pouring must be done on a levelled surface.
3 Agar overlay. Prepare 0.7% agar solution in Hank's saline containing 0.5 mg ml^{-1} of diethylaminoethyl (DEAE)−dextran (final concentration). DEAE−dextran (Appendix II) is used to prevent anti-complementary activity of the agar. Alternatively, use the more expensive agarose as in the previous section.

Materials and equipment
SRBC-immunised mice
2−4-week old sheep blood in Alsever's solution (Appendix II)
Agar overlay
Petri dishes containing agar underlay
Hank's saline, without phenol red indicator dye (Appendix I)
Water bath, 45°
Guinea-pig serum, as complement source (Appendix II)

Method
1 Wash SRBC three times in Hank's saline by centrifugation (300 g for 10 min at room temperature). Adjust to 20% v/v after re-suspension in Hank's saline.
2 Remove spleens from mice and prepare a single-cell suspension by teasing them apart with forceps into ice-cold saline (Section 1.15). Discard the fibrous connective tissue which remains.
3 Suck suspension in and out of a Pasteur pipette to disperse the cells, it is not usually necessary to let the cells stand to settle out the small aggregates. (To avoid loss and damage to the plasma cells do not filter cells through nylon wool and do not use a syringe and needle for cell dispersion.)
4 Adjust to a total volume of 2.5 ml in Hank's saline.
5 Dilute 1 ml of the spleen-cell suspension 1 : 10 and 1 : 100 with Hank's saline.

6 Pipette out 0.8 ml of overlay into small test tubes in a 45° water bath. Use a warm pipette.

7 Add 0.25 ml of the original or diluted spleen cell suspensions to each assay dish according to the Protocol.

Protocol

	Dish number		
	1	2	3
Spleen-cell suspension (ml)	0.25	0.25	0.25
(initial dilution)	(neat)	(1 : 10)	(1 : 100)
Agar overlay ⎱	0.80 ml ⎱		
SRBC (20%) ⎰	0.15 ml ⎰	————————→	
Fraction of spleen assayed	1/10	1/100	1/1000

8 Place dish on a levelled surface.

9 Add 0.15 ml SRBC suspension to each overlay tube just before use. Mix well by flicking the end of the tube.

10 Add overlay to dish and mix thoroughly with spleen cells.

11 Allow agar to set and add 1.0 ml of a 1 : 10 dilution of guinea-pig serum as a source of complement.

12 Incubate dishes at 37° for 1−1.5 h. If the plaques are not clear when the dishes are removed from the incubator, allow them to stand at room temperature for about 30 min before counting.

Although the plaques can be seen by holding the Petri dish up to the light (without its lid), counting is easier and more accurate if you use a low-power binocular microscope and draw lines on the bottom of the dish.

Only direct plaques (mainly IgM antibody) are detected by the method described above because of the high haemolytic efficiency of this antibody class. In theory, a single molecule of IgM can initiate the complement cascade and cause SRBC lysis. To detect IgG plaques it is necessary to increase the number of molecules binding to any one site (two adjacent molecules of IgG are required to activate the complement sequence via the classical pathway), plaques must, therefore, be developed with an antiserum against mouse immunoglobulin. This method of detecting so-called 'indirect' plaques can be used to assay each of the mouse IgG subclasses using appropriate subclass-specific antisera.

Indirect plaques

Materials and equipment
As preceding method, plus rabbit anti-mouse immunoglobulin, anti-Ig (Section 1.7.2 or Appendix II)

Method

1 Prepare a plaquing mixture as in the preceding method (steps 1–10) but instead of adding complement, add 0.1 ml of a 1 : 10 dilution of rabbit anti-mouse Ig and incubate at 37° for 45 min.

2 Wash away the developing antiserum by flooding the plate twice with Hank's saline.

3 Add 1 ml of 1 : 10 dilution of guinea-pig serum. Incubate for 45 min at 37°.

Again, the plaques may be clearer if the plates are left at room temperature for 30 min before counting. Under experimental conditions it is necessary to titrate the developing antiserum until the maximum number of plaques are obtained. The direct, or 'IgM', plaques are then subtracted from the total to give the number of 'IgG' plaques.

The technique as described can be used to enumerate antibody-producing cells in any species; however, in the case of chicken antibody-producing cells you must use an homologous serum as a source of complement. Chicken antibody does not fix the first component of mammalian complement (C1q). Alternatively, develop both IgM and IgG plaques using rabbit anti-chicken immunoglobulin class-specific antisera and guinea-pig complement.

Technical notes

1 If large numbers of SRBC are used for immunisation (10^6–10^9 per mouse) the peak of the direct plaque-forming-cell (PFC) response is 4 days; at lower doses (10^4–10^5 per mouse) the peak of the direct response is day 5. However, the numbers of indirect plaques peak at day 5–6 after immunisation. Day 5 is usually an acceptable compromise for measuring both the direct and indirect PFC response to SRBC. Other antigens may show different kinetics.

2 At doses of SRBC of 10^4 and below, the route of immunisation is important: intravenous injection gives more PFC than intraperitoneal injection. Above 10^5 SRBC per mouse both routes of administration give approximately the same number of plaques.

3 Use a spleen dilution giving approximately 200–300 plaques per assay plate. As cell density increases plaque size decreases and PFC number is not linear.

4 Some anti-immunoglobulin developing sera suppress IgM direct plaques while revealing IgG indirect plaques. Once the optimum dilution for plaque development has been determined, it is necessary to test for suppression of direct plaques by the serum using PFC 3 days after SRBC immunisation. The response is low but virtually all are IgM direct plaques.

The haemolytic plaque method can be extended using antigen coupled to erythrocyte-indicator cells. This, of course, allows more widespread application of the technique, especially in the technically more convenient Cunningham modification, which is described in Section 4.6.

4.5.3   ## Solid-phase detection of antibody-forming cells

ELISPOT (enzyme-linked immunospot)

This technique has been introduced as an alternative to the Jerne and Nordin plaque technique for antibody-forming cells. It is similar, in principle, to an ELISA, except that the antibody to be assayed is generated by secreting cells cultured in antigen-coated wells. The cells are allowed to settle on the antigen-coated surface and secreted antibody binds to the antigen in the immediate vicinity of the cell. The cells are then washed away and bound antibody is revealed by the addition of an enzyme-linked second antibody. The substrate is added in agarose to allow only limited diffusion of the coloured products so that visible 'spots', corresponding to plasma cells, can be counted.

Materials and equipment
Nunc−Linbro 24-well plates (Appendix II)
Antigen; for example, human serum albumin, HSA (Appendix II)
Phosphate-buffered saline, PBS (Appendix I)
PBS with 0.05% Tween 20
Mouse immunised with HSA
Alkaline phosphatase-conjugated anti-mouse immunoglobulin (Appendix II)
ELISA conjugate buffer (Appendix I)
5-bromo-4-chloro-3-indoyl phosphate, 2.3 mM in substrate buffer (10 mg in 10 ml)
ELISPOT substrate buffer (Appendix I)

Method
1 Coat each well of a 24-well plate with 500 µl of a 10 µg ml^{-1} solution of antigen in PBS.
2 Leave to incubate at 4° overnight.
3 Wash plate with PBS containing 0.05% Tween.
4 Wash plate twice with PBS alone.
5 Prepare a single-cell suspension from the spleen of the immunised mouse.
6 After washing in tissue culture medium containing 5% fetal bovine serum, prepare a series of dilutions of spleen cells (between 2×10^4 and 2×10^6 lymphocytes ml^{-1}) and add 500 µl of each spleen-cell suspension to different antigen-coated wells.
7 Incubate the plate, without disturbance, for 1 h at 37° in a humid atmosphere containing 5% CO_2 in air.
8 Wash plates with cold PBS−Tween until all adherent cells are removed.
9 Add 500 µl of appropriate dilution (usually 1:500 to 1:2000) of alkaline phosphatase-conjugated anti-mouse immunoglobulin in conjugate buffer.
10 Incubate at 37° for 1 h.
11 Wash three times with PBS−Tween.

12　Mix 4 volumes substrate (5-bromo-4-chloro-3-indoyl phosphate) with 1 volume molten 3% agarose and, before it sets, add 500 μl to each well.

13　Allow the agarose to set on a levelling table and then incubate at 37° for 1 h.

14　Visible blue spots should be seen, which correspond to the former positions of individual antibody-secreting cells. They are most easily counted with a microscope using low-power magnification (×6.4).

4.6　T—B cooperation with hapten—carrier conjugates

In the next chapter we will use *in vivo* techniques to examine the interactions between murine T and B lymphocytes responding to antigen (Section 5.6). Using similar transfer techniques it was established very early on that B lymphocytes alone transform to plasma cells and become glycoprotein-synthesising and -secreting factories. Surprisingly, however, it was found that newborn children or animals lacking a thymus (either because of a congenital failure of thymus development — thymic hypoplasia — or its experimental near equivalent — neonatal thymectomy, see Section 11.2.2) showed relatively poor antibody responses. It became clear that T—B lymphocyte cooperation was required for antibody production, especially for the generation of IgG plaque-forming cells (PFC).

Antigen-presenting cells
Several cell types show the ability to present surface antigen in an immunogenic form to T and B lymphocytes; for example, T lymphocytes with a helper phenotype recognise antigen on the surface of Langerhans' cells where it is presented in the context of MHC class II molecules. In contrast, follicular dendritic cells take up antigen in the form of immune complexes via their C3b receptors and are especially effective at stimulating B lymphocytes. B lymphocytes can also present antigen to helper T lymphocytes, having concentrated it via their antigen-specific immunoglobulin receptors and presented it as a complex with major histocompatibility (MHC) class II molecules. Intriguingly, the precise function expressed by a cloned T-cell line (Section 12.14) can be varied in response to the type of antigen-presenting cells used for *in vitro* stimulation.

There is an impressive array of anatomically or morphologically distinct cell types known to be able to present antigen: interdigitating cells in the thymus, Langerhans' cells in the skin which traffic to the lymph nodes to become dendritic cells, macrophages with 'professional phagocyte' propensities in the medullary region of the lymph node, as well as follicular dendritic cells and marginal zone macrophages. However, the majority of these observations have been made *in vitro* on isolated cell populations. Consequently, the true *in vivo* relevance of these potential cell—cell interactions remains to be established.

Chemical requirements for cooperation
The use of chemically defined antigens provides a powerful research tool with which to investigate the specific requirements of T—B cooperation. Mitchison showed very

convincingly that the antibody response to a hapten, for example dinitrophenyl, (DNP), depends on it being *chemically coupled* to a carrier molecule, for example fowl γ-globulin (FγG) or keyhole limpet haemocyanin (KLH). It is obvious that B cells recognise and respond to the hapten: in this experiment we will investigate the nature of the cells recognising the carrier.

PREPARATION IN ADVANCE

Throughout this experiment you will use mice primed to DNP−FγG or DNP−KLH. Prepare the hapten−carrier conjugates as described in Section 1.6.1 and adsorb them onto alum as in Section 1.8.

Inject groups of 15−20 inbred mice intraperitoneally according to the protocol below, for use 2−3 months after priming. If required, the mice may be boosted a second time according to the same schedule.

Protocol

Group	Antigen on alum	Amount (μg)	Adjuvant
I	DNP−FγG	400	4×10^9 B. pertussis
II	DNP−KLH	400	4×10^9 B. pertussis
III	FγG	400	4×10^9 B. pertussis

4.6.1 Assay for DNP plaque-forming cells

This assay was modified by Cunningham from the Jerne haemolytic plaque assay (Section 4.5) and can be used to enumerate antibody-forming cells against soluble antigens conjugated to the surface of indicator erythrocytes, in this case DNP or trinitrophenyl (TNP).

4.6.2 Preparation of DNP- or TNP-conjugated erythrocytes

Three methods are available to sensitise the indicator erythrocytes (for example, sheep or horse RBC):

(a) *Chemical*. TNP may be coupled directly to the erythrocytes. This is a more gentle reaction than dinitrophenylation, and TNP cross-reacts strongly with DNP.

(b) *Dinitrophenylated, non-complement fixing antibodies*. Chicken antibodies do not fix mammalian complement and so DNP−chicken anti-erythrocyte antibodies may be used to sensitise indicator cells at subagglutinating doses. However, in using this assay method for DNP plaques, one cannot then use FγG as a carrier molecule.

(c) *Dinitrophenylated fragments of mammalian anti-erythrocyte antibodies*. The addition of whole DNP−rabbit IgG anti-SRBC to the SRBC indicator cells, for example, would cause haemolysis and so the dinitrophenylated non-complement fixing Fab fragment must be used to sensitise erythrocytes. DNP−Fab will still bind to the erythrocytes but cannot induce agglutination or fix complement.

4.6.3 Trinitrophenylation of erythrocytes

Materials and equipment
Erythrocytes, horse or sheep (Appendix II)
2,4,6-trinitrobenzene sulphonic acid (Appendix II)
Glycyl glycine
Phosphate-buffered saline, PBS (Appendix I)

Method

1 Prepare a phosphate-buffer solution by dissolving 5.62 g sodium dihydrogen phosphate dihydrate and 16.19 g disodium hydrogen phosphate in 1 litre water. This solution is pH 7.2 and isotonic with sheep erythrocytes (SRBC) (289 mosmol) and so causes less SRBC lysis than the original method which used 0.28 M cacodylate buffer, pH 6.9.

2 Wash erythrocytes three times with PBS by centrifugation (300 *g* for 10 min at room temperature).

3 Re-suspend 4 ml of packed cells in 16 ml phosphate buffer, and react with trinitrobenzene sulphonic acid according to the Protocol.

4 Mix TNP solution with cells for 30 min on a magnetic stirrer at room temperature.

5 Add 50 ml of a solution of glycyl glycine (initial concentration 2 mg ml^{-1}) in phosphate buffer to each aliquot to react the free TNP sulphonate.

6 Wash three times in PBS by centrifugation (300 *g* for 10 min) and store at 4°.

Determine the optimum conditions for sensitisation according to Section 4.6.7.

Protocol

	Tube number			
	1	2	3	4
TNP in 2 ml buffer (mg)	25	30	35	40
20% suspension SRBC 5 (ml)	5 ————————————————→			

4.6.4 DNP–Fab' anti-sheep erythrocyte (SRBC) sensitisation

PREPARATION OF Fab' ANTI-SRBC
The antiserum prepared in Section 6.14 is suitable for this purpose. This method described works well but it is not the only route that may be used to prepare Fab or Fab' (see also Section 8.8).

Materials and equipment
Rabbit anti-sheep erythrocyte (anti-SRBC) hyperimmune serum (Section 6.14)
Other materials and equipment as in sections indicated

Method

1 Isolate the IgG fraction of the antiserum by diethylaminoethyl (DEAE)−cellulose ion-exchange chromatography (Section 8.5).
2 After concentration, dialyse the IgG anti-SRBC against 0.1 M sodium acetate and digest with pepsin (Section 8.8.2) to obtain the $F(ab')_2$ fragment.
3 Apply the digest to a Sephadex G-100 or G-150 column equilibrated with PBS, recover the $F(ab')_2$ peak (Section 8.8.2), concentrate and dialyse against PBS.

Store a small sample at −20° for testing later.

4 Reduce the $F(ab')_2$ fragments with 0.02 M dithiothreitol for 30 min at 37°.
5 Alkylate with 0.05 M iodoacetamide for 10 min at room temperature.
6 Dialyse Fab' mixture overnight against PBS.

Reduction and alkylation of the $F(ab')_2$ is usually sufficient to prevent haemagglutination and so it is not necessary to fractionate the mixture any further.

7 Dinitrophenylate the Fab' anti-SRBC as described in Section 1.6.1 and determine the average number of DNP groups per Fab' molecule.
8 Test each preparation by haemagglutination (Section 6.14) and haemolysis (Section 7.1) according to the Protocol.

Protocol

Preparation number	Description	Haemagglutinin titre	Haemolysin titre
1	Rabbit anti-SRBC whole serum		
2	IgG anti-SRBC		
3	$F(ab')_2$ anti-SRBC		
4	Fab' anti-SRBC		
5	Fab' anti-SRBC + goat or sheep anti-rabbit immunoglobulin		
6	DNP−Fab' anti-SRBC		
7	DNP−Fab' anti-SRBC + goat or sheep anti-rabbit immunoglobulin		

The haemagglutination and haemolysis test should be carried out after each stage of the procedure, and the procedure continued only if the results of the tests are satisfactory.

A typical haemagglutination result is shown in Fig. 4.5.

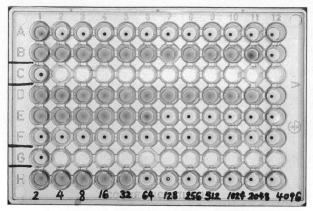

Fig. 4.5 Haemagglutination test with rabbit anti-sheep erythrocyte (anti-SRBC) serum. Doubling dilutions of antiserum along the tray starting at 1 : 2.

Row A: pre-immunization bleed showing low-titre 'natural' or heterophile antibodies, end point 1 : 2.

Row B: antiserum after two injections of 5×10^8 SRBC in Freund's complete adjuvant and five intravenous boosts with 10^8 SRBC. Antiserum collected 12 weeks after first challenge, end point 1 : 2048.

Row C: SRBC alone, control for spontaneous agglutination.
Row D: IgG fraction of antiserum isolated by DEAE-cellulose ion-exchange chromatography.
Row E: F(ab')$_2$ fraction.
Row F: Fab' fraction.
Row G: SRBC alone.
Row H: Fab' fraction plus 25 μl of 1 : 40 dilution goat anti-rabbit IgG.

4.6.5 Sensitisation of indicator cells

Materials and equipment
Sheep erythrocytes (Appendix II)
DNP—Fab' anti-SRBC
Phosphate-buffered saline, PBS (Appendix I)

Method

1 Wash SRBC three times in PBS by centrifugation (300 *g* for 10 min at room temperature) and adjust to a final concentration of 40% v/v.
2 Sensitise aliquots of SRBC according to the Protocol.

Protocol

	Aliquot number					
	1	2	3	4	5	6
DNP-Fab' anti-SRBC added (μl) (initial conc. 1 mg ml^{-1})	1	5	10	20	40	100
SRBC 40% v/v suspension (ml)	1 —————————————————→					

3 Incubate at 37° for 30 min, mixing occasionally.
4 Wash five times with PBS by centrifugation (300 *g* for 10 min at room temperature) to remove unbound protein.
5 Adjust cell concentration to 20% v/v and store at 4°.

Determine the optimum conditions for sensitisation as described in Section 4.6.7.

Technical notes

1 Use 2−3-week old SRBC, but fresh horse RBC.
2 The sensitised erythrocytes are stable for 1 week at 4°. It is, however, advisable to wash the cells each time before use.

4.6.6 Preparation of assay chambers

Materials and equipment
Glass microscope slides
Adhesive tape, double-sided (Appendix II)
Photographic roller

Method

1 Wash slides overnight in a strong solution of a free rinsing detergent and rinse thoroughly in distilled water. Soak overnight in absolute ethanol. Air dry the slides. Clean slides are absolutely essential to allow bubble-free filling of the assay chambers.
2 Place 20 slides in a line with their long edges adjacent and stick double-sided tape along each edge and along the centre of the row.
3 Remove the backing from the tape and add a second row of slides to complete the sandwich.
4 Roll the slides firmly with a photographic roller to seal the chambers.
5 Separate adjacent slides.

4.6.7 Anti-DNP assay

Materials and equipment
Dinitrophenyl−fowl γ-globulin, DNP−FγG-, or DNP−Keyhole limpet haemocyanin, KLH, primed mice (Section 4.6)
Trinitrophenyl, TNP-, or DNP-sensitised sheep erythrocytes, SRBC (Section 4.6.3 or 4.6.4)
Tissue culture medium (Appendix I)
Fetal bovine serum, BSA
Guinea-pig serum, as complement source (fresh or preserved serum Appendix II)
Assay chambers (Section 4.6.6)
50 : 50 mixture of paraffin wax and petroleum jelly on hot plate
Micro-titre tray, U-shaped (Appendix II)
Dropping pipettes (18 gauge needle with end cut square attached to 1 ml syringe barrel, delivers a constant but approximate 25 µl) or automatic pipette (Appendix II)

Method

1 Remove the spleens from two to three mice and prepare a single-cell suspension as described in Section 1.15.

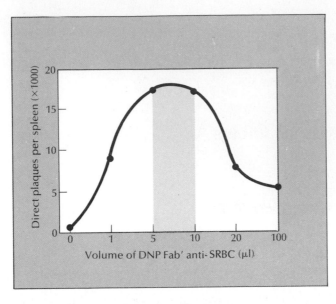

Fig. 4.6 Relationship between number of anti-DNP plaques and volume of DNP—Fab′ anti-SRBC used to sensitize indicator cells. The optimal volume for sensitization within the tinted area, would be used in routine assays.

2 Adjust to 10^7 lymphocytes ml^{-1}.
3 Place 25 µl of medium into each well of the micro-titre tray to be used.
4 Add 25 µl of 20% sensitised erythrocyte suspension.
5 Add 100 µl of spleen-cell suspension.
6 Add 25 µl of neat guinea-pig serum absorbed with SRBC (see Section 7.5.1, Technical note 2, p. 278).
7 Mix the suspension in each well of the tray and load into an assay chamber with a Pasteur pipette.
8 When both chambers are full, seal edges by dipping into paraffin wax — petroleum jelly mixture.
9 Incubate at 37° and examine at 30, 45, 60 and 90 min.
10 Remove all the assay chambers as soon as plaques are clearly visible to the naked eye.
11 Count the number of plaques per chamber using a low-power binocular microscope.
12 Calculate the number of plaques per total spleen for each group, and plot a graph of plaque-forming cells (PFC) against volume or concentration of sensitising agent, as shown in Fig. 4.6.

Use this optimum volume or concentration of sensitising agent in all future assays.

Technical notes
1 It is technically more convenient to remove clumps from the spleen suspensions by settling them through 1 ml of fetal bovine serum instead of filtering through nylon wool.
2 It is not necessary to perform replicates of each assay point, the major source of experimental variation is the likely difference between mice receiving the same immunogen or similar numbers of transferred cells. Immunisation relies upon cell proliferation and so the experimental error arises exponentially.
3 Use 37° incubator without forced air circulation, any vibration will prevent uniform settling of the RBC.

4   Use a low angle of incidence for the light when counting the plaques under the microscope. The plaques will appear as dark holes in the birefringent layer of erythrocytes.

In the assay described above, direct (mainly IgM) plaques were detected; indirect (mainly IgG) plaques may be detected by the addition of a developing serum; for example, anti-mouse immunoglobulin, as described below.

Indirect plaques

Materials and equipment
Optimally sensitised erythrocytes (Section 4.6.7 and Fig. 4.6)
Rabbit anti-mouse immunoglobulin (Section 1.7.2 or Appendix II)
Other materials and equipment as given for previous section

Method
1   Dilute the anti-immunoglobulin serum with PBS as shown in the Protocol.
Protocol

	Tube number				
	1	2	3	4	5
PBS (ml)	0.8	0.5 ——————————————→			
Antiserum (ml)	0.2				
		0.5 ml	0.5 ml		
Dilution	1 : 10	1 : 20	1 : 40	1 : 80	1 : 160

mix mix etc.

2   Add 25 µl of each dilution to corresponding wells of the micro-titre tray.
3   Repeat the assay as in previous section, but *omit* the 25 µl of medium from each well of the tray, this has been replaced by the anti-immunoglobulin serum.
4   Determine the dilution of developing serum giving the maximum number of plaques.

Technical notes
1   The IgG plaques are taken to be the difference between the total number of developed plaques and the number of direct plaques.
2   Some anti-Ig sera inhibit IgM plaques while developing IgG plaques. If this is found to be the case in your system, then no correction of the number of developed plaques is required.
3   Test for the inhibition of direct plaque formation as follows. Determine IgM (direct) plaques with and without anti-Ig using either: (a) spleen cells from an animal 4 days after antigen priming; or (b) spleen cells from an animal primed with a highly substituted carrier (see Section 1.6.1). This will prime for an IgM response but not allow IgG switching.

Having spent a great deal of time standardising reagents, application of the assay to an experimental situation is extremely rapid.

4.7 Hapten—carrier cooperation with a heterologous carrier

PREPARATION IN ADVANCE
Inbred mice must be primed to dinitrophenyl—keyhole limpet haemocyanin (DNP—KLH) or DNP—fowl γ-globulin (DNP—FγG), respectively, 2—3 months before this experiment (see Sections 1.9.2 and 4.6).

Materials and equipment
Mice primed as above
Inbred mice for X-irradiation (Section 1.19.1)
DNP—HSA, DNP—KLH, DNP—FγG and FγG soluble antigens (Section 1.6.1)
Materials for plaque assay (Section 4.6.7)

Method
1 Prepare spleen-cell suspensions from donor mice primed with DNP—KLH or FγG.
2 Treat 10^8 FγG-primed spleen cells with anti-Thy-1 and complement or irrelevant monoclonal of same isotype and complement at 37° for 30 min (see Section 7.5).
3 X-irradiate the recipient mice with 8—8.5 Gy and reconstitute them according to the Protocol.

Protocol

Group	X-irradiated recipients per group*	Number of cells given i.v. in 0.2 ml	Intraperitoneal challenge (soluble antigen)
1	3—5	2×10^7 DNP—KLH spleen	10 μg DNP—KLH
2	3—5	2×10^7 DNP—KLH spleen + 2×10^7 FγG spleen	10 μg DNP—FγG
3	3—5	2×10^7 FγG spleen	10 μg DNP—FγG
4	3—5	2×10^7 DNP—KLH spleen + 2×10^7 FγG spleen	10 μg DNP—HSA+ 10 μg FγG
5	3—5	2×10^7 DNP—KLH spleen + 2×10^7 anti-Thy-1 and complement-treated FγG spleen	10 μg DNP—FγG
6	3—5	2×10^7 DNP—KLH spleen + 2×10^7 irrelevant Mab and complement-treated FγG spleen	10 μg DNP—FγG
7	3—5	None	10 μg DNP—FγG or 10 μg DNP—KLH

* Never less than five mice per group for research purposes. Group 7 is the control for the efficacy of X-irradiation and may be omitted after the initial experiment.

4 Assay the mice for direct and indirect DNP plaques on the 7th day after cell transfer.
5 Calculate the total number of plaques per spleen for each recipient and the geometric mean for each group (see Section 5.2.1).

You should now be aware that B cells primed to a hapten on carrier 1 can respond to the same hapten on carrier 2 by cooperating with a second population of cells primed to carrier 2. Identify the experimental group which supports this statement.
(a) What is the nature of the cooperating cell in this second population?
(b) What is the chemical requirement for hapten−carrier cooperation (cf. groups 2 and 4).
(c) What is the rationale for including groups 3 and 6 in this protocol?

4.8

Effector T cells

The effector functions of T lymphocytes have been determined almost entirely from *in vitro* studies. It has been possible to dissect out lymphocyte populations and determine the role of each T-lymphocyte subset using monoclonal antibodies against cell-surface antigens which happen to correlate with a functional subset (undoubtedly the number of subsets and their functional attributes have not yet been exhausted but see Section 12.13 for range of available monoclonal antibody-defined cell-surface markers). Briefly, there are at least four functional subsets, and, although their function might change with time, at any one instant the cells are apparently mono-functional.

(a) *Cooperator T lymphocytes* provide antigen-specific 'help' for the activation of B lymphocytes (Section 5.6).

(b) *Cytotoxic T lymphocytes* are responsible for direct (cell-mediated) killing of foreign target cells (Section 4.11).

(c) *Lymphokine-secreting T lymphocytes*. After antigen stimulation, these cells secrete cytokines (see Chapter 13) which affect the function of different cell types; for example, they can support a mitogenic response in lymphocytes, cause an increase in vascular permeability, induce a local inflammatory response due to their chemotatic effect, etc. Cytokines may be produced by more than one phenotypic subset of lymphocytes.

(d) *Suppressor T lymphocytes* can suppress an immune response, either with or without regard to antigen specificity. They are probably negative regulators of immune reactivity (cf. 'helper' T lymphocytes) and are intimately associated with the induction and maintenance of tolerance (Section 5.7).

An antigen-induced T lymphocyte response *in vivo* undoubtedly involves these subsets acting alone or in concert. The soluble mediators produced in this way will affect other lymphoid and non-lymphoid cells not involved in the primary antigenic stimulation. The result is a complex series of cell and humoral changes at the site of antigen stimulation.

The classical example of cell-mediated immunity is the Mantoux reaction obtained by the injection of tuberculin into the skin of an individual, who has been previously exposed to the tubercle bacillus either by infection or vaccination. The reaction is characterised by a reddening of the skin and a localised injurious reaction which reaches its height at 24–48 h, hence the name of delayed-type hypersensitivity. In general terms, *in vitro* assays of delayed-type or cell-mediated immunity show an overall correlation with *in vivo* immune status. As yet, it has not been possible to relate even the most discriminatory measures of T cell-mediated immune function, for example limiting dilution analysis, to the detailed behaviour of T lymphocytes *in vivo*.

4.9   Mitogenic response

Like B cells, when T cells meet their specific antigen they are stimulated to undergo division. This mitogenic response is usually accompanied by a morphological change to a blast cell. The degree of lymphocyte activation may therefore be assayed either by determining the percentage of blast cells in the culture or by measuring the amount of radioactive DNA analogue incorporated into newly synthesised DNA. It is important to note, however, that blast transformation, DNA synthesis and cell prolif-eration are not synonymous. Several instances have been reported where incorpor-ation of DNA analogue has occurred without cell division. The *in vitro* mitotic response has been shown to have an approximate correlation with the *in vivo* situation; for example, a normal individual would have a lower mitotic response to PPD (purified protein derivative of tubercle bacilli) than a Mantoux-positive indi-vidual. In addition, an immunodeficient individual with poor Mantoux reactivity would have a low *in vitro* mitotic response to PPD.

Many plant substances, known collectively as lectins or phytomitogens have the ability to induce blast-cell transformation and mitosis in a manner similar to antigen. The mitogen binds to a specific cell-surface receptor, as does antigen, and the signal thus generated causes the nucleus to be de-repressed and the lymphocyte enters the cell cycle. Unlike antigens, however, mitogens stimulate a large proportion of lym-phocytes. Again, as for antigen stimulation of lymphocytes *in vitro*, it has been possible to show an approximate correlation between the *in vitro* response to mitogens and the immune status of the individual.

Phytohaemagglutinin (PHA) has been the most extensively studied of the phy-tomitogens. Available evidence suggests that soluble PHA stimulates only T cells, although the activated T lymphocytes secrete cytokines which in turn activate B lymphocytes. There are, however, mitogens available that stimulate both T and B cells (pokeweed mitogen) or B cells alone (lipopolysaccharides, such as *Escherichia coli* endotoxin). The ability of mitogens to stimulate T and/or B cells selectively varies not only with species but also with the cell source, suggesting that only a subpop-ulation of T and/or B cells are capable of responding to mitogen stimulation.

We will describe two *in vitro* techniques for the assay of the response of human peripheral blood to PHA. The first is a 'low tech' tube-based macro-assay which uses a lot of cells and is not convenient for large numbers of experimental groups; however, it requires very little in the way of specialised equipment. The micro-assay is based upon micro-culture wells. It uses very small quantities of cells and reagents and has been semi-automated, thus enabling many experimental groups with three to five replicates per group to be tested.

Materials and equipment
Human peripheral blood
Phytohaemagglutinin, PHA (Appendix II)
Density gradient for lymphocyte isolation (Section 1.14 or Appendix II)
Tissue culture medium containing antibiotics (Appendix I)
Fetal bovine serum (Appendix II)
^{3}H-thymidine (Appendix II)
5 ml plastic tubes, Falcon (Appendix II)
37° incubator
Cylinder of 5% CO_2 in air

All procedures must be carried out under sterile conditions.

Method
1   Mix the blood with an equal volume of serum-free tissue culture medium.
2   Layer an equal volume of de-fibrinated blood onto the density gradient and centrifuge at 400 g for 20 min at 4°. (For economy, it is possible to use a 2 : 1 ratio of diluted blood to density gradient.)
3   Most of the leucocytes will be found as a fuzzy white band at the serum–density gradient interface. Insert a Pasteur pipette into this band and aspirate the cells.
4   Wash the cells once with serum-free medium (250 g for 15 min at room temperature) and twice with medium containing 5% fetal bovine serum (150 g for 10 min at room temperature) by centrifugation.
4   Count lymphocytes and adjust to 2×10^6 ml^{-1}.
5   Set up lymphocyte cultures with PHA according to the Protocol.
6   Incubate the tubes in a 37° CO_2 incubator.

The maximum uptake of ^{3}H-thymidine occurs about 72 h after PHA stimulation. If you intend to conduct a complete experiment, it is essential that you investigate both the full dose–response curve and the kinetics of the response in your own culture system.

7   Four hours before harvesting, add 37×10^3 Bq of ^{3}H-thymidine to each culture.

Protocol

	Tube number (3–5 replicates of each tube)				
	1	2	3	4	5
1 ml PHA diluted to:	0	1 : 10	1 : 20	1 : 40	1 : 80
Volume of lymphocytes (ml) (2×10^6 ml^{-1} initial concentration)	1 ————————————————→				
Final PHA concentration	0	1 : 20	1 : 40	1 : 80	1 : 160

Harvesting and counting cultures

Filter papers, Whatman 3MM, 2.1 cm circle (Appendix II)
Phosphate-buffered saline, PBS (Appendix I)
Chloroform
Trichloroacetic acid, TCA, 10% w/v aqueous solution
Scintillation fluid (Appendix II)
Scintillation vials
β spectrometer

Method
1   Wash cells two to three times in PBS by centrifugation.
2   Re-suspend cell pellet in 0.4 ml PBS.
3   Support filter discs (one for each culture tube and numbered in pencil) on a pin in a cork board.
4   Place 0.2 ml of cell suspension onto the corresponding disc.
5   Air dry discs with a fan.
6   Wash all discs in 10% cold TCA to precipitate the protein. (At this stage all the discs may be combined).
7   Wash discs in PBS and then absolute alcohol.
8   Rinse in the chloroform and allow to dry.
9   Place each disc in a scintillation vial containing scintillation fluid and count β emissions in a scintillation counter.

Assessment of results
Calculate the geometric mean c.p.m. for each group of replicates (Section 5.2.1).
There are basically two ways of recording data:
(a)   By simply giving the mean c.p.m. for stimulated and unstimulated cultures or their difference (Δ c.p.m.).
(b)   As an index of stimulation; this is calculated by the following equation:

$$\text{index of stimulation} = \frac{\text{c.p.m. PHA cultures}}{\text{c.p.m. unstimulated cultures}}.$$

In the experiment described here, either method of data presentation is acceptable as we simply wish to compare the mitogenic response to different concentrations of PHA. If, however, we wished to compare different types of cells, each having their own unstimulated control, the situation is more complex. Cells from different tissues may have varying numbers of cells undergoing spontaneous division and often the serum supplement used for culture is itself mitogenic, sometimes more on some tissues than others. Consequently, unstimulated (i.e. not PHA stimulated, in this case) or 'background' radioisotope incorporation may be abnormally high in some cultures but not others. Spleen cultures, for example, show a much higher background incorporation than blood lymphocyte cultures. In this case an index of stimulation would not be a useful way in which to present the data as the background variation would be hidden.

Technical notes

1 It may be necessary to test several batches of fetal bovine serum as they vary in their ability to 'support' *in vitro* cultures.

2 ^{131}Iodo-deoxyuridine may be used instead of ^{3}H- or ^{14}C-thymidine. This DNA analogue has the advantage that it is not re-utilised in a culture and so is a measure of incorporation alone, without the complication of turnover. In addition, as it is a γ emitter, it does not require scintillation fluid for counting.

3 In the experiment above, we used only a 4 h pulse with ^{3}H-thymidine instead of the 16−20 h (overnight) pulse used by some investigators. We do this not only to shorten the time in culture after isotope addition, thus reducing any effect of bacterial infection, but also to avoid re-utilisation of isotope released from cells. This latter consideration is, however, minimal under these conditions as there is a vast excess of free thymidine.

4 Occasionally a high 'background' incorporation may be encountered when culturing cells from penicillin-sensitive individuals due to the antibiotic in the culture medium. Under these conditions use gentamycin alone (Appendix I).

4.10 **Micro-culture technique**

Although similar in principle to the macro-technique described above (Section 4.9), this technique uses a maximum of only 10^5 responding cells per culture. The reduced cell number allows a greater number of variables to be tested per experiment. In addition, the introduction of semi-automated procedures has greatly reduced the time required for plating out and harvesting.

Materials and equipment
Blood, containing heparin (10 iu ml^{-1}). The heparin must be preservative free
Tissue culture medium (Appendix I)
Lymphoprep (Appendix II)
^{3}H-Thymidine (Appendix II) use at 37×10^4 Bq ml^{-1} in tissue culture medium
Scintillation fluid
Micro-culture trays, 96 wells, flat bases (Appendix II)
Eppendorf multi-dispenser (Appendix II)
Cell-harvesting machine (Appendix II)
β spectrometer

Method
1 Mix the blood with an equal volume of serum-free tissue culture medium.
2 Carefully layer 6 ml of diluted blood onto 3 ml Lymphoprep or similar separation medium.
3 Centrifuge at 400 *g* (interface force) for 20 min at room temperature. A misty layer of lymphocytes will be visible at the plasma−density gradient interface.
4 Remove lymphocytes using a Pasteur pipette and mix with an equal volume of tissue culture medium.

5 Centrifuge at 250 g for 15 min at room temperature and remove the supernatant.

6 Wash twice in tissue culture medium by centrifugation (150 g for 10 min at room temperature).

7 Remove an aliquot of cells and determine the number of viable lymphocytes ml^{-1} (Section 3.4). Adjust to 2×10^6 lymphocytes ml^{-1}.

8 Prepare cultures in micro-wells according to the following Protocol.

Protocol

Controls wells	Stimulated wells
100 µl tissue culture medium	50 µl tissue culture medium
	*50 µl stimulant
50 µl lymphocyte suspension	50 µl lymphocyte suspension
50 µl autologous plasma	50 µl autologous plasma
200 µl total volume	*200 µl total volume*

* Mitogen, antigen or allogeneic cells, at optimum concentration.

9 Set up three to five replicate cultures of each treatment using an Eppendorf multi-dispensing pipette.

10 Replace the lid and place the culture tray in a humidified incubator gassed with 5% CO_2 in air.

11 The magnitude of the mitotic response is determined by the addition of 50 µl of ^{3}H-TdR to each well before harvesting.

As an approximate guide:
(a) *For PHA cultures* add ^{3}H-TdR 40–48 h after the initiation of culture, incubate for 4 h at 37° before harvesting.
(b) *For mixed lymphocyte (cf. Section 4.10.1) or antigen-stimulated (for example, Candida or PPD) cultures* add ^{3}H-TdR 5 days after the initiation of culture, incubate for 6 or 18 h at 37° before harvesting, depending on the sensitivity of the assays in your hands. Once the assay is highly reproducible, you will need fewer counts to detect a significant difference between experimental groups so a shorter 'pulse' time will be possible.

12 Harvest the cultures using a semi-automatic cell-harvesting procedure (for example, see cell-harvesting machines, Appendix II).

13 Dry filter strips from harvesting machine at 37° for at least 3 h.

14 Remove discs from the filter strips and place each disc in a counting vial containing scintillation fluid.

15 Count β emissions in a scintillation counter, assess results as in Section 4.9.1.

4.10.1   Mixed-lymphocyte reaction

A mitotic response is also obtained when cells taken from two inbred strains or from two outbred individuals of any species are mixed in *in vitro* culture. This so-called mixed-lymphocyte reaction (MLR) is an *in vitro* counterpart of the host versus graft (HvG) or graft versus host (GvH) reactions examined later (Sections 4.17 and 4.18). Like the GvH reaction (Section 4.18) the majority of the *responsive* (as opposed to responding) cells are T lymphocytes. Again, like the GvH reaction, it has not been possible to demonstrate unequivocally an effect of previous immunisation on the magnitude of the response between strains with a 'strong' H-2 difference. It is however, possible to increase the magnitude of the response by previous sensitisation across 'weak' H-2 differences.

It is important, in the context of the MLR, to distinguish between responsive and responding cells because of the phenomenon known as *back stimulation*. It was found that F_1 cells gave a mitotic response when mixed with X-irradiated or mitomycin-treated parental cells. In MLR genetics the F_1 should not recognise the parent cells as being foreign. The mechanism proposed to explain this back stimulation was that the blocked parental cells recognise the F_1 cells as foreign and produce 'mitogenic factors' (previously cytokines) which non-specifically induce proliferation in the immuno-logically unresponsive F_1 cells.

MLR cultures may be performed using culture conditions similar to those described for PHA (Section 4.10) but mix 10^6 cells from each of two donors to yield the total of 2×10^6 per culture. In this case a two-way MLR will result, i.e. donor A will recognise B and vice versa. In many situations it is an advantage to have a uni-directional response and so parent and F_1 mixtures can be used (cf. Section 4.18), or, more simply, the proliferation of either cell type may be blocked with X-irradiation or mitomycin C treatment.

A suggested experimental protocol is given in Section 4.12.1; these cultures are then used as a source of cytotoxic effector cells.

The ability to activate and expand T-lymphocyte populations on a clonal basis by antigenic stimulation and culture in interleukin 2 (Section 12.14) has provided a much more sensitive and precise method of quantitation of antigen-reactive T lymphocytes by limiting dilution analysis (Section 4.13).

4.11 Cell-mediated cytotoxicity

T lymphocytes will respond to foreign cell-surface antigens by blastogenesis. Later in this response, effector cells are generated that will specifically lyse relevant target cells *in vitro*. This *in vitro* killing is generally regarded as being analogous to one type of cell-initiated tissue damage *in vivo*.

Classically the phenomenon of T cell-mediated cytotoxicity was elucidated using lymphocytes sensitised to DBA/2 alloantigens and assayed on ^{51}Cr-labelled P815Y (DBA/2) mastocytoma cells. A similar system can be used to investigate T-cell killing against any system of alloantigens using PHA-transformed blast cells labelled with ^{51}CrO$_4$.

Effector cells may be generated by either: (a) immunising C3H mice; for example, with DBA/2 spleen cells; (b) initiating a GvH reaction (Section 4.18) in, for example, irradiated (DBA $\times$ C3H) F_1 using C3H cells; or (c) in the course of an MLR (Section 4.10.1).

4.12   **Mixed-lymphocyte reaction (MLR) and cell-mediated cytolysis (CMC)**

Materials and equipment
CBA or C3H and DBA/2 mice (Appendix II)
P815Y mastocytoma cells (Appendix II)
Sodium ^{51}chromate (Appendix II)
X-ray machine or γ source
γ spectrometer

4.12.1   Mixed-lymphocyte reaction

1   Prepare spleen-cell suspensions from C3H and DBA/2 mice.
2   Irradiate DBA/2 cells (30 Gy); these will be used as MLR-stimulator cells. Irradiate immediately before putting into culture. The stimulatory capacity of irradiated cells falls within a few hours if they are allowed to stand at 4°.
3   Prepare MLR cultures using irradiated DBA/2 and C3H cells (Section 4.10.1). Mix 10^6 of each cell type, culture in 3 ml of medium in 5 ml Falcon plastic tubes as in Protocol A.

Prepare sufficient replicates of each tube to provide cells for the CMC assay on the 4th day of MLR culture (see Protocol B) (viability of MLR cultures varies — this must be standardised for each laboratory) and, in addition, prepare three replicates of tubes 1–3 for the assay of DNA synthesis in the MLR culture.

4   On the 4th day of the MLR culture collect cells for the CMC assay (Protocol B).
5   On the 5th day of the MLR culture add ^{3}H-thymidine to three replicates of tubes 1–3 to assay for DNA synthesis (Section 4.9.1).

We have given absolute numbers of MLR cells rather than the usual lymphocyte: target ratio. In fact, the efficiency of target-cell killing is not ratio dependent over a wide range.

A   *MLR protocol*

	Tube number		
	1	2	3*
X-irradiated cells	2×10^6 DBA/2	10^6 DBA/2	10^6 C3H or CBA
C3H- or CBA-responder cells	0	10^6	10^6

* This is a better control than unirradiated cells alone as irradiated cells might exert a slight inhibitory activity upon the generation of possible CMC cells.

B *CMC protocol*

	Tube number (three replicates)					
	1	2	3	4	5	6
^{51}Cr-labelled mastocytoma cells	10^5	$\longrightarrow$				
MLR lymphocytes from tube number:						
1	50×10^5	—	—	—	—	—
2	—	50×10^5	20×10^5	10×10^5	—	—
3	—	—	—	—	50×10^5	—

4.12.2 Cell-mediated cytolysis

1 Label mastocytoma cells with ^{51}CrO$_4$ (Section 7.5.2).
2 Count number of viable lymphocytes recovered from MLR (Protocol A).
3 Prepare cell mixtures in 2 ml of medium as shown in Protocol B.
4 Culture for 6 h at 37° in a CO$_2$ incubator.
5 Re-suspend the cells after culture and centrifuge (150 *g* for 10 min at 4°).
6 Remove 1 ml of the supernatant from each tube for γ counting.

4.12.3 Calculation of isotope-release (= target-cell destruction)

1 Lyse an aliquot of 10^5 original ^{51}Cr-labelled mastocytoma cells either by freezing and thawing (three times at 37° and −20°) or with 10% w/v saponin.
2 Spin down insoluble material from the lysate and count radioactivity in the supernatant. Use this value as the maximum (100%) isotope release.
3 Calculate spontaneous release from the labelled mastocytoma (tube 6 in triplicate) as a percentage of the total counts released by saponin. The mean of these three determinations will be used to correct the release observed in lymphocyte–target mixtures (tubes 1–5).
4 Calculate experimental release for each lymphocyte–target mixture as a percentage of the total counts released by saponin (tubes 1–5, in triplicate).
5 Calculate specific release as follows:

$$\% \text{ specific release} = \frac{100\,[R_e - R_s]}{100 - R_s}$$

where:

R_e = mean % experimental release,
R_s = mean % spontaneous release.

6 Plot a graph of % specific release for each group against the number of MLR-derived cells used to lyse the mastocytoma cells. Calculate also the standard deviation of each group (Section 5.2.1).

Technical note
In experimental determinations of CMC it is advisable to assay at 4, 6 and 8 h to determine the optimum under your conditions, rather than at the single time-point as suggested here.

4.12.4 CMC with PHA blasts

As mentioned earlier, the applicability of CMC may be extended to any system of alloantigens using ^{51}Cr-labelled PHA blasts as targets cells.

PHA blasts may be produced *en masse* as follows.

Materials and equipment
As Section 4.9, but in addition:
Inbred mice
Tissue culture medium containing fetal bovine serum and antibiotics (Appendix I)
Plastic tissue culture flasks

Method
1 Prepare cell suspension from mouse lymph nodes.
2 Count cells and adjust to $3-5 \times 10^6$ ml^{-1}.
3 Add optimal concentration of PHA (determined in Section 4.9).
4 Add 20 ml of cell suspension to each bottle and gas for 60 sec with 5% CO_2 in air.
5 Place bottles on their sides in a 37° incubator.

The kinetics of the response are essentially similar to those seen in Section 4.9.

6 After 72 h, pool cells, wash three times in tissue culture medium and label with $^{51}CrO_4$ (Section 7.5.2).
7 Use for CMC as in Section 4.12.2.

Technical notes
1 The protocols above are technically less demanding when carried out with human peripheral blood lymphocytes, PBL. In general, PBL, even from the mouse, are much easier cells to culture and give a very low spontaneous background.
2 The ability to expand T lymphocytes to form large clonal populations using antigen stimulation and the cytokine interleukin 2 (IL-2) means that cytotoxic effector cells may be generated from even a single progenitor cell grown in limiting dilution culture (Section 4.13). Although the implications of this powerful cell technology are enormous, such refinements are natural developments of the techniques described here.

Estimation of antigen-specific lymphocyte-precursor frequency

One of the main factors which determines the magnitude of an immune response is the number of antigen-specific lymphocytes available to respond at the time of antigenic challenge. The effector cell assays described earlier in the chapter give no more than an overall impression of the quality of the immune response and have inherently poor quantitation. However, because of the clonality of the immune response, it is in theory a relatively trivial undertaking to modify these assays to estimate the number of clones generated and calculate the number of responding precursors.

For illustration of the principle of the theoretical basis of such assays, let us assume that one in 5000 T lymphocytes respond to any particular foreign major histocompatibility complex (MHC) gene product in a mixed-lymphocyte culture. Consequently, in a pool of 10^5 T lymphocytes we could expect to have on average 20 antigen-specific lymphocytes, so that if we dispersed our lymphocyte pool into 50 micro-cultures, each containing 2×10^7 lymphocytes, some of the wells would contain no antigen-specific lymphocytes, whereas others would receive one, two or more antigen-specific precursor cells. The frequency with which the wells containing zero, one, two or more responsive cells occurs within the micro-plate follows the Poisson distribution (Fig. 4.7), and so can be described by the equation:

$$F_x = \frac{u^x \cdot e^{-u}}{x!}$$

where:

F_x = fraction of wells containing x cells (x = 0,1,2, etc.),

x = number of antigen-specific precursor cells per well,

u = average number of antigen-responsive precursor cells per well,

e = base of the natural logarithm.

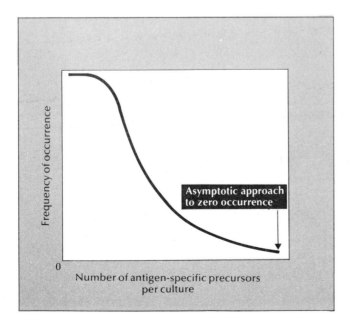

Fig. 4.7 The Poisson distribution. The Poisson distribution describes the relative frequency of occurrence of numbers of rare elements in each sample of a randomly sampled population. Where $u=1$, there is a relatively high frequency of samples containing 0 or 1 element, thereafter the frequency of samples containing 2 or more elements declines steeply.

If we were to set up a series of such mixed-lymphocyte micro-cultures and assay them 10–12 days later, when the proliferation of a single cell would have been sufficient to permit its clonal progeny to be detected, we would find that some cultures had responded whereas others had not. Because we are dealing with a cell suspension in liquid culture we cannot tell whether a responding culture had received one, two, three or more precursor lymphocytes; indeed, all that is known with confidence is the fraction of negative (non-responding) cultures which must have effectively received no antigen-specific lymphocytes.

The above equation can be applied to predict the expected fraction of negative wells for any frequency of responding cells: Substituting for the 'zero-term'

$$F_0 = \frac{u^0 e^{-u}}{0!}$$
$$F_0 = e^{-u}$$

where F_0 = fraction of negative wells, other terms as above.

Thus, we can calculate the frequency of responding cells from the observed fraction of negative cultures, as below.

Clearly, if we added too many responsive lymphocytes to each well all cultures would be positive, and the converse would apply if too few lymphocytes were added. As the frequency of responsive cells is the unknown we wish to measure, we cannot know how many cells to add to ensure that the assay is on the correct part of the 'information curve'. In practical terms, it is necessary to set up a titration series of assays with different numbers of total lymphocytes (only some of which can respond) and then record the fraction of negative cultures at different cell input numbers. These data can be used to calculate precursor frequency using the logarithmic transformation of the zero-term equation:

$$u = -\ln F_0$$

where symbols as above.

In other words, *the mean number of antigen-specific precursors is proportional to the negative value of the natural logarithm of the fraction of negative wells*. The data can be represented and analysed graphically as a semi-log plot, as in Fig. 4.8. Provided the data lie along a straight line the assay is said to show 'single-hit kinetics' and can be analysed to yield a frequency estimate. If the data show significant deviation from linearity (calculated by χ-square statistics and confidence limits for the slope, see Technical notes, p.169) then more than just the number of responding cells is limiting (for example, two cells may need to act together to give a response, culture conditions may be suboptimal, or many other things) and the calculated frequency would be meaningless.

Assuming that our curve was linear, then when we had on average one responding

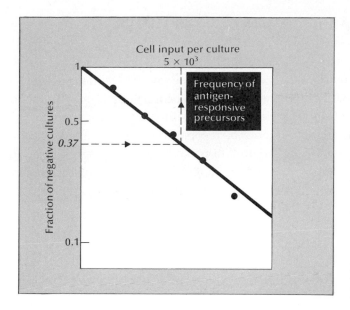

Fig. 4.8 Semi-log plot of cell input data and proportion of non-responding cultures from a limiting dilution assay. If only one element is limiting, in this case the specific antigen-reactive T lymphocytes, then data should approximate to a straight line. When there is on average, one responsive lymphocyte in the volume dispensed into each culture, 0.37 of the cultures should be negative. Interpolation from the point on the x axis (dotted line) to cell input numbers allows the frequency of antigen-responsive lymphocytes in the total population to be estimated.

cell per culture ($u = 1$), 37% of the cultures would be negative by random chance.

To confirm this, substitute $u = 1$ into the zero term of the Poisson formula:

$$F_0 = e^{-u}.$$

If $u = 1$ then

$$\underline{F_0 = e^{-1}}$$

Fraction of non-responding cultures, $F_0 = 0.37$ (or 37%).

Interpolation from the y axis at 0.37 (Fig. 4.8) onto the x axis gives an estimate of the numbers of normal human T lymphocytes that must be added to have, on average, one responding cell per culture; in this case, $1 : 5000$. (Remember, that the immune response to MHC antigens is special as it involves complex antigens recognised by a large number of pre-committed lymphocytes and shows little increase following deliberate immunisation. Frequencies to more 'conventional' antigens such as keyhole limpet haemocyanin or dinitrophenylated foreign protein antigens would show much lower frequencies — between $1 : 20000$ and $1 : 50000$ — which increase significantly after immunisation.)

The limiting dilution assay can be used to estimate the frequency of antigen-specific lymphocytes which undergo or mediate a wide range of immune transformations *in vitro*: proliferation, antibody production, B- and T-lymphocyte cooperation, suppression and cytotoxicity.

The utility of the assay as a route to functional quantitation of the immune response is constrained only by the experimenter's ingenuity to design appropriate assays. We will describe a technique based upon the estimation of the frequency of cytotoxic effector cells reacting to MHC antigens.

4.13.1 Limiting dilution analysis (LDA) assay

We will describe an assay to estimate the frequency of lymphocytes from the peripheral blood of one individual (responder) capable of differentiating into cytotoxic effector cells specific for the MHC antigens of a second individual (stimulator).

   In principle, we need only perform a one-way mixed-lymphocyte reaction (MLR, Section 4.10.1) with different numbers of responding cells to obtain the necessary data. The main practical attribute required to make these assays work reproducibly is the ability to dispense large numbers of replicates of very small volumes of cell suspensions accurately; remember to mix intermittently while dispensing.

Materials and equipment
As Sections 1.14 and 4.10, but in addition:
Interleukin 2, IL-2, as recombinant protein (Appendix II). Material should be pre-titrated for its ability to support the growth of T lymphocytes (Section 12.14.1, Technical note, p. 412)

MIXED-LYMPHOCYTE CULTURE

1 Prepare lymphocytes from heparinised whole blood taken from the 'stimulator' and 'responder' donors (assign status arbitrarily at the beginning of the experiment).
2 Irradiate 30×10^6 stimulator cells in 10 ml tissue culture medium with 35 Gy of γ- or X-irradiation to prevent their proliferation in culture.
3 Wash the irradiated stimulator cells once by centrifugation and re-suspend them to 4.0×10^6 lymphocytes ml^{-1} in complete tissue culture medium.
4 Add an equal volume of IL-2-containing medium, units ml^{-1} previously standardised for ability to support lymphoblast proliferation *in vitro* (Section 12.14.1).
5 While the stimulator cells are being irradiated, prepare a suspension of responder cells at 8.0×10^4 lymphocytes ml^{-1} and dilute with complete tissue culture medium to obtain a $1:2$ titration series according to the Protocol.

Protocol

	Tube number				
	1	2	3	4	5
Tissue culture medium (ml)	0	2.25			
Lymphocyte suspension (ml)	2.25	2.25			
Cells ml^{-1}	8×10^4	4×10^4	2×10^4	1×10^4	0.5×10^4

mix ——→ *mix* ——→ etc.
2.25 ml   2.25 ml

6 Dispense 100 µl volumes of the cell suspensions into micro-cultures (Fig. 4.9), and incubate at 37° in a humidified incubator gassed with 5% CO_2 in air for 7 days.

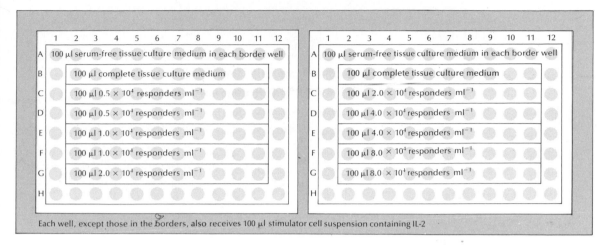

Fig. 4.9 Experimental design of a limiting dilution assay plate. Suggested layout of LDA assay plates for estimation of the frequency of MHC-reactive lymphocyte precursors in paired samples of human peripheral blood. The numbering and lettering correspond to that of conventional 96-well micro-culture plate. The border wells are filled with tissue culture medium and are not used for cultures in order to improve humidification, and therefore observed reproductibility, across the plate. In the cell-mediated cytolytic assay, which will be carried out on the clonal products of these micro-cultures, rows B of each plate provide the data for the calculation of the mean ± standard deviation of the spontaneous leakage of isotope from intact target cells. In assays employing conventional, rather than cell-based, antigens, the row B should also receive irradiated 'filler' cells as explained in the technical note to Section 4.13.1, p.168.

7 Examine the culture plate from below by eye to determine the degree of pro-liferation, visible as small white clumps (compare wells containing responding and stimulator cells with those containing stimulators alone).

8 If the medium has turned yellow at 7 days, add 50 µl of fresh tissue culture medium containing IL-2 to each well.

CELL-MEDIATED CYTOLYSIS

Materials and equipment
As for Section 4.9 and 4.12, but use heparinised human peripheral blood.

Method
1 Prepare PHA lymphoblasts from each of the 'stimulator' donors 3 days before the CMC assay, according to Section 4.12.4.
2 Harvest the lymphocytes and wash twice in serum-free tissue culture medium by centrifugation (150 g for 10 min at room temperature). You will need about 4×10^5 lymphoblasts as targets.
3 Re-suspend the cell pellet in 150 µl of medium containing 11.1×10^6 Bq of $^{51}CrO_4$ and incubate in a 37° water bath for 90 min with regular shaking.
4 Wash cells three times by centrifugation in tissue culture medium containing 10% fetal bovine serum and re-suspend in 5 ml of medium for a haemocytometer count. (*Take care, the cells should now be radioactive.*)

5 Prepare a 15 ml suspension containing 2.5×10^4 target cells ml^{-1} from each original donor.

6 Remove 100 μl of supernatant from each of the culture wells of the limiting dilution assay plates and add 100 μl of the target cell suspension.

7 Incubate for 4 h at 37° in a humidified incubator gassed with 5% CO_2 in air.

8 Remove 100 μl of supernatant medium from each well for counting in the γ spectrometer. Take care not to disturb the cell pellet during aspiration of the supernatant sample.

9 In order to determine an acceptable maximum for spontaneous $^{51}CrO_4$ release, calculate the mean and standard deviation of the radioactive content of the supernatant in rows B of plates 1 and 2 (Fig. 4.9).

10 Set the minimum threshold for a positive culture at the sum of the mean plus 3 standard deviations of the spontaneous release.

11 Score cultures as positive or negative according to this threshold, and determine the fraction of negative cultures at each input number of responder cells.

12 Plot the fraction of negative cultures on a log scale against the cell input, as in Fig. 4.8, and determine the cell input number giving 37% (0.37) negative cultures.

This corresponds to the input number required to give, on average 1 responder lymphocyte per well which is able to recognise the stimulator MHC molecules.

Technical notes

1 The protocol above has been designed to provide a simple robust assay by which to illustrate the important principles of limiting dilution analysis. Previous experiments have shown that the frequency of precursor cytolytic cells in human blood sample pairs lies in the range $1:500$ to $1:5000$, hence our ability to choose an arithmetic dilution series and so gain maximum information for the construction of the semi-logarithmic plot. In addition, the efficient generation of cytotoxic effectors by these antigens results in a high effector : target cell ratio thus increasing the sensitivity of the cytolytic assay by maximising the difference between the ^{51}Cr released spontaneously from intact target cells and that released by specific lysis. It therefore provides an excellent assay for teaching purposes.

In experimental situations with less favorable antigens, it is usual to perform an LDA in two cycles. In the first the cell input numbers vary logarithmically, and so only a fraction will show a useful proportion of negative cultures. The LDA should then be repeated with an arithmetic series of cell input numbers around the optimum of the logarithmic series.

2 The efficiency of the *in vitro* response of lymphocytes is cell-density dependent. If the density is too high, nutrients and culture conditions become limiting. More importantly, if the cell density falls too low then the linear relationship between cell numbers and observed effector function is lost. In the assay described above, we added a standard number of irradiated stimulator lymphocytes (4×10^5 per culture), these also acted as 'filler' cells to maintain optimum cell numbers. This 40-fold excess of filler stimulator cells renders the variations due to the fourfold

change in responder numbers insignificant. If an LDA assay is performed on a single lymphocyte population responding to a 'conventional' antigen then irradiated autologous 'filler' cells should be added, both to counteract the variation in cell number in the dilution series and also to provide sufficient antigen presenting cells.

3   At least two useful computer programmes have been published for statistical analysis of the curve and calculation of the precursor frequency: for the Texas Ti-59 calculator with the statistics module see Fazekas de St Groth *et al.* (1982) and for the BBC microcomputer Waldmann *et al.* (1987). Individuals requiring a deeper understanding of the potential and limitations of limiting dilution analysis should consult Lefkovits and Waldmann (1979).

4.14   Antibody-dependent cell-mediated cytotoxicity

Antibody-dependent cell-mediated cytotoxicity (ADCC) is a phenomenon in which target cells, coated with very small amounts of antibody, are killed by non-immune effector cells. The effector cells (K cells) have receptors for the Fc regions of the antibody and appear to recognise immune complexes specifically. The exact killing mechanisms are unknown, but it involves cell to cell contact and, in some of the effector cell types involved, might result from the release of lysosomal enzymes.

The spectrum of cell types able to mediate this killing remains to be elucidated, but it is known that different types of effector mediate the killing, depending upon the character of the target. With red-cell targets the effector cells tend to be of the granulocyte—macrophage lineage; but with tumour target cells, cells of the lymphocyte lineage predominate as effectors.

On present evidence, it seems certain that there is a large overlap between the progenitors of ADCC effector cells and those of LAK cells (lymphokine-activated killers, Section 4.15). Although some of these progenitors also show NK cell (natural killer, Section 4.15) activity, the overlap is almost certainly confined to cells of lymphoid lineage in this case.

It is possible to distinguish between the NK and LAK non-specific (non-antigen-specific) cytotoxic cells by the use of NK resistant or susceptible target cells. ADCC effector cells may be detected by their antibody dependence.

Materials

Mouse (Appendix II)

Chicken (Appendix II)

Rabbit anti-chicken erythrocyte serum (diluted 1 : 6000 in tissue culture medium plus 10% fetal bovine serum, Appendix I)

Tissue culture medium

Fetal bovine serum, FBS (Appendix II)

Sodium ^{51}chromate (Appendix II)

Sheep erythrocytes, SRBC (Appendix II)

4.14.1 Target cells

1 Take 0.2 ml of blood from the chicken into a heparinised syringe. The main wing vein is a convenient site for venepuncture to obtain small volumes of blood.
2 Dilute 0.1 ml of blood with 1.9 ml of Eagle's MEM containing 10% FBS.
3 Use 0.1 ml of diluted blood and add 0.1 ml of sodium $^{51}CrO_4$ (specific activity, see Appendix II).
4 Gas with 5% CO_2 in air.
5 Incubate at 37° for 1 h.
6 Wash four times with medium containing 5% FBS. Centrifuge at 90 g for 7 min at 4°.
7 Wash SRBC in tissue culture medium four times by centrifugation (450 g for 10 min).
8 Adjust SRBC concentration to 10^7 ml^{-1}.
9 Add 10^5 labelled chicken red cells to each ml of sheep red cells.

4.14.2 Effector cells

1 Remove the spleen from the mouse and prepare a single-cell suspension (Section 1.15).
2 Adjust to 2.5×10^6 leucocytes ml^{-1}.

4.14.3 Cytotoxic assay

1 Set up culture tubes according to the Protocol below.

Protocol

Tube (in triplicate)	Spleen cells (μl)	Antibody (μl)	^{51}Cr-labelled chicken red cells (μl)
A	100	100	100
B	100	0	100
C	0	100	100
D	0	0	100
E	100 μl distilled water	100 μl distilled water	100

2 Cap the tubes and incubate them, leaning at an angle of 30–45 degrees, in a gassed CO_2 incubator or a desiccator (5% in air) for 18 h.
3 Add 1 ml medium to each tube and then spin (90 g) for 10 min.
4 Remove 0.8 ml supernatant from each tube and assess this for ^{51}Cr release in a γ spectrometer.

Technical note
Tube A shows the ^{51}Cr release due to spleen cells plus anti-target antibody. The other cultures are controls. Tube B gives the amount of release due to spleen cells

alone, while C measures the release due to antibody. Spontaneous release of the label by the erythrocytes is monitored by tube D.

Calculation

The calculation of the amount of cytotoxicity is complicated as there is some difficulty in choosing the correct control value against which to calculate the experimental ^{51}Cr release. This is because spleen cells, in the absence of antibody, exert a protective effect over the chicken erythrocytes. It will be seen that the ^{51}Cr release in tube B is usually less than the spontaneous release in tube D. Therefore, for the control culture, one may choose either effectors plus target cells (B) or target cells plus antibody (C).

The calculation of percentage cytotoxicity may then be as follows:

$$\% \ ^{51}Cr \ release = \frac{A - C}{E - C} \times 100$$

or

$$= \frac{A - B}{E - B} \times 100.$$

Letters in formulae correspond to culture tubes in the Protocol (facing page).

4.15 Antibody-dependent cell-mediated cytotoxicity (ADCC), lymphokine-activated and natural killer cells

In ADCC, the apparent specificity of the killing reaction is superimposed on a non-specific effector cell by its acquisition of, or adsorption to, target cell-specific antibody. In the absence of antibody, a proportion of these non-specific killers can kill target cells directly and are referred to as *natural killer* (NK) cells. They are able to kill tumour cells without the need for previous immunisation or passive antibody, are greatly increased in numbers in mice carrying the *nu/nu* athymic mutation (where they presumably account for the resistance to spontaneous tumours shown by these T lymphocyte-deficient animals) and are virtually absent in the beige mutant of the C3H mouse. Treatment of human or murine normal (non-immune) lymphocytes with IL-2 greatly enhances their non-specific killing capacity to many tumour targets. This led to the definition of a third functional class of non-specific cytolytic cells known as lymphokine-activated killer or LAK cells. These cells may have clinical use for anti-tumour therapy.

At present the lineage of cytolytic cells is confused but their functional classification is clear:

(a)   There is a 'common pool' of antigen-specific and non-specific cytolytic effector cells, composed of several cell lineages.

(b)   T lymphocytes are the only cytolytic effector cells known to date to have clonally distributed endogenous receptors for specific target-cell antigens.

(c)   Some lymphocytes, the so-called *large granular lymphocytes*, identified by virtue of their morphology (Fig. 3.1c), are able to mediate NK- and LAK- cell activity *in vitro*.

(d) Additional, as yet incompletely characterised, non-lymphoid cells are able to mediate NK and LAK activity.

(e) LAK and NK cells may be functionally distinguished by the judicious choice of tumour target cells; most tumour targets used to date have been LAK sensitive, but only a few are NK sensitive. For example, the erythromyeloid leukaemia cell line K-562 is both NK and LAK sensitive, whereas T-24 (urinary bladder carcinoma), Daudi (Burkitt's lymphoma-derived B-lymphoblastoid cell line), ME-180 (cervical epidermoid carcinoma) and OVCAR-3 (ovarian adenocarcinoma) are all NK resistant or relatively so. T-24 seems to be an especially good target for LAK cells because of its production of IL-6, whereas LAK-resistant targets appear to produce TGFβ and so block LAK-cell induction.

(f) Most primary cultures of freshly excised tumours are NK resistant but LAK sensitive, as are hapten-modified normal cells.

Whatever their *in vivo* relevance or clinical utility, the LAK cells are a powerful *in vitro* killing system.

4.15.1 Assay of LAK- and NK-cell activity

Materials and equipment
Heparinised, human venous blood
Density gradient; for example, Lymphoprep (Appendix II)
Tissue culture medium containing 5% fetal bovine serum, FBS (Appendix II)
Recombinant IL-2 (Appendix II)
T-24 and K-562 cell lines (Appendix III)
Sodium $^{51}CrO_4$ (Appendix II)
U-shaped micro-culture plates (Appendix II)
Micro-plate carrier for centrifugation (Appendix II)
γ spectrometer

Method
1 Isolate peripheral blood mononuclear cells (PBMC) from heparinised venous blood by density-gradient centrifugation (Section 1.14.1) and wash three times in tissue culture medium by centrifugation (150 g for 10 min at room temperature).
2 Adjust the PBMC to 5×10^6 cells ml^{-1} with tissue culture medium containing 5% FBS.

For the assay of NK activity, no IL-2 or induction period is required, proceed to step 4.

3 For LAK-cell induction, supplement the PBMC suspension with recombinant IL-2 to 500 U ml^{-1} and dispense 100 μl aliquots into a U-shaped micro-culture tray as follows: allow for at least triplicate cultures at each dilution (see Protocol below), for each donor and each target (NK resistant and susceptible, see Technical notes) and leave five wells empty for each of the target cells for the

determination of spontaneous isotope release. Culture in a humidified 37° incubator gassed with 5% CO_2 in air.

The time for optimum induction of LAK activity will vary both with donor and type of assay for which they are intended. Typically use cultures at 48−72 h after induction; however, LAK cells are still detectable at 7 days. It is conceivable that the early and late LAK activity might be due to varying proportions of the different cell types known to mediate this effector function.

4 Label the T-24 and K-562 target cells with $^{51}CrO_4$ by mixing 37×10^5 Bq of isotope with 10^6 T-24 or K-562 targets and incubate in a 37° water bath for 1.5 h, mixing every 30 min.

5 Wash the target cells three times by centrifugation, re-suspend and count cells using a haemocytometer. Retain an aliquot of labelled cells for freeze−thaw determination of maximum isotope release (Section 4.12.3.)

For accurate determination of LAK activity it is necessary to determine isotope release over a range of different effector:target cell ratios.

6 Prepare a series of target-cell suspensions according to the Protocol, add 100 μl of each to separate assay wells.

7 Add 100 μl of the highest target suspension to each of the five empty wells allowed for the determination of spontaneous release and supplement with 100 μl of tissue culture medium.

8 Centrifuge the plate at 50 g for 15 min at room temperature in a micro-plate carrier.

Protocol

	Assay number			
	1	2	3	4
PBMC at 5×10^6 ml^{-1}	100 μl ⟶			
Target cells ml^{-1}, use 100 μl per culture	3×10^7	6×10^7	12.5×10^7	27×10^7
Effector:target ratio	6:1	12:1	25:1	50:1

9 Incubate for 4 h at 37° in a humidified incubator gassed with 5% CO_2 in air.

10 Remove 100 μl of supernatant into separate LP3 tubes, cap and count in a γ spectrometer.

11 Calculate specific lysis of each experimental well as follows:

$$\% \text{ specific lysis} = \frac{\text{experimental c.p.m.} - \text{spontaneous c.p.m.}}{\text{maximum c.p.m.} - \text{spontaneous c.p.m.}} \times 100.$$

12 Determine the mean ± standard error of each set of replicates (Section 5.2.1) and display each donor's titration curve graphically for ease of comparison.

Technical notes

1 LAK and NK effector functions are distinguished by differential killing of the two target cells used in the assay. T-24 cells are relatively NK resistant, whereas K-562 cells are both NK and LAK susceptible. LAK activity varies widely between normal donors, between 30 and 100% specific lysis.

2 As a guide, the maximum release from 10^4 target cells should be about 10 000 c.p.m. and the spontaneous release <10% at 4 h. High spontaneous release is often due to the batch of FBS used as a tissue culture supplement; batches should be screened before purchase. FBS and autologous human serum give comparable results.

3 It is also possible to generate LAK cells in bulk by culturing in flasks.

4 The relatively high concentration of IL-2 used to generate these cells excludes the use of cell supernatants, for example from MLA 144, as an IL-2 source.

5 Over a short induction period, <48 h, LAK activity is resistant to hydroxyurea, cyclosporine and steroid treatment. However, when longer induction periods are used, up to 7 days, there is a decrease in the rate of LAK induction, suggesting that the cells participating in the early expression of LAK activity might be different to those involved at later time points.

4.16 In vivo assays of delayed hypersensitivity

The magnitude of a localised delayed hypersensitivity reaction *in vivo* may be assayed by measuring one of the secondary consequences of lymphocyte activation in an experimental animal; for example, leakage of intravascular ^{125}I-albumin into the tissues, increase in foot volume or ear thickness (in mice) or the enlargement of the wattle in male chickens. Unfortunately, many of these assays have poor reproducibility or may be initiated by mechanisms that are not entirely mediated by T lymphocytes.

An extremely elegant assay has recently been described that relies on the localisation of isotopically labelled cells at the site of antigen administration. Although the magnitude of the response is low the reproducibility is impressive.

4.16.1 Localisation of isotopically labelled cells

PREPARATIONS IN ADVANCE
Sensitise mice with antigen using a regime known to stimulate good delayed hypersensitivity. For example, shave an area of skin of a mouse and paint it at three sites using 50 μl dinitrofluorobenzene (10 mg ml^{-1} in a 1 : 1 mixture of acetone−olive oil).

Materials and equipment
Mice, sensitised as above
2,4-dinitro-1-fluorobenzene (10 mg ml^{-1} in acetone−olive oil, 1 : 1)
5-iodo-2′deoxyuridine-^{125}I, ^{125}I-UDR (Appendix II)

0.14 M saline

γ spectrometer

Method

1   Paint the left ear pinna (outer flap of the ear) of the DNFB-sensitised and normal control mice with 5 μl DNFB in acetone—olive oil (as above).

2   Paint the right ear of all mice with 5 μl acetone—olive oil alone.

3   After 10 h inject 0.1 μl of saline containing 74×10^3 Bq ^{125}I-UDR into the tail vein of each mouse. (Warm the mouse under a heat lamp for 10 min before injection.) Before removing the needle, inject a small volume of saline intradermally at the injection site (this will collapse the vein and prevent leakage of blood and radio-isotope from the punctured vessel).

4   After 16 h, kill the mice by cervical dislocation and cut off the left (antigen-treated) and right (control) pinnae at the hair line.

5   Count the radioactivity in each pinna using a γ counter.

Calculation of the response

$$\text{Index of response} = \frac{\text{c.p.m. left ear}}{\text{c.p.m. right ear}}.$$

Technical note

If the mice have been primed with cellular or soluble antigens, elicit the secondary response with a 10 μl intradermal injection into the pinna.

4.17   Graft rejection

The cell-mediated immune response is very important in the apparently highly artificial system of transplant rejection. Although the mechanism of rejection of whole-organ grafts are many and varied, cell-mediated immunity is known to be instrumental in the rejection of foreign skin grafts. This is the easiest system in which to demonstrate the basic principles of cell-mediated immunity (*in vivo*).

4.17.1   Skin-graft rejection

In the experiment described below, tail-skin grafts will be transferred between inbred strains of mice to demonstrate the two fundamental principles of T cell-mediated immunity: its *specificity* and *memory*.

Materials and equipment

Mice from inbred strains with contrasting coat colours

Safety razor blades

4—5 cm glass tubes, internal diameter slightly larger than the mouse's tail

Michel clips

It is necessary to prepare a 'bed' for a skin graft before transplantation. In the technique described below with paired mice, the removal of the donor tail-skin graft automatically prepares the 'bed' for the recipient graft.

Method

1 Anaesthetise one of the pair of mice with ether.

2 Hold the mouse's tail over your forefinger with the mouse pointing away from you. Hold the razor blade horizontally on the tail, about 2 cm from the base of the tail, and press slightly to indent the skin. Draw the blade towards you with a slicing action. Do not cut too deeply or the tail will bleed — this will not make a good 'bed' for a recipient graft. Cut off a piece of skin about 0.5 cm long, and leave the skin graft on the blade.

3 Move about 1 cm down the tail and cut a second graft.

4 Replace one of the grafts (autograft) but turn it through 180° so that the hairs are facing the wrong way.

5 Use a gauze swab to press the graft firmly in place to exclude all the air. If there is bleeding around the graft, pressure must be applied until haemostasis is achieved.

6 Anaesthetise the second mouse and prepare two pieces of tail skin for grafting as above.

7 Again return one of the pieces of skin to the donor as an autograft. The skin graft of the first mouse (allograft) can now be placed on the second 'bed', again turning it so that the hairs face the wrong direction. Press the graft firmly in place.

8 The first mouse, which will need to be re-anaesthetised, can now receive the allograft.

9 The grafts are protected with glass tail tubes. These should be about 4—5 cm long and wide enough to slide easily over the mouse's tail. (The cut edges of the glass must be flame polished to avoid injury to the mouse.)

10 The tail tube is held in place by a Michel clip placed through the tail bones. (The tube must not be attached too near the base of the tail or it will become fouled with faeces and urine.)

11 Remove the tail tubes 24—36 h after grafting.

The grafts should be observed during the following 2 weeks and the time taken for necrosis and sloughing of the allograft recorded. This should occur within 11—14 days of grafting, although with some strain combinations this can be as soon as day 8. Other than for technical reasons, the autograft should become established, and continue to grow.

4.17.2 ## Immunological nature of graft rejection

The immunological nature of graft rejection may be established by observing rejection times in immunised and normal mice. This experiment involves the use of three inbred mouse strains.

PREPARATION IN ADVANCE

Recipient mice become immune when they have rejected a primary or first-set skin graft; however, transplantation immunity can be established more conveniently by transferring an allogenic spleen-cell suspension between the two strains to be tested as follows:

1   Prepare a spleen-cell suspension of CBA cells in tissue culture medium. Wash and count the cells (Sections 1.15 and 3.4).
2   Inject 10^7 CBA spleen cells intraperitoneally into adult BALB/c mice.

These BALB/c mice will be immune to CBA cells 2 weeks after injection.

Materials and equipment
As for Section 4.17.1, but in addition:
Recipient BALB/c mice, normal and previously injected with CBA cells
CBA- and C57BL-strain donor mice.

Method
1   Kill the CBA and C57BL donor mice and remove two skin grafts from each strain as previously described (Section 4.17.1, steps 1−3).
2   Anaesthetise the normal BALB/c recipient mouse and remove three sections of tail skin.
3   Return one piece of skin as an autograft and transplant the CBA and C57BL grafts to the other two 'beds'.
4   Protect the grafted areas by a tail tube held in place by a Michel clip.
5   Repeat the grafting procedure for the immune BALB/c mouse, again protecting the grafted areas with a tail tube.
6   Remove all tail tubes 24−36 h after grafting.

The rejection time for the grafts must now be observed. The normal BALB/c should reject the two allogeneic grafts within 11−14 days. The allografts on the immune BALB/c mouse should show differential survival times. The rejection of the CBA graft should be accelerated, about 7 days, whereas the C57BL graft should stay on for the full 11−14 days.

This experiment again demonstrates that the memory or anamnestic response is specific − both for B cells as seen previously, and for T cells as seen here.

4.18   Host rejection (graft versus host reaction)

In the previous experiments we saw that an immunologically mature animal was able to reject a foreign skin graft. There are, however, situations in which the graft, rather than the host, is immunologically competent and so the host is rejected by the graft. Clinically, such reactions have arisen during attempts to reconstitute immunodeficient children; for example, those with severe combined immunodeficiency, by bone marrow therapy or after allogeneic bone marrow grafting of leukaemia patients given whole-body irradiation. Human bone marrow, unlike that of the mouse, contains many immunologically competent cells which produce a florid graft versus host (GvH) reaction characterised by fever, rash, diarrhoea, splenomegaly, pancytopenia and death. An area of great current interest is the application of monoclonal antibody technology to the 'purging' of bone marrow: autologous bone marrow from leukaemic patients can be purged to remove tumour cells or allogeneic bone marrow can be purged of alloreactive T lymphocytes.

The degree of splenomegaly induced by a GvH reaction can be used experimentally in neonatal mice or chickens *in ovo* to quantitate the anti-host response following an injection of adult allogeneic lymphocytes.

A GvH reaction can also be induced in adult animals, in the absence of immuno-suppression, by injecting parental cells into an F_1 hybrid. Because the important transplantation antigens are codominant the F_1 hybrid will express and develop tolerance to both sets of parental antigens coded for by the major histocompatibility complex. Accordingly, parental cells will not be recognised as foreign by the F_1 cells, but the parental cells will recognise and react to the other parental component on the F_1 cells. The GvH reaction can be assayed in rats using lymph-node enlargement. In the technique described here the GvH reaction is limited to the popliteal lymph node by injecting parental cells into the foot pad of an F_1 hybrid (the popliteal node receives the lymph drainage from the foot-pad area). The lymph-node enlargement assay in rats has several advantages over the splenomegaly assay in mice; for example, the index of lymph-node enlargement (10−15 times) is much greater than that of splenic enlargement (2−3 times) and the contra-lateral node, which receives the same number of *syngeneic* cells, provides an excellent internal control for non-specific enlargement.

4.18.1   GvH assay in rats

Materials
Individuals of an inbred strain of rats and F_1 hybrids; for example DA, or Lewis and (DA × Lewis) F_1 (Appendix II)

Method
1 Remove the spleens from the parental and F_1 hybrid donors.
2 Tease out, wash and filter the cells (Section 1.15).
3 Count the cells and adjust to the required concentration (see Protocol in suggested experimental design Fig. 4.10).
4 Inject 0.1 ml of the parental and F_1 cells into the right and left foot pad, respectively.
5 After 7 days kill all the recipients and remove the right and left popliteal nodes (the nodes are in the muscle just behind the knee joint − remove the GvH node first as this is the easiest to find cf. Fig. 4.11).
6 Weigh each pair of nodes and calculate the index of enlargement as follows:

$$\text{index of enlargement (IE)} = \frac{\text{weight of node receiving parental cells}}{\text{weight of node receiving } F_1 \text{ cells}}.$$

Rats used:

4 DA donors

21 (DA × Lewis) F_1 hybrids. Donors and recipients

Recipients given lymphocytes in 0.1 ml into foot pad according to table below:

Right footpad — DA cells (GvH node)

Left footpad — F_1 cells (control node)

Lymph nodes assayed at 7th day post-injection

Number of lymphocytes transferred	Weight of GVH node	Weight of contra-lateral (control) node	Index of enlargement	Geometric mean
5.0×10^6				
1	49.43	4.80	10.3	
2	63.20	5.12	12.3	11.6
3	59.60	5.80	10.3	
4	68.35	4.91	14.1	
2.5×10^7				
1	110.10	7.93	13.9	
2	98.92	7.19	13.8	15.6
3	99.54	5.23	19.0	
4	120.61	7.44	16.2	
5.0×10^7				
1	89.96	5.83	14.4	
2	90.25	7.81	11.6	13.0
3	67.34	7.22	9.3	
4	75.43	4.10	18.4	
1.0×10^8				
1	80.31	5.00	16.0	
2	65.62	8.31	7.9	11.0
3	81.40	7.20	11.3	
4	73.60	7.21	10.2	

Fig. 4.10 **Graft versus host reaction dose—response curve**

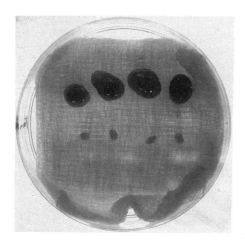

Fig. 4.11 **Lymph-node enlargement induced during a GvH reaction**. Popliteal lymph nodes taken from (DA × Lewis)F_1 rats receiving DA cells into the right foot pad (above) and an equal number of F_1 cells into the left foot pad (below).

An IE of up to 2 may be expected from the injection of syngeneic cells alone. The normal range for lymph node enlargement following GvH induction is 10−15.

7 Calculate the geometric mean for each group (Section 5.2.1).

8 Determine the optimum number of parental cells, i.e. the number giving maximum IE.

The observed increase in lymph-node weight during the local GvH reaction is due to an increased number of host, not donor, cells. Presumably, this host response is caused by mitogenic and chemotatic cytokines, released by the activated donor cells, which induce non-specific inflow and division of host cells. Several studies have now been published which have determined the number of alloreactive lymphocytes infiltrating a rejecting allogeneic organ (host versus graft) or the site of a GvH reaction using limiting dilution analysis (Section 4.13). In each case, although the actual frequency of alloreactive lymphocytes has risen following immune stimulation, suggesting an immunologically specific infiltrate, their absolute numbers have been very small. Presumably these cells are very active and much of the damage they induce is through recruitment of innocent bystander cells.

It is also possible to assay a host versus graft reaction in the system described above by transferring F_1 cells into parental recipients.

4.18.2 GvH reaction in other species

In mice, the degree of lymph-node enlargement produced by a local GvH reaction is much less dramatic and has low reproducibility. The index of enlargement is only in the range of 1.5−3.0. The reasons for this difference between the rat and mouse system are not known. A GvH reaction may be reliably quantitated in mice and chickens by measuring the degree of splenic enlargement induced by an intravenous injection of allogeneic cells into an immunologically incompetent host. Again, this incompetent situation is achieved by: (a) injecting adult lymphocytes into heavily irradiated adult recipients; (b) injecting parental cells into a F_1 hybrid; or (c) injecting adult cells into a new-born or embryonic recipient. In (c), it is necessary to use a group of age-matched, littermates as controls, and to inject them with an equal number of adult syngeneic cells. In both experimental and control groups, the GvH spleen weight is expressed as a fraction of the total body weight.

As has been seen, the GvH and mixed-lymphocyte reactions (Section 4.18 cf. 4.10.1) have several properties in common; it is not possible, for example, to demonstrate an effect of pre-sensitisation on the magnitude of the response to major histocompatibility differences, and in both reactions, specific effector T cells are generated which are able to lyse appropriate target cells (Section 4.12).

4.19 Summary and conclusions

This is a key chapter in the book. The cell assays examined here have been absolutely basic to our understanding of the specificity and adaptability of the cell-based immune response. Now that their analytical potential has been matched by simplification and standardisation of the lymphocyte populations for study — T- and B-cell lines and hybridomas (Chapter 12) — the future potential of these techniques far outweighs their historical achievements.

We still have much to learn about the way in which the specific elements of the immune response interact with the powerful, but non-specific, killing systems based on ADCC, LAK and NK cells. It is possible that amplification of these mechanisms *in vivo* might allow innate immunity to fulfill the earlier expectations of adaptive immunity in the control of tumours and tumorigenesis.

4.20
Further reading

Fazekas da St. Groth S (1982) The evaluation of limiting dilution assays. *J. Immunol. Methods* **49**: 11–23.

Gupta S, Paul W and Fauci A (editors) (1987) *Mechanisms of Lymphocyte Activation and Immune Regulation*. Plenum, London.

Herberman RB, Reynolds CW and Ortaldo J (1986) Mechanisms of cytotoxicity by NK cells. *Annu. Rev. Immunol.* **4**: 651–674.

Lefkovitz I and Waldmann H (1979) *Limiting Dilution Analysis of the Immune System*. Cambridge University Press, Cambridge.

Polak JM and van Noorden S (1987) *An Introduction to Immunocytochemistry: Current Techniques and Problems*. Oxford Science Publishers, Oxford.

Sternberger LA (1979) *Immunocytochemistry*, 2nd edition. John Wiley and Sons, London.

Waldmann H *et al.* (1987) Limiting dilution analysis. In *Lymphocytes*, Klaus GGB (editor). IRL Press, Oxford, pp. 163–188.

5 Cell Dynamics *In Vivo*

We are now at the stage where we can start to reconstruct the immune system of our animal model and try to gain some understanding of the complex interactions that actually occur in a 'real' immune response. Again, for ease of experimental manipulation, the animal will be responding to highly artificial antigens.

While being intrigued by the wonderful specificity and adaptation of lymphocytes, their progeny and highly polymorphic molecules such as antibody, we must also consider an area of immunity that shows only 'crude' specificity and virtually no adaptivity. This is innate, non-specific or natural immunity.

5.1 Innate immunity

The body has many mechanisms of defence against microorganisms that are of prime importance but do not concern lymphocytes at all. Indeed many potential pathogens are resisted and destroyed without the lymphoid system becoming aware of their existence.

At the body surface, for example, lactic acid in sweat and the fatty acids in sebaceous secretions are very potent anti-bacterial agents. In the tissues there are anti-bacterial enzymes; for example, lysozyme which splits the linkages between *N*-acetyl glucosamine and *N*-acetyl muramic acid in the bacterial cell wall. This enzyme is known to facilitate the disruption of bacteria after an antibody and complement-mediated lesion has been formed. Again we see that although the body has many potentially independent mechanisms of defence, they usually act in concert.

5.2 Particle clearance by the reticuloendothelial system

Microorganisms, or their experimental equivalent of carbon particles, are readily engulfed by circulating and tissue-fixed phagocytes. Neutrophils (polymorphonuclear leucocytes) and monocytes (Section 3.2.1.) together with histiocytes or tissue macrophages (microglia in the brain, kupffer cells in the liver, glomerular mesangial cells in the kidney, synovial macrophages in the joints, etc.) and vascular endothelial cells constitute the *reticuloendothelial system* (RES). The cells of the RES are all capable of ingesting foreign material and degrading it by means of intracellular enzymes in phagolysosomes. The term reticuloendothelial system is less restrictive than that applied to the so-called mononuclear phagocyte system, which is essentially confined to blood monocytes and specialised tissue macrophages. *In vivo* it is virtually impossible to predict which of the phagocytic compartments will be involved in the clearance of different particles.

Materials and equipment
Albino mice
Colloidal carbon (Appendix II)
Acetic acid, 1% v/v glacial acetic acid in water
Spectrophotometer or colorimeter

Method

1 Warm the mouse at 37° for 15—20 min.
2 Snip the end from the tail and collect 1 drop of blood onto a microscope slide. Immediately, lyse a 20 µl sample in 4 ml of acetic acid.
3 Inject 0.1 ml of colloidal carbon into the tail vein.
4 When the mouse's eyes have turned black (within 30 sec) collect 1 drop of blood and lyse a 10 µl sample (before it clots) in 2 ml of acetic acid.
5 Collect 1 drop of blood at the following times post-inoculation: 2, 5, 10, 15, 20, 30, 45, 60, 90 min, and lyse a 10 µl sample, before it clots, in 2 ml of acetic acid solution.
6 Observe the colour change of the mouse's eyes. Kill the mouse and examine the lungs, liver and spleen. (If you are not sure of the appearance of normal organs kill and examine a control mouse, which has not been injected with carbon.)
7 Using the original, pre-injection blood sample as a standard, read the density of all the lysed samples.

5.2.1   Data presentation

We have decided to use the data from this experiment, in which the underlying biological principles are relatively simple, to illustrate some of the methods of data presentation. However, the comments and methods of presentation are generally applicable.

By inspection of the data in Fig. 5.1, it can be seen that each mouse has a slightly different rate of clearance of carbon particles from the blood. This is due to many

Time (min)	0	2	5	10	15	20	30	45	60	90
Mouse	% transmission of lysed sample									
1	44	26	29	47	51	89	78	92	100	100
2	0	6	12	19	31	27	42	80	76	100
3	9	21	30	41	49	52	68	89	95	100
4	15	22	28	59	58	74	87	92	100	100
5	0	9	12	33	16	20	31	26	—	—
6	9	18	28	—	44	48	74	86	89	100
Arithmetic mean ($\bar{x}$)	13	17	23	40	42	52	63	78	92	100
Standard deviation (s.d.)	16	8	9	15	15	27	22	26	10	0

Fig. 5.1 Clearance of blood-borne colloidal carbon by the reticuloendothelial system.

184 / CHAPTER 5

biological variables, both uncontrolled and uncontrollable, such as age, blood volume, number and activity of phagocytic cells, etc., and also the technical error of the sampling method. We wish to present the data in a way that it can be:

(a) *Appreciated* — to discern any central tendency of the dependent variable (amount of carbon in the blood) relative to the independent variable (time).

(b) *Analysed* — we may ultimately wish to know whether mice treated in different ways vary significantly in their clearance times.

Arithmetic mean

This is the simplest description of the data, in that we are all used to using this value. The sample arithmetic mean, $\bar{x}$, may be calculated as follows:

$$\text{sample mean } \bar{x} = \frac{\Sigma x}{n}$$

where :

Σx = sum of all values of
n = number of observations.

1 Tabulate your data and calculate the mean transmittance value for each time point as in Fig. 5.1.
2 Plot a graph of (100−mean transmittance value), i.e. the relative amount of carbon remaining in the blood, against time as in Fig. 5.2. (It is conventional to plot the independent variable on the x or horizontal axis and the dependent variable on the y or the vertical axis.)

If the sample mean alone is recorded we are losing valuable information describing the distribution of the data around the mean. The simplest description of the spread

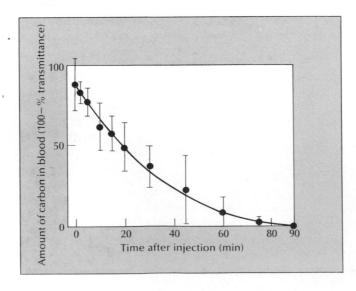

Fig. 5.2 Exponential clearance curve of colloidal carbon. The rate of carbon clearance is proportional to the excess of the residual blood concentration over a certain threshold value. Although the individual time points conform reasonably to the curve fitted by eye it is more accurate to fit a straight line to the log-transformed data.

The standard deviation of each group of observations is shown as bar lines above and below the arithmetic mean.

of the data is the *range*. However, this depends only on the extreme values of the dependent variable. In most cases the extreme values in a data set occur least frequently and so will be the least typical members of the distribution. One therefore defines the *standard deviation*.

Standard deviation

This value gives an estimate of the dispersion of the data which takes into account the frequency with which each value occurs and its distance from the mean.

$$\text{Standard deviation, s.d.} = \sqrt{\frac{\Sigma (x - \bar{x})^2}{n - 1}}$$

where:

x = value of each observation,
$\bar{x}$ = sample mean,
n = number of observations.

For ease of calculation, this equation may be re-written:

$$\text{s.d.} = \sqrt{\left\{\Sigma x^2 - \frac{(\Sigma x)^2}{n}\right\}\frac{1}{n - 1}}.$$

The standard deviation has been calculated for the amount of carbon remaining at each time point in Fig. 5.1. The sample mean ± standard deviation uniquely defines each set of data. The standard deviation (above and below the mean) is shown on the graph (Fig. 5.2) as vertical bar lines. It can be shown that 68% of the data lie within the limits of one standard deviation above and below the sample mean.

The data in this experiment do not lie in a straight line but instead form a smooth curve. This is known as an *exponential clearance curve* where the rate of carbon clearance is proportional to the excess of the concentration over a certain threshold value. Fitting such a curve mathematically, especially when the measurements contain random variation can be a very elaborate statistical exercise. In addition, we wish to determine the slope of the curve, as this will give us the rate of carbon clearance. It is, therefore, necessary to transform the data logarithmically by plotting it on semi-log graph paper as shown in Fig. 5.3. The points now approximate to a straight-line curve which can be fitted more accurately than the exponential curve. The slope of the line, and, therefore the rate of carbon clearance may be determined using the following formula:

$$r = \frac{dc}{dt}$$

where:

r = slope of line,
dc = amount of change in blood carbon,
dt = time taken to observe this change.

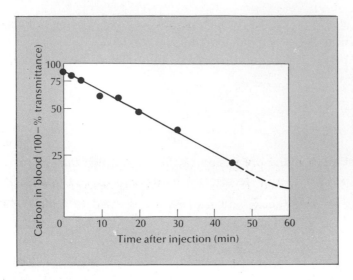

Fig. 5.3 Clearance of colloidal carbon from blood (log transformed data). After logarithmic transformation, the data should conform to a straight line. At sample times later than 50 min there is a bend in the straight line showing that other variables are exerting an effect on the rate of clearance. The slope of the line, i.e. the rate of carbon clearance, is determined only for those observations before the point of inflexion.

The values for dc and dt may be obtained by extrapolating two conveniently spaced time points from the x to the y axis in Fig. 5.3 and then calculating the difference between the two sets of values. As the concentration is decreasing with time, the slope will be negative.

Geometric mean

In the above data there was less than one log variation between the highest and lowest values in the data set. In many biological systems depending, for example, upon cell proliferation, the error arises exponentially and so the data can show much greater variation. Such dispersion of data is shown by a haemolytic plaque assay (Section 4.5.2) or a mitogenic response (Section 4.9). Under these conditions an arithmetic mean is biased towards the extreme values of the distribution and so a *geometric mean* is used. It is calculated as follows:

Geometric mean, $g = \sqrt[n]{x_1, x_2, \ldots, x_n}$

For ease of calculation this may be re-written as:

$$\log g = \frac{\sum\limits_{i-1}^{n} \log x_i}{n}$$

where:

x_i = values of x
n = numbers of observations.

Standard error

Many workers represent their data by a mean value ± the standard error of the mean. This is a description of the oscillation of the sample mean around the true or population mean and is calculated as follows:

standard error, s.e. $= \dfrac{\text{s.d.}}{\sqrt{n}}$

where s.d. = standard deviation,
  n = number of observations.

As a rule of thumb, if the mean and s.e. of two normal distributions do not overlap they are likely to belong to different distributions and achieve statistical significance on student's t test.

The standard error is, of course, smaller than the standard deviation and reduces as the size of the sample is increased. It does not, however, describe the distribution of the data around the sample mean, and should not be used to replace standard deviation purely for aesthetic appearance.

5.3 Neutrophil function tests

In vitro assays are available for many of the key neutrophil activities shown in Fig. 5.4; for example, chemotaxis, phagocytosis and microbicidal activity. However, the precise relationship between the parameter being measured and its *in vivo* expression is not always clear.

The nitroblue tetrazolium reduction assay described below can be used to measure both phagocytosis (this is the only way in which the dye enters the cell) and one of the metabolic pathways responsible for microbial killing (hexose monophosphate

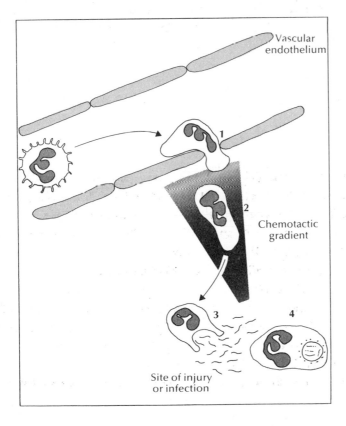

Fig. 5.4 Action of neutrophils. Neutrophils leave the blood and congregate at the site of tissue injury or infection. Dysfunction in any of the stages shown would adversely affect the ability of neutrophils to perform their rôle as front-line defenders against microbial infection. The important stages in the development of an inflammatory response are: (1) attachment to and migration through, the vascular endothelium; (2) locomotion, which may be chemotactic or more strictly chemokinetic (undirected); (3) phagocytosis; and (4) digestion of microbes.

shunt activation). The assay for measurement of respiratory burst described for human neutrophils in Section 14.3.5 uses a dye whose uptake is not phagocytosis dependent.

5.3.1 Nitroblue tetrazolium (NBT) test

The addition of the yellow NBT dye to plasma results in the formation of a NBT–heparin or NBT–fibrinogen complex, which may be phagocytosed by neutrophils. Normal neutrophils show little incorporation of the complex unless they are 'stimulated' to phagocytic activity; for example, by the addition of endotoxin. This assay may be used, therefore, to measure the degree of 'stimulation' of untreated cells or their capacity for phagocytosis after stimulation.

Stimulated neutrophils incorporate the dye complex into phagosomes and, after lysosomal fusion, intracellular reduction results in the formation of blue insoluble crystals of formazan. The percentage of phagocytic cells may be determined using a light microscope or, as described below, the total dye reduction may be quantitated spectrophotometrically after dioxan extraction.

Materials and equipment
Sample of venous blood in heparin (20 iu ml^{-1})
Distilled water
Phosphate-buffered saline, PBS (Appendix I)
Escherichia coli endotoxin (Appendix II) (1 mg ml^{-1} in PBS)
4 mM nitroblue tetrazolium, NBT, dye (Appendix II) in PBS containing 340 mM
    sucrose
Dioxan
0.1 M HCl
Nylon wool (Appendix II), 100 mg in siliconised pasteur pipette
Water bath at 70°
Spectrophotometer

Method
1 Obtain blood sample in heparin (20 iu ml^{-1}) by venepuncture. Use a sample for total and differential leucocyte counts (Sections 3.2.1 and 3.4.2). The NBT reduction activity of the sample must be determined within 60 min of venesection.
2 Add 15 µl of endotoxin solution (1 mg ml^{-1} in PBS, initial concentration) to 1.5 ml of blood and incubate at 37° for 10 min.
3 Add 0.1 ml of freshly prepared NBT dye solution and mix gently.
4 After 20 min at 37°, add blood dropwise to a nylon-wool column.
5 Once the sample has entered the column wash twice with 2 ml of PBS and then 2 ml of distilled water. The distilled water will lyse any residual erythrocytes.
6 Add 2 drops of the HCl to the column, to stop further reduction of the intra-cellular dye, and wash with 2 ml of distilled water.
7 Remove the nylon wool with forceps and place in 5 ml dioxan (in a glass container).

8 Incubate at 70° with occasional vigorous shaking until the nylon wool returns to its original white colour (about 20 min).

9 Centrifuge the dioxan extract to remove any precipitate or nylon fibres (1000 g for 10 min at room temperature).

10 Measure the extinction at 520 mm using a spectrophotometer (use a dioxan standard).

The unstimulated control value is obtained by a parallel incubation of untreated blood, i.e. add 15 µl PBS alone at step 2, then assay as 3–10.

Technical notes

1 All glassware must be siliconised to prevent adherence of phagocytes (Section 1.16).

2 Both neutrophils and monocytes ingest NBT by phagocytosis.

3 The conversion factor for the calculation of moles of formazan from extinction coefficient must be calculated for a sample of each batch of dye, after chemical reduction, as below.

5.3.2 Determination of conversion factor

Materials and equipment
Ascorbic acid
4 mM nitroblue tetrazolium, NBT, in distilled water containing 340 mM sucrose
0.1 M sodium hydroxide containing 24 mM sodium bicarbonate
Distilled water
Dioxan
Waterbath at 70°
Spectrophotometer

Method

1 Add 150 µmol ascorbic acid to 0.2 ml of NBT solution and mix.

2 Add 2 ml of 0.1 M sodium hydroxide containing 24 mM sodium bicarbonate.

3 Incubate for 10 min at room temperature and add 5 ml distilled water.

4 Centrifuge at 1000 g for 15 min at room temperature.

5 Wash once in water by centrifugation (1000 g for 15 min at room temperature). Remove the supernatant and re-suspend the blue insoluble formazan precipitate in 10 ml dioxan.

6 Dilute 1 ml of the suspension with 9 ml dioxan and incubate at 70° for 20 min.

7 Cool to room temperature, and measure the extinction at 520 nm using a spectrophotometer (use a dioxan blank).

8 Calculate the conversion factor from the extinction value. As a rough guide, the conversion factor should be approximately 1 extinction unit = 40 nmol of formazan.

5.3.3 Calculation of NBT uptake by phagocytes

1 Using the conversion factor determined above, determine the number of moles of formazan extracted from the untreated and endotoxin-stimulated blood.
2 Calculate the number of potential phagocytes used per assay (the percentage of the absolute count due to neutrophils and monocytes).
3 Express results as moles of formazan per phagocyte.
   Normal range: untreated blood, 0.92–3.62 fmol per phagocyte,
   Normal range: endotoxin-stimulated blood, 2.52–4.90 fmol per phagocyte.

5.3.4 Reticuloendothelial blockade

The foreign material taken into phagocytic cells is not invariably degraded and lost. It is known that the antibody response to many antigens is dependent upon 'non-professional' phagocytes such as dendritic cells and monocytes. This may involve some form of 'antigen presentation' to the B cells via these cells. This has been discussed in more detail in Section 4.6.

The rate of uptake of foreign material into phagocytes varies under different conditions. It has been shown that an acute malarial infection will cause a reticulo-endothelial (RE) blockade, presumably because of release and subsequent phago-cytosis of malarial organisms, toxins and red-cell fragments. This blockade may be mimicked by loading the reticuloendothelial system (RES) with colloidal carbon and then observing the clearance of a second material; for example, heat-aggregated protein.

Materials and equipment (see also Section 2.5.1 or 2.5.3, for iodination techniques)
Albino mice
Bovine serum albumin, BSA
Colloidal carbon (Appendix II)
γ spectrometer

Method
1 Heat the BSA solution at 60° for 40 min to form soluble complexes. Centrifuge off any precipitate. Iodinate the soluble aggregated protein as in Section 2.5.1 or 2.5.3.

Protocol

	Mouse number															
	1	2	3	4	5	6	7	8	9	10	11	12	13	14	15	16
Colloidal carbon (ml)	0 ⟶			0.1 ⟶					0.2 ⟶				0.4 ⟶			
^{125}I-BSA (mg)	5 ⟶															
Sample times (min post-BSA injection)	0	20	40	60	0	20	40	60	0	20	40	60	0	20	40	60

2 Inject groups of four mice with 0.1, 0.2 and 0.5 ml of colloidal carbon, respectively (see Protocol, p. 190).
3 Three hours later inject 5 mg of heat-aggregated ^{125}I-BSA intravenously.
4 Collect 20 μl blood samples (Section 5.2) at the times shown in the Protocol. (The sample does not need to be lysed.)
5 Determine the radioactivity in each sample by γ counting.
6 Calculate the percentage of radioactivity remaining in the blood for each time point and plot a graph of the data as for Section 5.2.1.

Analysis of data

In the above experiment you have compared the activity of phagocytic cells in normal animals with cells in animals undergoing 'RE blockade'. We wish to ask the question: has the blockade been effective, i.e. has the phagocytic ability of the cells been altered after carbon treatment? In this case the answer should be clear by simply inspecting the slopes of the two graph lines. In many experiments, however, the difference between control and experimental animals is not so clear. In such cases it is necessary to use statistical tests to evaluate the significance of the difference between groups.

In this case, where we are comparing the mean values of two treatments, it is useful to determine the standard error of the mean. As a rule of thumb: if the standard errors of two means do not overlap, the difference between the means is likely to be statistically significant.

5.3.5 Microorganism clearance

This determination of RE activity is similar, in principle, to that described in the previous section. However, the number of bacteria remaining in the blood at each time point is determined by dilution plating and colony counting and so is more time consuming than the spectrophotometric method demonstrated above.

Materials and equipment
Rabbit
Suspension of *Escherichia coli* (Appendix II)
McConkey agar (Appendix II)
Culture broth (Appendix II)

Method
1 Inject the rabbit intravenously with 10^6 *E. coli* organisms.
2 Take 0.5 ml blood samples at the following times post-injection: 0, 5, 10, 20, 30, 60, 90 min.
3 Dilute the blood 1:10 and 1:100 with broth and plate 1.0 ml aliquots onto McConkey agar.
4 Kill the rabbit at the end of the experiment and grind up the lungs, liver and spleen individually in broth. Dilute a sample of each 1:1000 and plate 1.0 ml aliquots onto agar as before.

5 Count the number of bacterial colonies (circular colonies with a smooth convex surface — red—pink on McConkey agar).
6 Plot a graph of number of colonies against time and calculate the rate of clearance of microorganisms from the blood.

Interaction between innate and adaptive immunity

Innate immunity may be usefully viewed as that non-specific component(s) of the immune response whose intrinsic characteristics are not affected by prior contact with the antigen of interest or an invading microorganism. As with many biological systems, the discrimination *in vivo* is by no means so neat and tidy. If the simple measurements made in Section 5.3.5 were repeated in an animal previously immunised against *Escherichia coli*, the rate of bacterial clearance would be dramatically enhanced compared with the unimmunised control. This does not represent an intrinsic change in the innate system, but rather a potentiation of its action by the adaptive or specific immune system.

There are numerous points of contact between the non-specific and specific arms of the immune response. For example, in the days of pre-antibiotic medicine, bacterial infection was a serious affair and the fate of the patients was often decided in relation to the so-called crisis. This represented a mobilisation of the specific B-lymphocyte immune response to augment a previously ineffective non-specific response. We now understand these events in molecular terms: phagocytosis of bacteria requires that the organisms first adhere to the surface of the phagocyte. Several species of pathogenic bacteria possess anti-phagocytic 'coats' and so grow unrestrained for the first week or so, until the production of specific antibody in sufficient quantities. Thereafter, the bacteria are incorporated into an immune complex with antibody and complement components and are easily phagocytosed.

Similar interactions occur between T lymphocytes and phagocytes. Some microbes such as *Listeria*, *Pasteurella*, *Trypanosoma cruzi* or *Toxoplasma gondii* are actively taken up by macrophages but then evade their intracellular microbicidal mechanisms and thrive in this unlikely environment. However, if the macrophages are activated via T lymphocyte-derived macrophage-activating cytokines, then they are both resistant to new infections and able to kill established infections.

There is a whole range of chemical mediators produced by cells of the immune system (Chapter 13). Even though many of the factors remain to be fully characterised *in vivo*, it is already possible to appreciate the precision of 'fine tuning' of the immune response that can be achieved by these positive and negative regulators.

Immune elimination

As has been seen in Section 3.8, it is possible to lyse T and B lymphocytes directly using anti-lymphocyte serum (ALS) with complement. It is unlikely, however, that this is the main mechanism by which ALS suppression is achieved *in vivo* because, especially for clinical use, much lower concentrations of ALS (as γ-globulin or IgG fractions) are used than are required to fix enough complement for cell lysis. At the lower antibody concentrations enough complement is bound to bring about immune adherence to macrophages (and erythrocytes in primates) via C3. The ALS-coated cells can then be removed by the reticuloendothelial system (RES).

Materials and equipment
Anti-lymphocyte serum, ALS, and normal rabbit serum, NRS (Section 3.8)
Other materials as in Section 5.3.4.

Method
1   Prepare a lymphocyte suspension and label with $^{51}CrO_4$ as in Section 4.14.1.
2   Treat labelled lymphocytes with ALS or NRS according to the Protocol. Total final volume 0.5 ml.
3   Wash the cells twice by centrifugation and re-suspend in 1.0 ml of medium.
4   Inject 5×10^6 cells intravenously, and retain an aliquot of 5×10^6 cells from tube 1 for γ counting.
5   Kill the mice 4 h post-injection and count the γ emissions from spleen and liver. Count also the 5×10^6 cells from tube 1.
6   Calculate the amount of radioactivity in each organ as a percentage of the original counts injected. Calculate also the spleen : liver ratio.

Protocol

	Tube number					
	1	2	3	4	5	6
ALS or NRS final dilution	0	1 : 50	1 : 100	1 : 200	1 : 400	1 : 800
Lymphocytes- ^{51}Cr (10^8 ml^{-1})	0.5 ml ——————————————————————→					

Interpretation of results
The % radioactivity per organ is an estimate of the proportion of lymphocytes localising in that organ. The ratio of counts localising in the spleen relative to the liver is a good estimate of the viability of the original lymphocyte suspension. If the suspension has a high viability the index is high, and vice versa. The ratio of spleen : liver localisation also changes if cells are coated but not necessarily killed with anti-membrane antibodies (due to *in vivo* immune adherence and possibly opsonisation).

5.5   **Lymphocyte circulation**

Lymphocytes do not circulate in a random manner. It is known, for example, that there is a functional division of lymphocytes into the so-called re-circulating and non-re-circulating pools. Hence a full knowledge of the parameters affecting the passage of cells from one pool to the other during the immune response is essential. In addition, cells show set migration patterns during ontogeny, moving, for example, from the central to the peripheral lymphoid organs.

The traffic pattern of lymphocytes may be followed using radioisotope or fluorescein-labelled cells as detailed below.

5.5.1 Ontogenic migration patterns

Dividing cells in the bursa or thymus may be labelled by an intraorgan infusion of ^{3}H-thymidine or ^{131}I-iododeoxyuridine. In this procedure it is essential to minimise the effect of 'spill over' of the labelled material into the peripheral tissues, and so the animal is 'flooded' by an intravenous injection of non-radioactive DNA analogue.

Isotopically labelled cells in the peripheral lymphoid organs may then be identified by autoradiography of tissue sections as described in Section 3.5.4.

5.5.2 Lymphocyte 'homing'

If lymphocytes are removed from an animal, isotopically labelled *in vitro* and returned to a syngeneic recipient, they show definite migration patterns, localising within different organs at different times.

Materials and equipment
Inbred mice (Section 1.19.1 and Appendix II)
Sodium ^{51}chromate (Appendix II)
γ spectrometer

Method
1 Prepare a lymph-node suspension from two to four donor mice (Section 1.15).
2 Count and adjust the suspension to 10^8 viable lymphocytes ml^{-1}.
3 Incubate 1 ml of cells with 11.1×10^5 Bq Na^{51}CrO$_4$ for 30 min at 37° in tissue culture medium buffered with HEPES (20 mM) and containing 5% fetal bovine serum.
4 Wash the cells five times by centrifugation and re-suspend in 2 ml of medium.
5 Inject 5×10^6 cells intravenously into each of 12 recipients, and retain an aliquot of 5×10^6 cells for γ counting.
6 Kill three recipient mice at 4, 24, 48 and 72 h post-injection.
7 Remove the thymus, spleen, mesenteric lymph nodes and liver from each recipient and count the amount of isotope in each organ. (^{51}Cr is a high-energy γ emitter and therefore whole-organ counting is possible.) Count also the aliquot of 5×10^6 original cells.
8 Calculate the amount of radioactivity in each organ as a percentage of the original counts injected.
9 Plot a graph of % radioactivity against time for each organ.

Time after intravenous injection (h)	Number of recipients	Mean % radioactivity			
		Liver	Spleen	Thymus	Lymph node
4	3	6	35	0	9
24	3	7	18	0	17
48	3	7	15	0	13
72	3	8	13	0	12

Fig. 5.5 **Organ distribution of ^{51}Cr-labelled lymphocytes injected into syngenic recipients.**

Interpretation of results

The % radioactivity per organ is an estimate of the proportion of lymphocytes localising in that organ. The ratio of counts localising in the spleen relative to the liver is a good estimate of the viability of the original lymphocyte suspension. If the suspension has a high viability the index is high, and vice versa. The ratio of spleen : liver localisation also changes if cells are coated but not necessarily killed, with anti-membrane antibodies (due to *in vivo* immune adherence and possibly opsonisation) (Section 5.4.1).

Lymphocyte suspensions with high viability pass from the blood and localise predominantly in the spleen. Eventually cells leave the spleen and enter the lymph nodes, as shown by the change in radioactivity of each organ with time. As expected, no re-injected cells were detected in the thymus; the thymus is virtually excluded from the re-circulation pathway of immunocompetent lymphocytes once they have left the thymic cortex. Although there is a population of mature T lymphocytes in the thymic medulla, this seems to be a long-term resident population, members of which re-circulate only rarely. Compare your data with that shown in Fig. 5.5.

These data were obtained with thoracic-duct lymphocytes which have almost 100% viability. It is necessary to combine dead-cell removal (Section 1.16) with the method outlined in the text to obtain comparable results.

5.5.3 ## Intraorgan distribution of cells

A similar technique can also be used to examine the distribution of labelled cells within each organ. It is necessary, however, to use a different isotope as high-energy γ emissions cannot be efficiently captured by a photographic emulsion.

Materials and equipment

Inbred mice (Section 1.19.1 and Appendix II)

Tritiated uridine (Appendix II)

Materials for autoradiography (see Section 3.5.4)

Method

1 Prepare a lymph-node suspension from two to three donor mice.
2 Count cells and adjust to 5×10^7 cells ml^{-1} in tissue culture medium buffered with HEPES (20 mM) and containing 5% fetal bovine serum.
3 Add ^{3}H-uridine to a final concentration of 92.5×10^4 Bq ml^{-1} and incubate at 37° for 30 min.
4 Wash the cells three times by centrifugation and inject 1×10^7 cells intravenously into each of four recipients.
5 Kill recipients at 0.5, 4, 8 and 24 h post-injection.
6 Remove the spleen and mesenteric lymph nodes from each recipient and fix for histological sectioning.
7 Prepare sections of each organ and dip in photographic emulsion for autoradiography (Section 3.5.4).
8 After development of the autoradiographs, stain the tissue sections in haematoxylin and eosin.

Labelled cells may be identified by the presence of black grains of silver over their nucleus and cytoplasm. Examine the slides at low power and determine the change in distribution of labelled cells within the spleen and lymph node with time.

This technique can be used to determine the differential localisation of any pure cell-line populations.

5.5.4 Fluorescent label for *in vivo* studies

Radioisotopes and autoradiography may be avoided by using one of the new generation of intensely fluorescing dyes that bind to the cytoplasmic proteins (for example, carboxy-fluorescein diacetate) or DNA (for example, the bis benzimide H33342) of viable cells. These dyes do not impair the migration or localisation pattern of cells and are diluted only at cell division (small lymphocytes divide only rarely). They can be visualised under the fluorescent microscope in viable cell suspensions or histological sections, either frozen or after formaldehyde fixation.

Materials and equipment
Inbred mice (Section 1.19.1 and Appendix II)
H33342 dye (Appendix II)

Method

1 Prepare a stock solution of the dye at 600 μg ml^{-1} in distilled water at 4°.
2 Prepare a lymph-node suspension from two to three donor mice as in Section 1.15.
3 Count cells and adjust to 5×10^7 cells ml^{-1} in tissue culture medium buffered with HEPES (20 mM) and containing 5% fetal bovine serum.
4 Dilute the stock solution of the dye 1:100 into the cell suspension, final dye concentration 6 μg ml^{-1}.

5 Incubate for 15 min at 37° in a water bath.
6 Dilute in tissue culture medium and wash twice by centrifugation.

5.6 ## T—B lymphocyte cooperation

In previous chapters we have examined the T- and B-lymphocyte systems reacting independently to antigen. However, in the intact immune response this seldom, if ever, happens. The production of antibody by B cells depends not only on an interaction with antigen-presenting cells but also on an interaction with T cells. Accordingly, although T cells never secrete antibody they are essential for the production of antibody in response to the majority, but perhaps not all, antigens, by the process known as *cooperation*.

Cooperation involving T and B cells cannot be easily demonstrated using thymus and bursa cells from the chicken as they are essentially immunoincompetent cells, and the experiment would require the use of relatively rare inbred chickens. In the mouse the bone marrow behaves as though it were a source of B cells devoid of T cells and it is therefore operationally equivalent to the avian bursa.

Materials and equipment
6-month old inbred mice for X-irradiation (Section 1.19.1 or Appendix II)
3—4-week old inbred mice as thymus and bone marrow donors
Sheep erythrocytes (Appendix II)
X-ray machine or γ source
Materials for haemolytic plaques (Section 4.5)

We will use X-irradiated (immunosuppressed) mice as 'living test tubes' to examine the response of T and B cells, separately and together, to sheep erythrocytes.

Protocol

Group	Number* of mice	Cells for transfer	No. ml i.v.	Sheep-cell challenge
A	3	Bone marrow	0.1	10^8 i.p
B	3	Thymocytes	0.1	10^8 i.p.
C	3	Bone marrow + thymocytes	0.1+0.1	10^8 i.p.

* For experimental purposes it is better to use five or more mice per group.

Method
1 Give nine mice 8 Gy of irradiation (see Technical notes in Section 1.19.1).
2 Remove the femurs from six untreated donor mice.
3 Cut each end off the bones and 'blow out' the marrow with tissue culture medium using a hypodermic syringe with an 18 gauge needle.
4 Disperse the cells gently with a Pasteur pipette.
5 Count the cells and adjust to 2×10^8 ml^{-1}.
6 Remove the thymus from each of four donors and tease the cells into medium.

7 Wash the cells twice by centrifugation (150 g for 10 min at 4°), count and adjust the cells to 10^9 ml^{-1}.

Reconstitute and challenge the X-irradiated recipient mice as shown in the Protocol.

8 After 8 days assay the recipient spleens for direct haemolytic plaques as described in Section 4.5.2.
9 Calculate and tabulate the number of plaque-forming cells per spleen for each group of mice.

Technical notes
1 No control group is included to show that the X-irradiation was successful in suppressing the immune response of the recipient mice.
2 Bone marrow is a relatively poor source of B cells. In the regime described you will obtain a maximum of $4.0-6.0 \times 10^3$ plaques per spleen. More satisfactory results may be obtained using 'B' spleens, prepared either by reconstitution of X-irradiated, thymectomised recipients (Section 11.2.1), nude mice (T-lymphocyte deficient) (Fig. 1.4) or, more conveniently, by anti-Thy-1 treatment of normal spleen (Sections 1.15 and 7.5.1). Using 2×10^7 'B' spleen cells + 10^8 thymus cells you can expect at least 3.0×10^4 plaques per spleen.

In this experiment we have demonstrated the basic requirement for T cells in antibody production. The mechanism and specificity of this requirement were demonstrated in Section 4.7.

5.7 Tolerance

In chemical terms all antigens are equal; in immunological terms some are more equal than others. As we do not now question that an animal will react to foreign antigens, we must therefore ask why does it not react with itself? Burnet suggested that lymphocytes must go through a 'learning phase' in ontogeny when they learn to distinguish between 'self' and 'non-self'. He postulated that potential antigens present during this 'learning phase' in some way suppress the development or expression of specific antigen-reactive clones. Thus, the animal will be rendered tolerant to any antigen, 'self' or otherwise, present during the perinatal period. Tolerance is known to exist in both T- and B-lymphocyte populations but may be demonstrated more simply in assays involving the latter.

Materials and equipment
Neonatal mice
Bovine serum albumin, BSA (Appendix II)
Freund's complete adjuvant (Appendix II)
Sheep erythrocytes (Appendix II)

Material for Farr assay (Section 6.2.1)
Materials for haemagglutination (Section 6.14.4)

Method

1   Prepare a 10 mg ml^{-1} solution of BSA and centrifuge at $100\,000\,g$ for 3 h. Antigens are more immunogenic if they are insolubilised (Section 1.8); conversely, they are more tolerogenic if used in a soluble form completely free of aggregates.

2   Inject ten 1−2-day old mice with 1 mg of ultracentrifuged BSA intraperitoneally. Keep an equal number of uninjected littermates as controls.

3   Inject the mice with the same antigen dose each week for a total of 6 weeks.

4   On the 8th week, inject all mice intraperitoneally with 1 mg of BSA in Freund's complete adjuvant and 10^8 sheep erythrocytes.

5   Bleed all the mice on week 9, separate and store the sera at $-20°$ for testing.

TESTS ON SERA

1   Perform a Farr assay for antigen-binding capacity to BSA as in Section 6.2.1.

2   Perform a haemagglutination test for anti-sheep erythrocyte antibodies (Section 6.14.4).

Data and observations

Calculate and compare the average antigen-binding capacity of the sera from tolerised and normal mice. Record and compare the end-point haemagglutinin titre for each group. The tolerance should be antigen specific.

5.7.1   Tolerance versus selective unresponsiveness

It is essential to establish a clear difference between tolerance and selective unresponsiveness. It is useful to reserve the term tolerance for the complete mechanism by which self-unresponsiveness is established and maintained. All experimental attempts to reproduce this mechanism have merely concerned a selective unresponsiveness.

Two mechanisms have been proposed to explain the experimental finding:

(a) *Immunoparalysis.* This may be envisaged as a deletion or switching-off of selected T and B antigen-reactive clones. This mechanism would be passive or recessive and could be over-ridden by the addition of normal antigen-reactive cells.

(b) *Positive suppression.* In this case the unresponsiveness would be dominant and could suppress the response of normal antigen-reactive lymphocytes. Evidence indicates that suppression may be mediated via a subpopulation of T cells.

Mitchison has shown that selective unresponsiveness may exist at two levels dependent upon the dose of antigen used to induce the unresponsiveness. He termed these two states *low-* and *high-*zone tolerance (our italics). Low-zone tolerance is induced by antigens which fail to immunise with an injection of 1 µg (weak immunogens). High-zone tolerance may be established and maintained with repeated injections of antigens in excess of 1 mg. Weigle *et al.* (1973) have shown that at low antigen

ls alone are rendered unresponsive, whereas both T and B cells are
unresponsive at high antigen levels. It has been argued that the depressed
antibody response to an immunogenic challenge seen after an injection of a non-
immunogenic concentration of the same antigen (low-zone tolerance) may in fact be
due to switch away from humoral to cell-mediated immunity. If this were the case,
then the initial challenge would have generated 'cytotoxic/suppressor' rather than
'cooperator' T cells. In other words, in this experimental situation, unresponsiveness
may simply reflect a change in the immune response away from the parameter being
measured.

The two mechanisms for the induction of experimental unresponsiveness mentioned above may or may not operate together; however, it is apparent that whatever
mechanism(s) operates to establish and maintain self-tolerance, it must act on all the
sectors of the immune response.

5.8 Lymphocytes and disease

Although the immune system has evolved to provide us with an effective defence
against infection, and possibly against the development of tumours, there are
well-recognised instances where this immune protection can go wrong. Often with
disastrous consequences.

5.8.1 Experimental autoimmunity

When the normal 'self'-tolerance situation is either not established or breaks down,
autoantibodies are produced. It is, however, often difficult to establish a causal role
for autoantibodies in the so-called autoimmune diseases. Indeed, many investigators
have suggested that autoantibodies may be 'normal', aiding the disposal of altered
self-components released from dead or dying cells.

Several clinical situations in which autoantibodies may be detected are described
in Section 14.5.3. Experimentally, the New Zealand black (NZB) mouse presents an
excellent model for autoimmune disorders. Among several other autoantibodies (Fig.
1.4) this strain produces anti-erythrocyte antibodies; these may be detected by a
haemagglutination assay.

Materials and equipment
New Zealand black, NZB, mice (Appendix II)
Rabbit anti-mouse immunoglobulin serum (Section 1.7.2 or Appendix II)
Micro-titre trays and equipment for haemagglutination (Section 6.14)

Method
1 Bleed the mice by severing the axillary vessels (see Fig. 1.2). Collect the blood in
heparin.

2   Wash the blood cells three times with phosphate-buffered saline by centrifugation (300 g for 10 min) and prepare a 2% suspension.

3   Determine the highest dilution of antiserum giving complete haemagglutination with erythrocytes of individuals of different ages (Section 6.14.4).

Technical notes

1   The sensitivity of the haemagglutination technique as described can be increased: set the test up as above and after 1 h incubation at room temperature, centrifuge the plates at 150 g for 1 min. Then stand the trays at an angle of 45° for 20 min; the unagglutinated cells will roll away from the apex of the V. This modification is said to increase assay sensitivity by two or more dilutions.

2   Specificity controls as in Section 6.26.

5.8.2   Hypersensitivity states

After primary contact with antigen an individual is immunised or primed, and exists in a state of so-called *hypersensitivity*. The types of hypersensitivity states recognised by Coombs and Gell may be listed as follows:

Type 1   Anaphylactic hypersensitivity.
Type 2   Cytotoxic hypersensitivity.
Type 3   Immune complex-mediated hypersensitivity.
Type 4   Delayed (cell-mediated) hypersensitivity.

Types 1–3 initially involve the interaction of antibody with antigen. Type 4 is cell mediated and involves the reactions of the T-cell system encountered throughout this book. It is important to remember that the example given, macrophage-migration inhibition (Section 5.8.6), is only one manifestation of a T lymphocyte-initiated response.

5.8.3   Anaphylactic hypersensitivity

Animals given repeated intravenous injections of soluble antigen become immune but they also tend to die due to a reaction known as *acute anaphylaxis*.

Anaphylaxis in vivo

Guinea-pigs are extremely sensitive to anaphylaxis. If primed by an intravenous injection of 1 mg of ovalbumin they will die due to anaphylactic shock upon a second injection 2–3 weeks later. At post-mortem examination the animal will characteristically show intense constriction of the bronchi, thus accounting for death by asphyxia.

Anaphylaxis in vitro

The sensitivity of guinea-pigs to anaphylaxis may be demonstrated less dramatically but more humanely *in vitro*.

Materials and equipment
Guinea-pigs
Ovalbumin (Appendix II)
Freund's complete adjuvant (Appendix II)
Hank's saline (Appendix I)
Apparatus as in Fig. 5.6.

PREPARATION IN ADVANCE
Sensitise the guinea-pigs by an intramuscular injection of 500 μg of ovalbumin in Freund's complete adjuvant 3—4 weeks before the experiment.

Method
1 Kill the guinea-pig and remove the ileum into Hank's saline at 37°.
2 Remove a strip of muscle and mount it in the organ bath at 37° (Fig. 5.6).
3 Allow the muscle to relax for 20—30 min.
4 Add the antigen in solution and observe the contraction of the muscle.

Suggested experiments (use fresh muscle preparation for each experiment)
1 Add increasing concentrations of antigen to the bath starting at 1 μg ml^{-1} (final concentration) in steps of 5 μg. Determine the minimum concentration required to elicit contraction. After contraction, add further antigen in the mg range to stimulate a second contraction. Observe the magnitude of the first and second contractions in relation to the concentration of antigen added.
2 Use bovine serum albumin to test the specificity of the response.
3 Soak muscle from normal animals in sensitised guinea-pig serum for varying times at 37°. Test for passive sensitisation.

In humans, anaphylaxis is known to be mediated by membrane-bound IgE antibodies. Unlike membrane-bound immunoglobulin-receptor molecules (Section 3.5.1) which are inserted into the membrane after endogenous synthesis, this antibody is attached via its Fc portion to the Fc-binding site on the plasma membrane of mast cells. When antigen combines with the IgE antibody, the mast cell is caused to degranulate releasing the pharmacological mediators of anaphylaxis, the best known of which is histamine.

5.8.4   ## Cytotoxic hypersensitivity

Antibodies to cell-surface components may bring about cell death by promoting phagocytosis via opsonic adherence (binding to receptors for immunoglobulin Fc

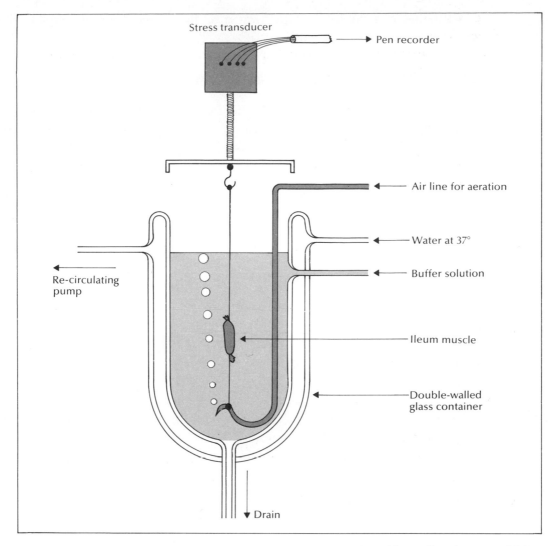

Stress transducer

Pen recorder

Air line for aeration

Water at 37°

Buffer solution

Re-circulating pump

Ileum muscle

Double-walled glass container

Drain

Fig. 5.6 Organ bath and recording apparatus for the demonstration of immediate hypersensitivity *in vitro*.

regions or activated components of complement, see Section 3.8.2) or by the activation of the complement system for direct cell lysis (Section 7.5). The result of cytotoxic hypersensitivity is seen in transfusion reactions or in haemolytic disease of the newborn due to rhesus incompatibility (Section 6.14.7).

5.8.5 Immune complex-mediated hypersensitivity

Circulating immune complexes have been detected in a wide variety of clinical conditions, from chronic parasitic infections, for example malaria, to autoimmune diseases; for example, systemic lupus erythematosus and rheumatoid arthritis. (In rheumatoid arthritis, recent experimental evidence suggests that the immune complexes found in synovial fluid are formed by the reaction of antiglobulin antibodies with self-immunoglobulin molecules.)

The formation and deposition of immune complexes usually initiate complement fixation with the consequent release of anaphylatoxins and chemotactic factors. Anaphylatoxins mediate histamine release and consequently induce increased vascular permeability and oedema. Chemotactic factors attract neutrophils, which release their proteolytic enzymes and cause local tissue destruction at the sites of immune-complex deposition in the skin, vascular endothelium, joints and kidney glomeruli. Chemotactic factors are more strictly acting via a chemokinetic effect, i.e. causing all-round increase in the phrenetic activity of affected cells.

Immune complex-mediated tissue damage is usually a self-limiting condition which resolves once the source of antigen for complex formation has been removed.

See Section 7.4 or 14.6 for assay of immune complexes.

Experimentally this condition is characterised by oedema and necrosis at the site of antigen injection in a hyperimmune animal.

5.8.6 Delayed hypersensitivity

If the Gell and Coombs' classification of immune hypersensitivity states was compiled today, when we understand much more about the intricacies of delayed-type hypersensitivity (DTH) or cell-mediated immunity, it is likely that this category would have been subdivided, thus giving relatively less weight to antibody-mediated hypersensitivities. The true diversity of cell-mediated immunity may be appreciated with reference to the T-lymphocyte assays described in Section 4.8. The example given here, macrophage-migration inhibition, has been chosen because it illustrates the interaction between T lymphocytes and macrophages *in vivo* reacting to BCG (*Mycobacterium tuberculosis*), an antigen which, in the human, elicits the classic example of a DTH response — the Mantoux reaction.

Macrophage migration inhibition

Materials and equipment
Guinea-pigs, normal and immunised with BCG (*M. tuberculosis*)
Purified protein derivative, PPD, of *M. tuberculosis* (Appendix II)
Tissue culture medium with 10% fetal bovine serum (Appendix I)
Siliconised 0.75 mm capillary tubes
Mackaness-type culture chambers
Paraffin wax or 'seal ease' (latter, Appendix II)
Silicone grease

Method

1 Obtain a suspension of peritoneal exudate cells from normal and immune guinea-pigs (Section 1.18).
2 Count cells and adjust to 5×10^7 nucleated cells ml^{-1}.
3 Fill capillaries with cell suspension and seal one end with softened paraffin wax or 'seal ease' dental plasticine.
4 Pack capillaries into flat-bottomed plastic tubes and centrifuge at 150 g for 5 min at 4°.
5 Meanwhile, prepare chambers by placing a small amount of silicone grease against the inside edge of the chamber and smear rim with silicone grease.
6 Half fill chambers with medium containing the appropriate antigen dilution (see Protocol).

Protocol

	Chamber number (five replicates)				
	1	2	3	4	5
PPD concentration ($\mu g\ ml^{-1}$)	0	50	100	250	500
Immune cells or normal cells	$\longrightarrow$				

7 Cut capillary just to the cell side of the cell−medium interface.
8 Place sealed end of capillary into silicone grease in migration chamber. *Check that the whole tube is on the bottom of the chamber.*
9 Fill the chamber with medium and antigen, and seal with a coverslip. Exclude all air bubbles.
10 Incubate the chamber at 37° overnight.
11 Place the migration chambers in a photographic enlarger and trace area of migration onto a sheet of paper.
12 Cut out the pencilled area and weigh.

The degree of migration inhibition is calculated as follows:

$$\% \text{ migration} = \frac{\text{weight of migration area immune cells}}{\text{weight of migration area normal cells}} \times 100.$$

A value of less than 80% is considered as a significant inhibition.

Technical notes

1 There is a wide scatter of data within replicates with this technique. At least five replicates must be used for each antigen dilution.
2 Because of the danger of bias in tracing the area of migration, it is essential that the whole experiment should be coded and read blind.
3 Many antigens are stimulatory or inhibitory depending on dose. It is therefore essential to perform a full dose−response curve at each test. Because of this it is advisable to use immune cells without antigen as a control.

5.9

Summary and conclusions

Although the innate or non-specific immune system is generally thought to be non-adaptive, recent evidence has shown that macrophages from a hyperimmune animal have an increased rate of phagocytosis *in vitro*. It is therefore possible that a primitive capacity for adaptation may exist at this level, although it is difficult to exclude some long-term effect of soluble mediators derived from the lymphoid system.

Macrophages are known to be required during antigen stimulation of T and B lymphocytes. For example, the removal of glass-adherent cells from lymphocyte populations reduces the *in vitro* immune response to soluble antigens or allogeneic cells. It is important to note, however, that although the majority of glass-adherent cells are monocytes and neutrophils, the glass-adherent population certainly contains other cells; for example, B lymphocytes.

Most soluble antigens are rapidly degraded after phagocytosis, but not, for example, pneumococcal polysaccharide or D amino acids. Approximately 1–3% of the ingested material is said to remain undegraded and eventually appears on the surface of the macrophage where it may have enhanced immunogenicity.

It has been suggested that macrophages may have a role to play in at least one form of tolerance induction. As demonstrated earlier (Section 5.7), soluble, de-aggregated antigens tend to be tolerogenic, but are immunogenic if aggregated, rendered insoluble or given in combination with Freund's complete adjuvant. Soluble antigens are not readily phagocytosed and so may confront the B cells directly to induce tolerance (this is especially true of T-dependent antigens). Insoluble antigens in Freund's complete adjuvant are rapidly phagocytosed and therefore only a relatively small amount eventually reaches the B cell — via the macrophage surface.

The role proposed for macrophages in antigen presentation to B cells is essentially non-specific; in contrast, the role played by T cells is highly specific.

5.10

Further reading

Dale MM and Foreman JC (1988) *Textbook of Immunopharmacology*, 2nd edition. Blackwell Scientific Publications, Oxford.

Klempner MS, Styrt B and Ho J (editors) (1987) *Phagocytes and Disease*. MTP Press, Lancaster.

Lachman P and Peters DK (editors) (1982) *Clinical Aspects of Immunology*, 4th edition. Blackwell Scientific Publications, Oxford.

Weigle WO (1973) Immunological unresponsiveness. *Adv. Immunol.* **16**: 61.

6 Antibody Interaction with Antigen

Plasma cells produce antibody which binds specifically to its corresponding antigen and may activate secondary mechanisms such as the complement system. In this and in the following chapter we are going to study some of the different ways in which this interaction can be demonstrated.

The combination of antigen with antibody to form a complex is a dynamic equilibrium as the bonds formed are non-covalent and reversible. The proportions of each reactant in a complex may also vary as antibodies are at least divalent, and antigens multi-valent (i.e. they may have many different immunogenic epitopes per molecule). Therefore, the amount of reaction observed depends upon the proportions of reactants used.

There are usually two stages in most antigen−antibody reactions. The *primary interaction* is the specific recognition and combination of an antigenic determinant with the binding site of its corresponding antibody. This step is usually very rapid especially when dealing with the interaction of antibody with the small molecules ($\approx 300-500$ Da) known as haptens. There usually follows a *secondary interaction* which activates some effector function. This can be, for example, complement fixation, macrophage binding or simply agglutination or precipitation. It is the manifestation of these secondary events which is usually observed in the laboratory. It must be remembered, however, that this secondary effect is only a reflection of the primary antigen−antibody interaction and does not directly correspond to it, especially with antigens having few antigenic determinants. With monovalent haptens, for example, although the primary interaction occurs there is no precipitation or complement fixation.

6.1 Antibody specificity

The specificity of the immune response is manifested at many levels; for example, in combating a virus infection the immune system is able to distinguish one virus from another. Viewed in molecular terms the specificity of the immune system is even more impressive and can recognise very subtle changes in conformation; for example, antibodies raised against meta-substituted aminobenzene sulphonate show virtually no reactivity against the same hapten when substituted in the para position.

The cellular basis of this specificity is invested in those lymphocyte clones selected and expanded after interaction with the specific antigens. These lymphocytes are specific by virtue of their surface receptors which are highly polymorphic molecules with a range of shapes of antigen-binding sites, potentially sufficient to cope with the whole of the antigenic universe.

Immunoglobulin molecules react with their specific antigens via precisely the same short-range forces governing any protein−protein interaction. However, the specific antigen—antibody interaction is quantitatively greater because of the complementary three-dimensional shapes of the antibody-combining site and its antigenic determinant. Thus, the interacting molecules are able to come closer and react over a greater area. The total strength of the interaction is dependent upon a combination of attractive (hydrogen bonds, hydrophobic bonds, coulombic interactions and van de Waals' forces) and repulsive forces (interpenetration of antigen- and antibody-electron clouds, chance apposition of opposite charges, etc.). Almost half of the binding force which holds antibody on its specific antigen comes from the entropy-driven process of hydrophobic bonding, wherein water molecules are excluded from between interacting hydrophobic surfaces.

Spatial considerations ('goodness of fit') are very important in the determination of antibody—antigen or receptor—antigen specificity as the forces of attraction and repulsion are inversely proportional to the distance between the interacting groups; for example, ionic forces are inversely proportional to the square of the distances of separation whereas van de Waals' are proportional to the sixth power of this distance. Steric repulsive forces are even more dependent upon 'goodness of fit' as they decline with the 12th power of the distance between the corresponding interacting groups.

6.2 Primary binding reactions

As we discussed earlier, tests based on secondary mechanisms, such as precipitation, do not necessarily measure the degree of primary binding of antigen to antibody. Figure 6.1. shows the general form of the precipitin curve obtained when a horse antiserum is reacted with the immunising antigen. Although antigen—antibody interactions occur for all proportions of antigen and antibody, in the region of antibody excess there is very little precipitate; the complexes form but remain soluble. Techniques such as the Farr assay (see below) were designed to overcome these problems and so are more direct measures of the primary binding reaction.

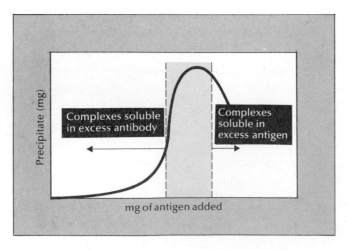

Fig. 6.1 Quantitative precipitin curve of horse antibody with antigen. The point of maximum precipitation is sharply defined because of the solubility of horse antibody—antigen complexes in both antibody and antigen excess. Accordingly the curve has quite a different profile to that found with rabbit antibodies (Fig. 6.6) where the complexes are soluble in antigen excess alone.

6.2.1 Ammonium sulphate precipitation (Farr assay)

In Chapter 1 immunoglobulins were prepared from whole serum by precipitation with ammonium sulphate. If ammonium sulphate is added to diluted serum to 50% saturation, most of the immunoglobulin is precipitated, while other serum proteins such as albumin, remain in solution. This is the basis of the Farr assay, which in its original form was only suitable for antigens soluble in 50% saturated ammonium sulphate solution.

Antigen, for example albumin, is radiolabelled and allowed to react with antibody, generally in antigen excess, so that soluble complexes are formed. An equal volume of saturated ammonium sulphate is added and all the immunoglobulin is precipitated. Only that antigen complexed with antibody is precipitated under these conditions. The precipitates are washed with 50% saturated ammonium sulphate solution to remove any free antigen and their radioactive content determined. The amount of radioactivity in the precipitate is proportional to the amount of antigen bound by the antibody and so results are expressed in terms of the antigen-binding capacity ml^{-1} of serum. For accurate determinations in research procedures, the results need to be calculated to the same degree of antigen excess for each antiserum. Therefore, in the original form of the assay, constant amounts of antigen are added to a series of dilutions of serum and the antigen-binding capacity determined at each dilution.

Figure 6.2. shows a typical binding curve. It has become the convention to calculate all results on the 33% end point, i.e. the dilution of serum which binds 33% of the added antigen. For many purposes a simpler assay can be used at a single antiserum dilution. This modified assay has been used as a research technique in many laboratories and is known to yield reliable results.

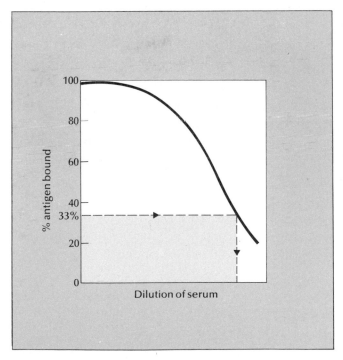

Fig. 6.2 Antigen-binding capacity of an antiserum determined by the ammonium sulphate (Farr) assay. In the original Farr assay all results were calculated on the 33% end point and so a full binding curve was required for each serum assayed. In the modified assay a large excess of antigen is used with a single antiserum dilution, thus approaching the total binding capacity of the sample.

Modified ammonium sulphate precipitation assay

Radiolabelling of antigen

Antigens may be labelled by several techniques (Section 2.5 *et seq.*); the following procedure is satisfactory for many antigens.

Materials and equipment
Sodium ^{125}I, carrier free (Appendix II)
Phosphate-buffered saline, PBS (Appendix I)
Protein antigen; for example, albumin (4 mg in PBS)
Chloramine T (1 mg ml^{-1} in PBS)
Sodium metabisulphite (2 mg ml^{-1} in PBS)
Sephadex G-25 column, disposable (Section 1.5)
Dextran blue dye (Appendix II)
Scintillation monitor for ^{125}I

Method
1 Pour a G-25 Sephadex column and calibrate as detailed in Section 1.5.
2 Dispense 0.5 ml aliquots of albumin solution (2 mg total protein) into a small test tube.
3 Add 18.5×10^5 Bq Na^{125}I.
4 Add 30 μg chloramine T.
5 Mix and leave for 2 min at room temperature.
6 Add 60 μg sodium metabisulphite.
7 Place the sample on the Sephadex column and collect the radiolabelled protein after the void volume has left the column. Collect fractions of 0.5 ml and monitor each one for the first appearance of radioactivity. This gives an accurate determination of the position of the protein front.
8 Allow 2 or 3 drops to go to waste after radioactivity has been detected, then collect a sample volume equivalent to the original sample volume added to the column. This will avoid unnecessary dilution of the sample, but will limit the theoretical recovery to about 60% of the radioactivity added to the column.
9 Measure the absorbance of the labelled protein at 280 nm in a UV spectrophotometer and calculate the protein concentration. For human serum albumin: at 280 nm, an absorbance of 1.0 (1 cm cell) = 1.88 mg ml^{-1}.
10 Dilute 2 μl of the radiolabelled protein solution in 2 ml of PBS and add 50 μl to a tube for γ spectrometry. Determine the c.p.m. of this sample.
11 Having determined both the protein and ^{125}I content of the sample, calculate its specific activity in c.p.m. mg^{-1} of protein (Section 2.5.2)

Technical notes
1 If radioactivity is detected impossibly early in the column effluent this means that the column was not correctly packed and the labelled protein is running down between the gel and the column wall. This may be prevented by ensuring that the

internal wall of the column is free from grease and that the gel is packed under pressure (Section 1.5).

2 Although free ^{125}I may be removed from the protein sample by exhaustive dialysis against PBS using dialysis tubing, this is more likely to lead to contamination of the environment because of the technical problems of pipetting into and out of the dialysis tubing.

3 Dialysis should remove virtually all the free iodine. However, if the efficiency of removal is suspect, a more accurate determination of protein-bound radioactivity may be obtained after precipitation of the sample with cold trichloroacetic acid (Section 2.5.2).

Assay

Materials and equipment
Radiolabelled ^{125}I-albumin (2 mg ml^{-1}), specific activity 7.4–29.6×10^5 Bq mg^{-1} protein
Test anti-albumin sera, diluted 1:10 with PBS
Control serum diluted 1:10, to determine background binding
Saturated ammonium sulphate solution (Section 1.3.1)
γ spectrometer

Protocol

	Tube number (in duplicate)	
Solution to be added	1	2 . . . . n
Serum diluted 1:10 with PBS	0	20 µl ⟶
^{125}I-albumin, 2 mg ml^{-1}	100 µl ⟶	
	Incubate and then add:	
PBS	0	400 µl ⟶
Saturated ammonium sulphate	0	520 µ ⟶

Repeat for each test antiserum and normal serum control.

Method

1 Add 20 µl of each diluted serum to tubes preferably in duplicate (see Protocol).
2 Add 100 µl of ^{125}I-albumin to each tube. Cap the duplicate tubes labelled number 1, these are for determining the c.p.m. in the original aliquot.
3 Incubate with occasional shaking at 37° for 2 h, then 2 h in the cold.
4 Add 400 µl PBS to each test tube.
5 Add an equal volume (520 µl) of saturated ammonium sulphate solution to each tube, mix rapidly and thoroughly. Allow to stand for 15 min.
6 Spin at 3000 g for 10 min.
7 Remove and discard the supernatant.
8 Wash precipitate twice with 50% saturated ammonium sulphate solution by centrifugation.

9 After removing final wash supernatant, count the precipitate and the tubes labelled 1 (containing ^{125}I-albumin alone) in a γ spectrometer.

Calculation of results

$$\text{Specific activity of albumin, c.p.m } \mu g^{-1} = \frac{\text{no. c.p.m. in 100 } \mu l \times 10}{\text{protein concentration (} \mu g \text{ ml}^{-1}\text{)}}.$$

Antigen content of precipitate =
$$\frac{\text{no. c.p.m. of antiserum precipitate } - \text{ no. c.p.m. of normal serum precipitate}}{\text{specific activity of the albumin}}.$$

Antigen-binding capacity per ml of serum = antigen content of precipitate $\times$ 50 $\times$ original serum dilution.

The antigen-binding capacity is expressed as μg albumin bound ml^{-1} of original serum.

Technical notes

1 Specific activity is quoted in Bq, rather than c.p.m mg^{-1} as this enables standardisation. Determination of c.p.m. depends upon the efficiency of the counting equipment and so would vary from laboratory to laboratory.

2 For demonstration purposes, the incubation times in step 3 above may be reduced to 15 min at 37° and 30 min on ice, and still yield useful data.

3 With some antigens it is necessary to use precipitating agents other than ammonium sulphate to ensure that the antigen remains in solution unless bound to antibody. A mixture of ethanol and ammonium acetate has been found useful for several assays of antibody binding to hormones, and polyethylene glycol for peptide and immunoglobulin antigens.

4 The technique can be modified to yield qualitative as well as quantitative information. With ammonium sulphate each immunoglobulin isotype is precipitated; however, it is possible to induce selective precipitation by adding an excess of anti-isotype serum. For example, anti-IgG precipitation of IgG antibodies would allow the determination of the antigen-binding capacity of this isotype in a polyclonal serum. This can be repeated with specific antisera for each class and subclass. The response in the different classes is found to differ markedly with different of immunisation schedules.

6.3 Determination of antibody affinity

So far we have considered antibody–antigen interaction in terms of the quantity of antibody produced or able to bind to a specified amount of antigen. For each antigenic determinant a range of different antibodies are formed, some of which will 'fit' the antigen better than others. Those with a better 'fit' will bind the antigen more strongly than the poorer fitting molecules. This leads to the concept of *antibody affinity*.

Affinity is a measure of the strength of antibody−antigen combination. More correctly, affinity refers to the interaction between monovalent antigenic determinants, i.e. haptens, and single antibody-combining sites. When dealing with multi-valent antigens and antibodies the interaction is more complex and the term *avidity* is usually used. Although the thermodynamic description of avidity is complex, it may be thought of in simple terms as the increased strength of binding gained because of the interdependence of binding sites. The fact that one arm of an IgG antibody molecule has bound to a multi-valent antigen greatly increases the chance that the second arm will also bind. Having bound, both arms would then be required to release simultaneously if the immune complex is to be broken. For example, the avidity of IgG is related to its affinity by the product of the two interacting binding forces. Consequently, it is easy to see why for the same affinity IgM has a much greater avidity than IgG.

6.3.1 Mathematical basis of affinity

The combination of antigen and antibody to form a complex is a reversible reaction:

$$Ab + Ag \underset{K_d}{\overset{K_a}{\rightleftharpoons}} Ab \cdot Ag$$

where K_a and K_d are the association and dissociation constants, respectively.

The law of mass action can be applied to this reaction with the affinity being given by the equilibrium constant K. As mentioned at the beginning of the section, although the law of mass action is used in general here, strictly it applies only to homogeneous systems such as monoclonal antibodies, from hybridomas or plasma-cytomas, reacting with monovalent haptens. In the real world, antibodies in serum are polyclonal and therefore heterogeneous.

By the law of mass action:

$$K = \frac{K_a}{K_d} = \frac{[Ab\cdot Ag]}{[Ag][Ab]}$$

where:

K, K_a and K_d are as defined above,
$[Ab\cdot Ag]$ = moles of immune complex (products),
$[Ab]$ = moles of antibody (reactant),
$[Ag]$ = moles of antigen (reactant).

Remember that Ag refers to monovalent antigenic determinants and Ab to independent antibody-combining sites. As can be seen the amount of complex formed is proportional to the value of K. As each reactant is expressed in mol litre^{-1} the overall units of K are litre mol^{-1}.

If K is determined with respect to total antibody-binding sites, Ab_t, the following form of the *Langmuir adsorption isotherm* may be derived from the mass action equation:

$Ab + Ag \rightleftharpoons Ab \cdot Ag$.

By the law of mass action

$$\frac{[Ab \cdot Ag]}{[Ab][Ag]} = K \text{ (equilibrium constant)},$$

therefore

$$[Ab \cdot Ag] = K[Ab][Ag]. \tag{1}$$

Make

$$[Ab_t] = [Ab \cdot Ag] + [Ab],$$

therefore

$$[Ab] = [Ab_t] - [Ab \cdot Ag]. \tag{2}$$

Substituting (2) in (1):

$$[Ab \cdot Ag] = K[Ag]([Ab_t] - [Ab \cdot Ag]),$$

therefore

$$[Ab \cdot Ag] = K[Ag][Ab_t] - K[Ag][Ab \cdot Ag]$$
$$[Ab \cdot Ag] + K[Ag][Ab \cdot Ag] = K[Ag][Ab_t]$$
$$[Ab \cdot Ag](1 + K[Ag]) = K[Ag][Ab_t]$$
$$\frac{[Ab \cdot Ag]}{[Ab_t]} = \frac{K[Ag]}{1+K[Ag]}. \tag{3}$$

Make $[Ab.Ag] = b$, then (3) may be re-written as

$$\frac{b}{[Ab_t]} = \frac{K[Ag]}{1+K[Ag]}$$

$$\frac{b(1+K[Ag])}{[Ab_t]K[Ag]} = 1$$

$$\frac{1}{b} = \frac{1 + K[Ag]}{K[Ab_t][Ag]}$$

$$= \frac{1}{K[Ab_t][Ag]} + \frac{K[Ag]}{K[Ab_t][Ag]}$$

$$= \frac{1}{K[Ab_t][Ag]} + \frac{1}{[Ab_t]}. \tag{4}$$

when $\frac{1}{[Ag]} = 0$ in (4)

$$\frac{1}{b} = \frac{1}{[Ab_t]}.$$

As

$b = [Ab \cdot Ag]$
   $= $ bound Ag concentration

and

$[Ag] = $ free antigen concentration

then a plot of $1/b$ against $1/[Ag]$ can be extrapolated to obtain $[Ab_t]$. This is the total of antibody-combining sites.

Note

The concentrations expressed in the above equations are molar equivalents; hence, for example, when $[Ab \cdot Ag] = $ bound Ag concentration, this is a molar equivalence and not a weight equivalence.

The determination of the total antibody-combining sites, although theoretically straightforward, is often difficult to determine experimentally. With a monoclonal antibody of high affinity there will be no problem obtaining a straight line for the Langmuir plot experimentally; thus, the extrapolation back to the ordinate is valid and accurate. However, with a heterogeneous antiserum there can be considerable deviation from linearity. This is often the case when a small amount of high-affinity antibody is present in an antiserum which is predominantly low-affinity antibody. Under these conditions the Langmuir plot can curve upwards as it nears the ordinate. In these situations, it is essential to have the maximum possible number of points along the linear part of the curve so that the best estimate of the intercept of this linear portion on the ordinate can be made. It is possible to circumvent some of these practical problems by using an independent method for determining the total anti-body; for example, quantitative precipitation (Section 6.4.1) or elution from immuno-adsorbants (Chapter 9). Unfortunately these alternatives also present their own problems.

To return to the mass action equation:

$$K = \frac{[Ab \cdot Ag]}{[Ab][Ag]}.$$

If increasing amounts of antigen are reacted with a fixed amount of antibody, a point is reached where half the antibody-combining sites are occupied by antigen. At this point

$[Ab] = [Ab \cdot Ag],$

therefore in the mass action equation,

$$K = \frac{[Ab \cdot Ag]}{[Ab][Ag]}$$

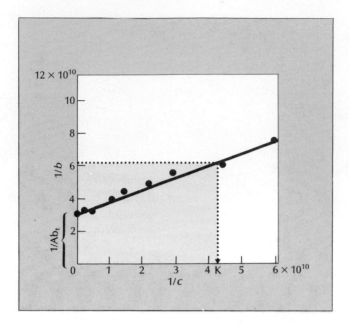

Fig. 6.3 Langmuir plot of reciprocal of bound (1/b) versus reciprocal of free antigen (1/c or 1/ Ag) of a serum, from a baboon immunized with human chorionic gonadotrophin. The regression coefficient, $r = 0.98$. The value for Ab_t obtained by extrapolation to infinite antigen concentration is 3.21×10^{-11} mmol litre^{-1}. Antibody affinity $K = 4.3\times10^{10}$ litre mol^{-1}.

$$K = \frac{1}{[Ag]}.$$

In other words, *affinity is equal to the reciprocal of the free antigen concentration when half the antibody sites are occupied by antigen.*

The value of K can be obtained from the plot in Fig. 6.3 by calculating the value of 50% Ab_t and reading off from the graph the value of K.

In experimental systems this value can also be obtained from a plot of the logarithmic transformation of the Sip's equation as follows: If

$$\frac{r}{n} = \frac{(K[Ag])^a}{1 + (K[Ag])^a}$$

where:

r = moles of antigen bound per mole of antibody,
n = antibody valency,
a = heterogeneity index (see below).

Then

$$\log \frac{r}{n - r} = a\cdot\log K + a\cdot\log[Ag]. \tag{5}$$

For IgG, $n = 2$, therefore

$$\text{moles of antibody} = \frac{[Ab_t]}{2}$$

and

$$r = \frac{b}{[Ab_t]/2}$$

where

$$b = [Ab \cdot Ag].$$

Substituting for n and r in (5),

$$\log \frac{b}{[Ab_t] - b} = a \cdot \log K + a \cdot \log[Ag].$$

If

$$\log \frac{b}{[Ab_t] - b} \text{ is plotted against } \log[Ag]$$

when

$$\log \frac{b}{[Ab_t] - b} = 0$$

then

$$K = \frac{1}{[Ag]}.$$

The *heterogeneity index*, a, is a measure of the number of different molecular species of antibody. It can range from a value of 0 to 1. Low values represent a large degree of heterogeneity, whereas monoclonal antibody should theoretically have an index of 1. These relationships have been derived on the assumption that the distribution of antibody affinities in a polyclonal population is random and symmetrical about the mean. There is now good experimental evidence to suggest that the distribution of affinities is often skewed or even bi-modal.

6.3.2 Equilibrium dialysis

This technique was devised in 1932 as a direct method for studying the primary interactions between antibody and hapten. The method is generally regarded as the standard method for affinity determination against which the other methods are judged. Unfortunately it is rather cumbersome to perform and uses up large amounts of antibody and antigen. As many haptens (but not oligosaccharides) bind to albumin, it is necessary to work with antibody isolated by ammonium sulphate precipitation, though further purification is not usually required.

Constant amounts of antibody (approximately the reciprocal of the expected equilibrium constant) are placed in dialysis bags and allowed to equilibrate with various concentrations of hapten over an antigen excess of one to 40. Free hapten will enter the dialysis bag along its concentration gradient (Fig. 6.4). Some of the hapten will complex with antibody and so will not contribute to the free-hapten concentration.

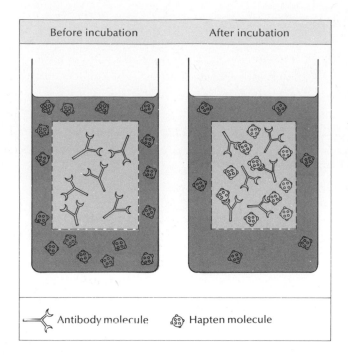

Before incubation   After incubation

— Antibody molecule   Hapten molecule

Fig. 6.4 Schematic representation of equilibrium dialysis showing relative distribution of the antibody and hapten molecules at time zero and after the equilibrium is established. Cell to left shows distribution at the beginning of the experiment, cell to right shows distribution at equilibrium. There is greater concentration of hapten molecules in the inner cell of the diagram on the right because of the hapten molecules bound to the antibody.

At equilibrium, the free-hapten concentration will be the same on either side of the dialysis membrane, but the total hapten concentration will be relatively greater inside the dialysis bag. For each experimental point on the binding curve the following samples, each in triplicate, are required:

(a) Antibody immunoglobulin.

(b) Irrelevant immunoglobulin, for the determination of non-specific binding.

(c) Buffer alone, to check that an equilibrium has in fact been established.

Typically each sample of protein or buffer solution (about 0.5 ml) is placed in a small dialysis bag. For each concentration of free hapten on the binding curve, nine sample bags can be equilibrated against a single pool of radioactive hapten, usually in a 50 ml bottle. The bottles are left in a water bath with mixing for 24−48 h and then triplicate volumetric samples are taken from each free-hapten solution and each dialysis bag.

The free-hapten concentration at equilibrium may be determined directly from the c.p.m. of the samples taken from the bottles. The bound hapten concentration may be calculated as follows:

Antibody-bound hapten, $Hb = (H_{Ab}) - (H_f + [H_N - H_f])$

where:

H_{Ab} = c.p.m. of sample from antibody bag,

H_f = c.p.m. of free hapten in bottle,

H_N = c.p.m. in bag containing irrelevant immunoglobulin.

The association constant may then be calculated using the Langmuir plot as detailed in the following section.

6.3.3 Ammonium sulphate precipitation

Determination of antibody affinity can be simplified by using a variation of the Farr assay described earlier in this chapter. A constant amount of antibody is reacted with increasing concentrations of antigen and left to equilibrate. The concentration of bound antigen is detected in the complex after ammonium sulphate precipitation and the concentration of free antigen determined in the supernatant. If the reciprocal of bound antigen is plotted against the reciprocal of the free antigen concentration and the line extrapolated to $1/[Ag] = 0$, the reciprocal of the bound antigen will equal the reciprocal of the total antibody-combining sites.

Materials and equipment

Radiolabelled antigen; for example, ^{125}I human serum albumin, HSA (Appendix II, Section 6.2.2)

Antiserum; for example, anti-HSA

Normal serum, as control

Saturated ammonium sulphate solution (Section 1.3.1)

Conical centrifuge tubes, 0.4 ml capacity (Appendix II)

Beckman 152 Microfuge (or equivalent)

γ spectrometer

Protocol

	Tube number							
	1	2	3	4	5	6	7	8
Antiserum or control serum	50 µl —————————————————————————→							
PBS	50 µl —————————————————————————→							
^{125}I Ag µg in 100 µl PBS	2.5	5.0	10	20	40	80	160	320

Method

1 Set up 16 tubes (eight each for antiserum and normal control serum) as shown in Protocol.
2 Mix the contents of the tubes thoroughly and incubate for 1 h at room temperature.
3 Add 0.2 ml saturated ammonium sulphate solution and mix immediately.
4 Incubate for 1 h at room temperature.
5 Spin the tubes at 10 000 g for 5 min.
6 Remove and keep 0.1 ml of supernatant.
7 Wash each precipitate twice with 50% saturated ammonium sulphate.
8 Determine the c.p.m. of radioactivity in the supernatant samples and precipitates using a γ spectrometer

Data required

Free antigen concentration = total radioactivity (c.p.m.) in the supernatant, i.e. radioactivity in 100 µl sample from step 6 multiplied by 4.

Bound-antigen concentration = (c.p.m. antiserum precipitate − c.p.m. control precipitate), for each antigen concentration.

Calculation of results

All the values should be expressed as molar concentrations, 1 pmole of HSA = 0.068 µg.

1 Record and calculate the results as in Fig 6.5a and b.
2 Plot $1/b$ (column 9) against $1/[Ag]$ (column 10). Extrapolate the graph line to $1/[Ag] = 0$, i.e. the intercept on the $1/b$ axis, this is the value of $1/[Ab_t]$.
3 Use the value for $[Ab_t]$ to calculate the values shown in Fig. 6.5b.
4 From Fig. 6.5b, plot:

$$\log \frac{b}{Ab_t - b} \text{ (column 3) against } \log[Ag] \text{ (column 4).}$$

The intercept on the $\log[Ag]$ axis, i.e. when

$$\log \frac{b}{[Ab_t] - b} = 0,$$

equals $1/K$, therefore

$$K = \frac{1}{[Ag]}$$

The units of K are litres per mole.

Low-affinity antibodies have K values around 10^5 litres mol^{-1}, whereas high-affinity antibodies often have K values of 10^{12} litres mol^{-1}.

Technical notes

1 Errors always occur during the washing of precipitates, particularly as dissociation may take place on removal of the free antibody and free antigen. A procedure to avoid this has been introduced using radioactive sodium as a buffer tracer. This is described below (Section 6.3.4).
2 There has been discussion as to how quickly the addition of ammonium sulphate freezes the equilibrium. Most authors assume that this is immediate and so calculate the concentrations, at equilibrium, on the volumes prior to adding ammonium sulphate, but it has been suggested that calculating the concentration on the basis of the volume after adding the precipitating agent is more accurate.
3 It must be recognised that the high salt concentrations used to precipitate the immunoglobulin might also dissociate some of the complexes, particularly those involving low-affinity antibodies. The use of polyethylene glycol as a precipitating agent avoids this problem.

221 / ANTIBODY INTERACTION WITH ANTIGEN

Column number

1	2	3	4	5	6	7	8	9	10
Tube no.	μg albumin per tube	c.p.m. in supernatant free [Ag]	c.p.m. antiserum precipitate	c.p.m. control precipitate	Bound antigen	Moles of Ag bound (b)	Moles of free Ag	$1/b$	$1/[Ag]$
	pmoles of albumin				c.p.m. col. 4 − c.p.m. col. 5	c.p.m. col. 6 ÷ specific activity*	c.p.m. col. 3 ÷ specific activity*	Reciprocal of col. 7	Reciprocal of col. 8
1	2.5	1 pmole = 0.068 μg							
2	5								
3	10								
4	20								
5	40								
6	80								
7	160								
8	320								

* Specific activity of antigen $= \dfrac{\text{c.p.m.}}{\text{molar concentration of antigen}}$.

Fig. 6.5a Table for calculation of Ab_t.

Tube no.	Column number			
	1	2	3	4
	pmoles of antigen	$\dfrac{b}{[Ab_t] - b}$	$\text{Log} \dfrac{b}{[Ab_t] - b}$	Log [Ag]
1			Log_{10} col.2	Log_{10} free-antigen concentration, i.e. log col. 8 Fig. 5.4a.
2				
3				
4				
5				
6				
7				
8				

Fig. 6.5b Table for calculation of K.

6.3.4 Double isotope modification to avoid washing

A major problem with the ammonium sulphate method is the need to wash the precipitates. If this is carried out thoroughly there is always the danger of losing precipitate or dissociating some of the complex. A useful development, introduced by Steward, is the incorporation of $^{22}NaCl$ as a marker of buffer volume. Most of the supernatant can then be removed, without accurate measurement, and the amount of free radioactive antigen remaining in the precipitate estimated from the ^{22}Na counts which will indicate the amount of buffer solution remaining with the precipitate. The technique is possible as ^{22}Na and ^{125}I have substantially different radiation energy emission spectra and so can be counted separately in a two-channel γ counter. There is some overlap of ^{22}Na counts into the ^{125}I channel, this is determined as part of the experimental design and is allowed for during the calculations.

The method is as above (Section 6.3.3) except for the incorporation of $^{22}NaCl$ into the assay and the inclusion of tubes containing $^{22}NaCl$ alone, or $^{22}NaCl$ plus antigen to estimate the spillover of ^{22}Na counts into the ^{125}I channel.

Materials and equipment
These are as for the ammonium sulphate affinity determination (Section 6.3.3) but in
    addition:
$^{22}NaCl$ (Appendix II)
Two-channel γ spectrometer

Method
1 Set up five microfuge tubes with the same amount of $^{22}NaCl$ in each tube (about 50 000 c.p.m. in 50 µl PBS should be sufficient) to provide replicate determinations of the total sodium counts.
2 Set up the 16 assay tubes for antiserum and control serum as in the Protocol

above (Section 6.3.3). In addition to adding varying amounts of ^{125}I-antigen also add the same amounts of ^{22}NaCl in 50 µl PBS, to each tube as in step 1. This takes the place of the PBS mentioned in the Protocol, p. 219.

3 Mix and incubate for 1 h at room temperature.

4 Add an equal volume of saturated ammonium sulphate solution and mix immediately.

5 Incubate for 1 h at room temperature.

6 Spin the tubes at 10 000 g for 5 min.

7 Aspirate the majority of the supernatant taking great care not to disturb the precipitate.

8 Count the radioactivity of the ^{22}NaCl, ^{22}NaCl plus antigen, and precipitate tubes in a two-channel γ counter.

Calculation

For each antigen calculate the total ^{125}I counts added per tube corrected for ^{22}Na spillover):

$$I = I' - \frac{Nx}{y}$$

where:

I' = total counts in ^{125}I channel including ^{22}Na spillover (for tubes containing ^{125}I antigen plus ^{22}Na),

N = total counts in ^{22}Na channel (for tubes containing ^{125}I antigen plus ^{22}Na).

x = counts in ^{125}I channel in tubes containing ^{22}Na only.

y = counts in ^{22}Na channel in tubes containing ^{22}Na only.

Counts in ^{125}I channel of experimental tubes (corrected for spillover from ^{22}Na):

$$i = i' - \frac{nx}{y}$$

where:

i' = counts in ^{125}I channel of experimental tubes including spillover from ^{22}Na.

n = counts in ^{22}Na channel of experimental tubes.

In the experimental tubes containing precipitate:

(a) The ^{22}Na counts allow a calculation of the carry over of free antigen (by determining the amount of buffer carried over).

(b) The ^{125}I counts allow a calculation of the concentration of antigen, both free and bound to antibody.

Therefore, at each of the eight antigen concentrations,

$$\% \text{ antigen bound} = \frac{Ni - nI}{I(N-n)} \times 100$$

where terms of the equation defined as above.

Antigen bound specifically to antibody =

$$\frac{100}{\% \text{ Ag bound by antiserum} - \% \text{ Ag bound by control serum}} \times \text{total Ag}$$

(thus correcting for non-specific uptake by the control serum)

Free antigen = total antigen − bound antigen.

Calculate antibody affinity graphically as in Section 6.3.1 above.

6.3.5   ## Determination of functional antibody affinity by ELISA

Absolute affinity determinations are complex and time consuming. Useful information on relative affinity can be obtained by performing ELISA assays in the presence and absence of diethylamine. This chaotropic agent has a much greater effect in inhibiting the binding of low-, compared with high-, affinity antibodies. In a study of a panel of monoclonal antibodies, diethylamine inhibition produced the same ranking of relative affinity as was seen with a full-affinity determination. This technique is especially useful for comparing the relative affinities of different immunoglobulin subclasses.

Materials
As for ELISA (Section 10.6)
Diethylamine
Phosphate-buffered saline, PBS (Appendix I) containing 0.25% gelatin and 0.05% Tween

Method
1 Prepare coated wells for the ELISA assay (Section 10.6).
2 Instead of a single serum dilution, make serial dilutions of the antiserum in PBS/0.25% gelatin/0.05% Tween in the presence and absence of diethylamine. (A concentration between 1 and 50 mM should be suitable depending on the affinity range of the antibody. A 20 mM solution is worth trying first.)
3 proceed as for ELISA.
4 Plot the OD on the ordinate against $\log_{10}$ serum dilution for the two curves.
5 Measure the degree of left displacement of the dose−response curve in the presence of diethylamine at 50% of the maximum OD.

Results are expressed as $\log_{10}$ of this displacement. The higher the value of the displacement the lower the functional affinity.

6.4   ## Secondary interactions: precipitation

6.4.1   ## Quantitative precipitin test

This test, developed by Heidelberger and Kendall, is the basis of all quantitative studies of antigen−antibody interaction. Increasing amounts of antigen are added to a constant amount of antibody and the weight of precipitate formed in each tube is determined. Originally precipitation was thought to result simply from the build up of a large three-dimensional lattice formed by combining site cross-linking of epitopes on different antigen molecules, but it is now known to also depend upon the presence of an intact Fc region in the antibody. Precipitation is far less efficient with F(ab′)$_2$ fragments of antibody, even though they are divalent. The procedure outlined below is suitable for most antisera and antigens.

Materials
Antiserum; for example, anti-human serum albumin
Human serum albumin, HSA (1 mg ml^{-1}) (Appendix II)
Phosphate-buffered saline, PBS (Appendix I)
0.1 M sodium hydroxide

Method

1 Add antigen, PBS and antiserum to a series of numbered tubes (suitable for centrifugation), according to the Protocol. (For antisera with high or low antibody content it will be necessary to increase or decrease the range of antigen concentrations used.)

Protocol

Reagent	1	2	3	4	5	6	7	8	9	10
Antigen (μl)	0	10	20	50	100	150	200	250	350	450
PBS	450	440	430	400	350	300	250	200	100	0
Antiserum (μl)	100									→

2 Mix the reactants thoroughly.
3 Incubate at 37° for 1 h and then at 4° overnight. (For accurate determinations, these incubations can be extended for up to 10 days at 4°. However, for demonstration purposes using high-titred and high-avidity antisera; illustrative curves may be obtained with only 30 min incubation at 37° and 30 min at 4°.)
4 Spin at 3000 g for 5 min and remove supernatant. An angle-head rotor should be used as the precipitate is then formed at the side of the tube, thus facilitating removal of the supernatant.
5 Check each supernatant for free antigen and antibody using a sensitive technique; for example, single radial immunodiffusion (Section 6.6).
6 Wash the precipitate twice by centrifugation with cold PBS.
7 Re-dissolve the final precipitate in 0.1 M sodium hydroxide (the volume to be used depends on the spectrophotometer cuvettes available, but should be about 1 ml for the amounts of reagents used here).
8 Measure the absorbance at 280 nm and plot a graph of the absorbance units of the re-dissolved precipitate against the amount of antigen added (see Fig. 6.6).

Calculations
(a) Determine the antibody content per ml of antiserum.

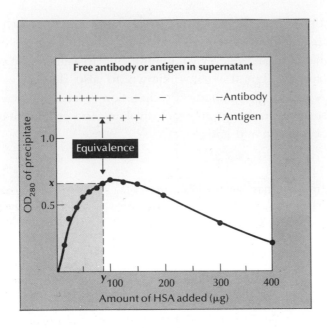

Fig. 6.6 Precipitin curve of human serum albumin (HSA) with anti-HSA. An increasing amount of antigen was added to a fixed concentration of antiserum and the optical density of the precipitate (in sodium hydroxide) determined. The supernatant was assayed for the presence of free antibody or antigen by single radial immunodiffusion. The equivalence point (arrowed), when all the antibody and antigen is complexed in the precipitate, occurs just before the point of maximum precipitation.

To determine the equivalence point exactly, it is frequently necessary to repeat the assay using smaller steps in antigen concentrations around the concentration required to give maximum precipitation.

(b) Calculate the number of antigenic determinants on each antigen molecule (i.e. antigenic valency).

Theoretical basis of the calculations

ANTIBODY CONTENT OF THE SERUM

If the supernatant from each tube is examined for the presence of excess antibody or antigen, there will be one point at which no free antibody or antigen can be detected. This is the point of *equivalence* which occurs just before maximum precipitation (Fig. 6.6). The amount of precipitate increases after the equivalence point because of continued incorporation of antigen into the complex. Eventually soluble complexes are formed in antigen excess and the amount of precipitate decreases (Fig. 6.7).

In Fig. 6.6, at equivalence, the precipitate contains x µg of total protein, if this includes y µg of antigen then there is $(x-y)$ µg of antibody. This is the total amount of antibody in the volume of serum used.

Specimen calculation (from Fig. 6.6)

The precipitate was dissolved in 1 ml of 0.1 M sodium hydroxide and absorbance measurements made in 1 cm light-path cells.

IgG absorbance of 1.0 at 280 nm in 1 cm cell = 0.695 mg ml^{-1}.
HSA absorbance of 1.0 at 280 nm in 1 cm cell = 1.886 mg ml^{-1}.

From the graph, at equivalence absorbance of precipitate x = 0.65.

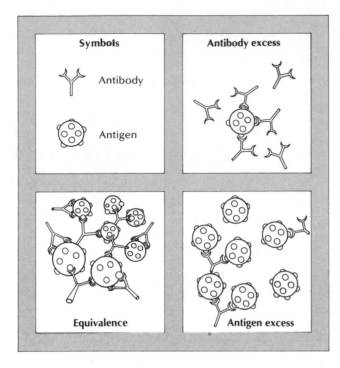

Fig. 6.7 Complexes formed at varying antigen : antibody ratios. Diagrammatic representation of complexes formed between a multi-valent antigen and a divalent antibody at antibody excess, equivalence and antigen excess.

In this case, maximum precipitation occurs at equivalence when a lattice is formed, producing a complex too large to remain in solution.

The precipitate contains 87.5 µg HSA, which if dissolved alone in 1.0 ml of sodium hydroxide would give an absorbance of 0.004 (calculated from the extinction coefficient). Hence,

absorbance of antibody component of the precipitate = OD precipitate − OD due to HSA
= 0.65 − 0.04
= 0.61.

Hence,

$$\text{total antibody content of serum, mg ml}^{-1} = \frac{\text{absorbance} \times \text{extinction coefficient}}{\text{sample volume}}$$
$$= \frac{0.61 \times 0.695}{0.1}$$
$$= 4.24 \text{ mg ml}^{-1}.$$

This antiserum has a relatively high antibody content.

Determination of antigenic valency

For this determination some theoretical aspects of the precipitation curve must be considered. When the antigen concentration is low there is a relative antibody excess (Fig. 6.6). At the other extreme, at high antigen concentrations, there is free antigen and so each combining site of the antibody is occupied. At either of these extremes

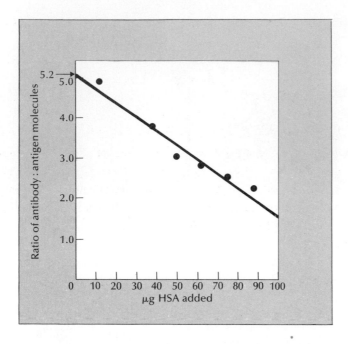

Fig. 6.8 Ratio of antibody : antigen molecules at different levels of antibody excess. The regression line calculated from the antibody : antigen ratios over a range of antigen concentrations, all in antigen excess, gives an intercept of 5.2(→), indicating that there are five antigenic determinants detected on the HSA molecule by this anti-serum. This antiserum differs from that used in Fig. 6.6.

the complexes are relatively small. At equivalence, however, there is much cross-linking between molecules and large complexes are formed.

Every antigenic determinant is likely to be covered by a separate antibody molecule at extreme antibody excess. If we calculate the amount of antibody in the precipitate at this point, in the same way as above, we can determine the ratio of antibody : antigen, and so the relative numbers of molecules of each in the precipitate, i.e.

$$\frac{\text{weight of antigen}}{\text{molecular weight antigen}} : \frac{\text{weight of antibody}}{\text{molecular weight antibody}}.$$

In a hyperimmune serum the major proportion of antibody will be of the IgG class with a molecular weight of 150 000. The molecular weight of HSA (the antigen in this case) is 68 000.

To obtain the best estimate of antigenic valency, the ratio of antibody : antigen in the precipitate should be plotted against the amount of antigen added, as in Fig. 6.8. If the plot is extended to the antibody : antigen axis, the intercept will give the ratio at infinite antibody excess.

Specimen calculation (from Fig. 6.8)
Absorbance of precipitate = 0.15
Absorbance of HSA (calculated as above) = 0.005 (10 μg).

Hence absorbance of antibody in the precipitate = 0.145 which is equivalent to 101.5 μg ml^{-1} IgG. Therefore the molar ratios are

$$\frac{10}{68\,000} : \frac{101.5}{150\,000}$$

$$= \underline{0.000147 : 0.000677}.$$

Therefore the ratio of antibody : antigen molecules = 4.6 : 1. This antiserum recognises between four and five determinants on the HSA molecule.

The quantitative precipitin test is particularly useful as it can be carried out without antibody standards; only known concentrations of antigen are required. The shape of the curve varies with different antigens: with protein antigens a sharp peak is usually obtained, but with polysaccharides there is usually a broader peak. In addition, the various antisera have different properties. Rabbit antisera give the typical curve shown in Fig. 6.6, whereas horse antisera give precipitates which have relatively greater solubility in *both* antigen *and* antibody excess (see Fig. 6.1). Both types of precipitin curve may be obtained with human antisera.

One of the properties of complement is to maintain immune complexes in solution and to re-solubilise insoluble complexes. Therefore, if fresh sera are used to produce the precipitin curve, little precipitation will occur unless they are heated to 56° for 30 min to destroy complement prior to assay. Most stored or commercially obtained antisera have already lost this activity.

6.5 Precipitation in gels

Although the precipitin test gives a great deal of basic information, it is lengthy to perform and requires relatively large quantities of reagents. In addition, it does not provide an easy basis for a qualitative comparison of antisera or antigens. Many gel precipitation techniques have been developed for qualitative analysis, based on the simple but effective principle that if antigen and antibody are placed in two adjacent wells in agar, they will diffuse into the agar and set up two opposing concentration gradients between the wells; at a point of optimal proportions between these gradients a line of precipitation will form. Thus, the analysis will be carried out with the reactants at their equivalence point, without the need for empirical determination.

Buffered agar and agar-coated slides may be prepared as described below for use in the procedures described in this section.

6.5.1 Buffered agar

Materials and equipment
Barbitone buffer (Appendix I)
Agar (Appendix II)

Method
1 Mix 2 g of agar with 50 ml of distilled water and dissolve in a microwave oven.
2 Add 50 ml of hot barbitone buffer and mix well. The agar may be stored at 4° for many weeks.

Note
The agar must be bought specifically for electrophoresis; many of the culture agars are not suitable for this purpose.

Pre-coating glass slides

Gel precipitation techniques may be conveniently performed on glass microscope slides and the gel then dried down onto the glass for convenient and permanent storage. To ensure good adhesion of the gel to the slide it is necessary to first coat the slide with a thin layer of agar which is allowed to dry, before layering on the analytical agar gel.

Materials and equipment
Glass microscope slides
Agar (Appendix II)

Method
1   Dissolve 0.5 g of agar in 100 ml of distilled water as in 6.5.1.
2   Pipette the agar solution on to clean, dry slides. Add enough to just cover one surface of the slide.
3   Dry the slides and store at room temperature until required.

Single radial immunodiffusion (SRID)

Diffusion reactions in gels have been used since 1905 and have been developed into highly sophisticated techniques. Oudin originally used analytical techniques involving the diffusion of antigens into an antibody-containing gel (single diffusion in one direction). Feinberg and later Mancini, Carbonara and Heremans extended this technique by incorporating the antiserum into a thin layer of agar and placing the antigen in wells cut into the agar. As the antigen diffuses radially a ring of precipitation forms around the well and moves outwards, eventually becoming stationary at equivalence. At equivalence, the diameter and area of the ring is related to the antigen concentration in the well. Using standard antigen concentrations a calibration curve may be constructed to determine unknown concentrations of the same antigen.

Materials and equipment
2% agar in barbitone buffer (Section 6.5.1)
Pre-coated slides (Section 6.5.2)
Antiserum; for example, anti-human IgG (Appendix II)
Standard antigen solution; for example human IgG (Appendix II)
Phosphate-buffered saline, PBS (Appendix I)
Flat level surface (use a spirit level)
Gel punch (Appendix II)
Humid chamber (plastic box with wet filter paper)

Method
1   Melt the agar in a microwave oven and transfer to 56° water bath. This temperature will keep the agar molten but is low enough to avoid denaturation of the antibody.

2   Dilute the antiserum with PBS. (The optimal dilution will, of course, depend upon the strength of the antiserum and antigen as the diameter of the precipitation ring is inversely proportional to the antiserum concentration. In practice, with rabbit antisera to human IgG, we find that a final dilution of approximately 1 : 40 in the agar is suitable for measuring IgG concentrations in the range of 50−200 μg ml^{-1}. However, this is only a guide; a standard curve should be determined for each antiserum.) Typically, add 75 μl of an antiserum to 1.9 ml of PBS and warm to 56°.

3   Add the diluted antiserum to 1 ml of agar at 56° and mix well.

4   Layer the agar on to a pre-coated slide standing on a levelled surface and allow to set.

5   After the agar has set, use a gel punch to cut about eight wells per slide. The wells should be 2−3 mm in diameter, and must have vertical sides.

6   Remove the agar plug with a Pasteur pipette attached to a water vacuum pump.

7   Fill each of four wells with standard solutions of 50, 100, 150 and 200 μg ml^{-1} IgG. Use the other wells for the IgG solutions of unknown concentrations. Maintain a standard volume by filling the wells quickly until the meniscus just disappears. Alternatively a measured volume, such as 10 μl, may be accurately pipetted into each well.

8   Leave the slide in a humid box to equilibrate. (Although a satisfactory standard curve may be obtained by overnight equilibration, the points will better approximate to a straight line if the slide is allowed to equilibrate longer: IgG and IgA 48 h, IgM 72 h. IgG concentrations may also be determined by incubation at 37° for 4 h.)

6.6.1   Measurement of precipitation rings

The diameter of each ring may be measured either directly using a magnifying glass with a μm scale or, after staining, with a plastic ruler.

Direct measurement

Hold the slide over a black background and illuminate it from the side. Measure the rings from the reverse side through the glass plate, do not rest the magnifying glass on the gel. If the rings are not distinct, soak the slides in 4% tannic acid for 1 min to increase resolution. (This is not a permanent preparation.)

Stained preparations

1   Wash the slide for 24 h in several changes of PBS to remove free protein from the agar.

2 Cover the slide with good-quality, lint-free, filter paper and dry overnight.
3 Remove the filter paper after dampening it slightly.

The slide may then be stained with any protein dye, but we suggest Coomassie blue.

Mixture for staining solution

Coomassie brilliant blue (1.25 g) (Appendix II)
Glacial acetic acid (50 ml)
Distilled water (185 ml)

Method
1 Dissolve the Coomassie dye in the glacial acetic acid and distilled water.
2 Stain the slide for 5 min and differentiate in the same solution without the dye. Staining with this dye is reversible so do not leave the slide too long in the de-staining solution.
3 Place the dry, stained slides in a photographic enlarger and measure the diameter of the precipitation rings with a ruler.

The staining solution may be stored for several weeks in a stoppered bottle. The de-staining solution can be regenerated by passing through powdered charcoal.

Calculation of results

Figure 6.9 shows a typical determination. The diameters of the rings were measured and plotted on a linear scale against the log of the antigen concentration. (With a semi-log transformation, the points should approximate to a straight line. If the assay has been allowed to reach equilibrium the areas of the rings should be calculated and plotted against the antigen concentration on a linear scale.)

Technical notes
1 The assay can be made more sensitive by incorporating from 2 to 4 % polyethylene glycol in the agar to enhance precipitation.
2 If chicken antisera are used, 7–8 % NaCl should be added to the agar to improve precipitation.
3 Although single radial immunodiffusion is now used as a quantitative technique, its first use was to compare the identities of different antigen solutions. If two antigens, placed in neighbouring wells close together, are identical in terms of their antigenic determinants then the two rings of precipitation fuse completely. If the antigens share no determinants recognised by the antiserum then each ring forms independently. Since the work of Ouchterlony, simpler procedures have been introduced to test the relationships between antigens or antibodies.

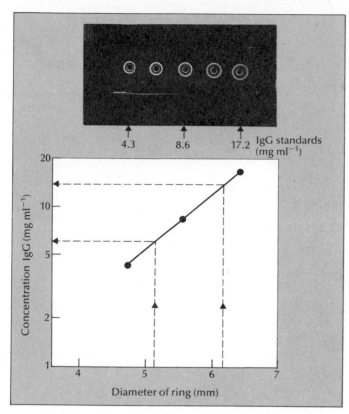

Fig. 6.9 Measurement of IgG concentration by single radial immunodiffusion. A calibration curve is constructed from the diameter of the precipitation rings formed at equilibrium by IgG standards of known concentration. The concentration of unknown samples can then be determined with reference to the standard curve.

6.7 Double diffusion in two dimensions

In this procedure antigen and antibody are allowed to migrate towards each other in a gel and a line of precipitation is formed where the two reactants meet. As this precipitate is soluble in excess antigen, a sharp line is produced at equivalence, its relative position being determined by the concentration of the antigen and antibody in the agar. The local concentration of each reactant depends not only on its absolute concentration in the well, but also on its molecular size and therefore, the rate at which it is able to diffuse through the gel.

Multiple lines of precipitation will be present if the antigen and antibody contain several molecular species. Consequently, this technique has the particular advantage that several antigens or antisera can be compared around a single well of antibody or antigen.

Materials and equipment
2% agar in barbitone buffer (Section 6.5.1)
Antigen and antibody solutions (see procedure for details)
Gel punch (pattern, for example, as in Fig. 6.10, see also Appendix II)

Method
1 Melt the agar in a microwave oven.
2 Pour agar on to pre-coated slides; use a levelled surface.

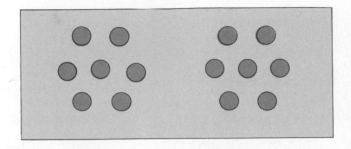

Fig. 6.10 Typical well pattern in agar for qualitative comparison of antisera or antigens. The number, size and distance between wells depends upon the number and strength of the antisera and antigens.

3 Punch pattern required (see Fig. 6.10).
4 Suck out agar plugs with a Pasteur pipette connected to a water vacuum pump.
5 Fill the wells with antibody or antigen until the meniscus just disappears.
6 Place the slide in a humid chamber and incubate overnight at a constant temperature.

Suggested antibody and antigen patterns
A straightforward demonstration of identity and non-identity can be shown using the antigen mixtures as in Fig. 6.11. In addition, this technique may be used to show the relationships between IgG molecules and their enzymic digests prepared in Chapter 8. Arrange the wells as shown in Fig. 6.12.

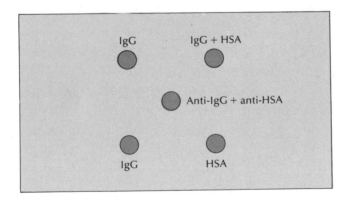

Fig. 6.11 Design of Ouchterlony plate to show reactions of identity and non-identity. IgG and albumin (HSA) with their respective antisera.

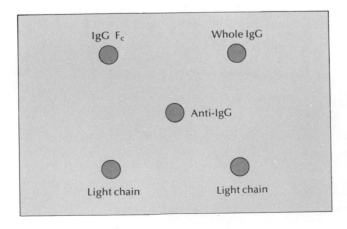

Fig. 6.12 Well arrangement to demonstrate spur formation, lines of identity and lines of non-identity. IgG Fc prepared by papain digestion of IgG (Section 8.8.1). Light chains prepared by reduction and alkylation of IgG (Section 8.7.).

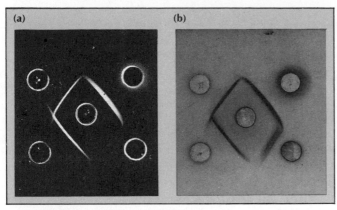

Fig. 6.13 The relationship of human IgG subclasses. In (a) and (b) wells 1−4 contain human IgG1, IgG2, IgG3 and IgG4, respectively, and the central well contains rabbit anti-human IgG. (Antisera prepared by immunising rabbits with IgG obtained from normal human serum by ion-exchange chromatography, see Section 8.5.)

Antiserum (a) recognised subclass differences between IgG1 and IgG4, hence the double spur, but failed to recognise IgG3. Antiserum (b) recognized subclass differences associated with IgG1 alone and so produced a single spur. Both antisera were raised against the same pool of antigen, the variation is due to the rabbits used for immunisation.

Antigen concentration: initially use 1 mg ml^{-1}, but vary the concentration to obtain optimal results.

Antiserum: use whole anti-IgG, non-absorbed. Specific anti-IgG sera available commercially are absorbed with light chains to render them class specific (Section 8.7).

Technical note

The rate of diffusion is temperature dependent. Precipitin lines can often be seen within 3 h at 37°.

Interpretation of results

There are three basic patterns of precipitation as shown in Figs 6.13 and 6.14.

(a) *Reaction of identity*. This occurs between identical antigenic determinants, the lines of precipitation fuse to give one continuous arc.

(b) *Reaction of non-identity*. Where two antigens do not contain any common antigenic determinants the two lines are formed independently and cross without any interaction.

(c) *Reaction of partial identity*. This has two components: (i) those antigenic determinants which are common to both antigens give a continuous line of identity; (ii) the unique determinant(s) recognised on one of the antigens gives, in addition, a line of non-identity so that a spur is formed. Of course, the antiserum may recognise unique determinants in both antigens, this would give rise to two spurs.

All these concepts of identity and non-identity are in terms of recognition by the antiserum. An antiserum recognising many determinants on the antigen molecules is necessary for the demonstration of all these features.

6.8   **Turbidimetry and nephelometry**

Although single radial immunodiffusion is technically simple, it is cumbersome for the examination of multiple samples. For this reason many laboratories now quantitate

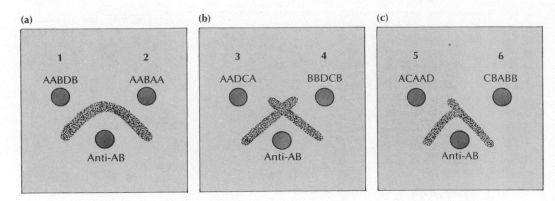

Fig. 6.14 Explanation of basic patterns of precipitation obtainable in Ouchterlony immunodiffusion. A−D represent antigenic determinants present within a series of protein molecules, 1−6, used as antigens. An antiserum has been raised against two of these determinants, A and B. **(a)** The precipitation lines have fused completely showing the presence of identical determinants in proteins 1 and 2. Note that the detection is mainly qualitative, although the relative position of the equivalence line gives some indication of relative antigen to antibody concentration and, in addition, does not give any information on any other determinants that may be present which are not recognized by the antiserum. **(b)** The two precipitation lines cross without any interaction. Proteins 3 and 4 do not, therefore, share any determinants detectable by the antiserum. **(c)** The two precipitation lines have fused, but in addition a spur has formed towards the well containing protein 5. Hence, proteins 5 and 6 share some common determinants but protein 6 has additional unique determinants detected by the antiserum.

immune complexes formed by the interaction of antigen and antibody using the techniques of turbidimetry or nephelometry. In these techniques monochromatic light is used to illuminate a cuvette containing a suspension of the immune complex. Light is both absorbed and deflected by the complexes. In turbidimetry the amount of light absorbed is measured in a spectrophotometer; whereas in nephelometry the amount of light scattered is measured by a detector mounted at an angle to the original light path. In both cases the measurements are proportional to the quantity of complex. The most sensitive instruments, incorporating laser light sources, are able to detect nanogram quantities of complex. Many of the machines are automated so that many hundreds of samples may be processed each day.

6.9 Immunoelectrophoretic analysis

So far we have studied antibody−antigen interaction solely by simple diffusion. This is possible if there are only a few components in the system but, if there are multiple antigens reacting with several antibodies, the precipitin lines become difficult to resolve and impossible to interpret. Increased resolution can be obtained by combining electrophoresis with immunodiffusion in gels, in the technique known as immuno-electrophoresis. The increased resolution thus obtained is of great benefit in the immunological examination of serum proteins. Serum proteins separate in agar gels, under the influence of an electric field into albumin, α_1-, α_2-, β- and γ-globulins. If you are not familiar with this electrophoretic separation of serum proteins, it is advisable to perform a simple agar gel electrophoresis as this will aid your understanding of the patterns obtained with the later techniques.

6.9.1   ## Agar gel electrophoresis

Materials and equipment
2% agar in barbitone buffer (Section 6.5.1)
Barbitone buffer (Appendix I)
Pre-coated microscope slides (Section 6.5.2)
Normal and myeloma sera (see Appendix II for myeloma sera)
10% glacial acetic acid in water (v/v)
Electrophoresis tank and power pack (Appendix II)
Gel punch (pattern as in Fig. 6.15) (Appendix II)

Method
1   Melt the agar in a microwave oven.
2   Mark the end of the slide that will be positive during the electrophoresis. If required, number the slides.
3   Pour 3–5 ml of agar on to the slide on a levelled surface.
4   When the agar has set, punch the pattern shown in Fig. 6.15. (Smaller wells than used for immunodifusion are required. A fine Pasteur pipette or a hypodermic needle with a square cut end may be used.)
5   Suck out the agar plugs.
6   Fill the wells with serum to which a small amount of bromophenol blue dye has been added.
7   Fill the electrophoresis tank with full-strength barbitone buffer.
8   Place the slide in the electrophoresis tank and connect each end of the slide to the buffer chambers with rayon or filter paper wicks. Close the tank.
9   Apply a current of about 8 mA slide^{-1}. The voltage drop will be about 5–7 V cm^{-1}.

The bromophenol blue dye binds to the serum albumin and as this is the fastest migrating band it serves as a marker throughout the electrophoresis. If excess dye has been added, however, a bright blue band of free dye will run in front of the albumin towards the anode.

10   When the albumin band (blue) nears the end of the slide — after about 60 min — remove the slide and fix the proteins by immersing the slide in 10 % glacial acetic acid.
11   Cover the slide with fine filter paper and leave to dry.
12   Dampen the paper and remove, then stain the slide with Coomassie brilliant blue (Section 6.6.1).

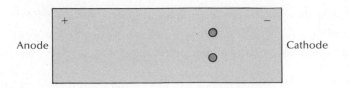

Fig. 6.15 Basic well pattern for agar gel electrophoresis.

Suggested design

One well should contain normal serum and the other serum from a patient with multiple myelomatosis (a disease in which a single clone of antibody-forming cells becomes malignant and produces large amounts of monoclonal antibody). If you are using mouse reagents, then ascitic fluid or serum from a hybridoma-bearing animal will do equally well.

Results

The main serum proteins should show clearly as oval bands. Identify each band (albumin, α_1-, α_2, β- and γ-globulins), and assign the abnormal monoclonal band to one of these (cf. Fig. 6.16).

Technical note

The negative charge on the agar generates an electroendosmotic flow of water through the gel. This flow, and not the potential difference, is responsible for most of the

Fig. 6.16 (*Facing page*) **Electrophoresis of serum samples.**
(a) Agar gel electrophoresis.
Well 1: normal serum.
Well 2: serum from patient with multiple myeloma.
Myeloma patients show an over-production of antibody, often of a single clone, in this case running in the γ-globulin region. You can see by inspection that there is an apparent decrease in the albumin content of the myeloma serum.
(b) Electrophoresis on cellulose acetate membranes.
Sample 1: normal serum as in (a).
Sample 2: myeloma serum as in (a), two preparations.
The principle of this separation of serum proteins is basically similar to that described for agar gel electrophoresis, except that the sample is applied onto the membrane as a band rather than via a well. The advantages of this technique are: (a) it is easier to discern the individual protein bands; and (b) it is possible to clear the membrane either with glycerol or one of the commercially available clearing oils. Thus, the protein content of each band can be determined by scanning photometry.
   The 'hawk-shaped' band seen in sample 3 is often observed with myeloma protein and is probably caused by overloading of this band.
(c) The traces obtained from scanning samples 1 and 2 of (b) are shown here. By integrating the area under each peak (this is usually done automatically by the scanner) it is possible to determine the total protein content of each band, and so confirm the observation made in (a), that there is indeed an albumin—γ-globulin reversal in the myeloma serum.
Sample 1: normal serum, above — albumin : globulin ratio 4.5
Sample 2: myeloma serum, below — albumin : globulin ratio 0.7.

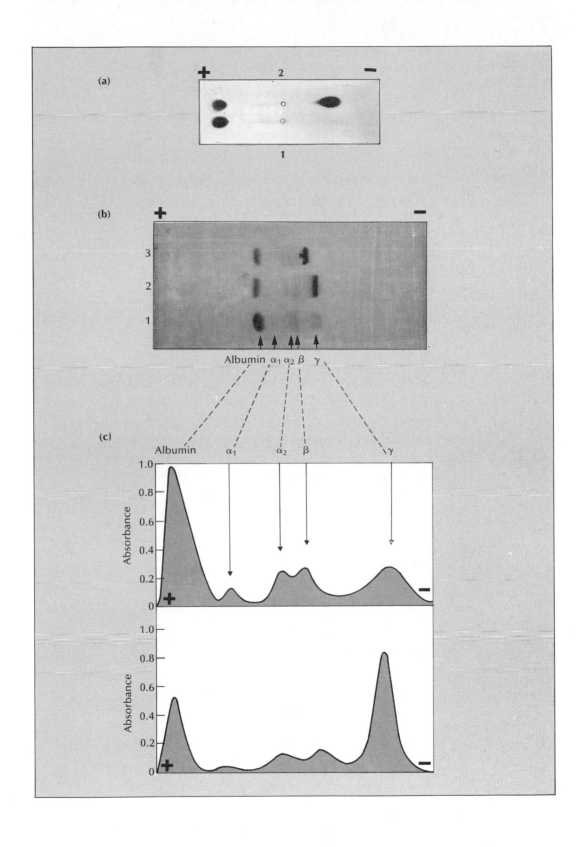

separation seen with some of the globulins, which are near their isoelectric point under the conditions used. This is discussed in more detail later.

6.9.2 Immunoelectrophoresis

Immunoelectrophoresis is a powerful analytical technique with great resolving power as it combines prior separation of antigens by electrophoresis with immunodiffusion against an antiserum (see Fig. 6.17).

Materials and equipment
As for agar gel electrophoresis (Section 6.9.1)
In addition:
Anti-human whole serum (Appendix II)

Method
1 Prepare slide as for agar gel electrophoresis (Section 6.9.1).
2 Cut the pattern shown in Fig. 6.18. (Although cutters and moulds are available commercially for many different patterns, the holes can be made with hypodermic needles (cut square and sharpened) and the trough with razor blades.)
3 Suck out the agar wells but do not remove the agar from the trough as this may cause abnormalities in protein banding during electrophoresis.
4 Fill one well with normal human serum and the other with myeloma serum.
5 Electrophorese as before (Section 6.9.1).

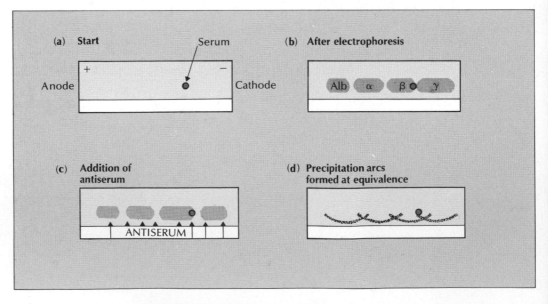

Fig. 6.17 Theoretical basis of immunoelectrophoresis. The antigen diffuses from a point source after the initial electrophoresis and interacts with the antiserum advancing on a plane front thus producing an arc of precipitation at equivalence.

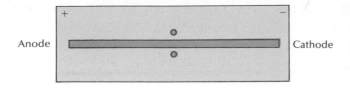

Fig. 6.18 Pattern for immunoelectrophoresis. It is convenient to mark the positive end of the slide before pouring on the agar. Alternatively mark the agar itself with a carbohydrate binding dye; for example, alcian blue (1% solution). Do not remove the central agar trough before electrophoresis. Up to three wells and two troughs can be cut into agar on an ordinary microscope slide.

6 Remove the agar trough and fill with anti-whole human serum.

7 Leave the slide to incubate overnight in a humid chamber at a constant temperature. (Again lines will appear within 2–3 h if the slide is incubated at 37°.)

8 Examine the lines produced and identify the IgG, IgA and IgM bands, and the bump in the precipitation arc typical of monoclonal immunoglobulin in the myeloma serum. The result obtained should be similar to that shown in Fig. 6.19, although the relative distribution of the bands will depend on the batch of agar used and the initial electrophoresis distance. At the pH of the barbitone buffer (pH 8.2) the γ-globulins are close to their isoelectric point and so would not migrate appreciably in the applied electric field. However, as mentioned earlier, the negative charge on the agar generates an electroendosmotic flow of water in the gel which sweeps the γ-globulins towards the cathode. Often agarose is used as a supporting medium. This has less charge and so generates a lesser electroendosmotic flow.

6.9.3 ## Counterimmunoelectrophoresis

γ-globulins are exceptional in their cathodic migration; most other proteins move to the anode. This property is used to advantage in counterimmunoelectro-

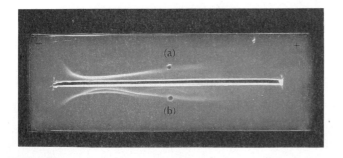

Fig. 6.19 Immunoelectrophoresis of human serum. Sample (**a**): normal human serum showing normal IgG precipitation arc. Sample (**b**): serum of a patient with multiple myeloma, in this case the monoclonal protein is identified as IgG because of the 'bump' in the IgG precipitation arc towards the antiserum well. *Antiserum in central trough*: rabbit anti-human immunoglobulin. (Photograph of unstained preparation.)

phoresis to cause antibody and antigen to migrate towards each other in the gel and form lines of precipitation. The technique is similar to a one-dimensional Ouchterlony immunodiffusion but much faster as it is electrically driven, and more sensitive as all the antigen and antibody are driven towards each other.

Materials and equipment
As for agar electrophoresis (Section 6.9.1)
Human serum albumin, HSA (Appendix II)
Anti-HSA serum

Method
1 Prepare slide as for agar gel electrophoresis (Section 6.9.1).
2 Punch two wells as in Fig. 6.20.
3 Place anti-HSA in the anodal well and HSA in the cathodal well.
4 Run the slide in an electrophoresis tank as before (Section 6.9.1).
5 Examine after 10–15 min.

This technique lends itself to the rapid processing of many antisera or antigens.

6.10 Electrophoresis in antibody-containing media

Just as counterimmunoelectrophoresis is related to Ouchterlony immunodiffusion, electrophoresis in antibody-containing media is related to the single radial immuno-diffusion (SRID) test. Again the speed of counterimmunoelectrophoresis is utilised to provide a fast quantitative assay. As in the SRID test, the antiserum is incorporated into agar and wells are cut into the agar to hold the antigen. When an electric current is applied, the antigen migrates anodally into the agar while the antibody migrates cathodally. At first, soluble complexes are formed in antigen excess. As the antigen migrates further, it becomes more dilute, because antigen is held back in complexes, eventually equivalence is reached and an insoluble precipitate is formed. The precipitate re-dissolves and moves forward as more antigen reaches it. Finally, when no more antigen remains to enter the precipitate, a stable arc is formed which becomes

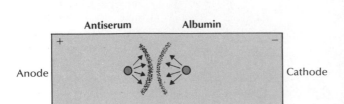

Fig. 6.20 Cross-over electrophoresis. As seen in Section 6.9.1 IgG moves towards the cathode at pH 8.2 because of the electroendosmotic flow; if a negatively charged antigen is used this will move towards the anode and precipitate on contact with the antiserum IgG.

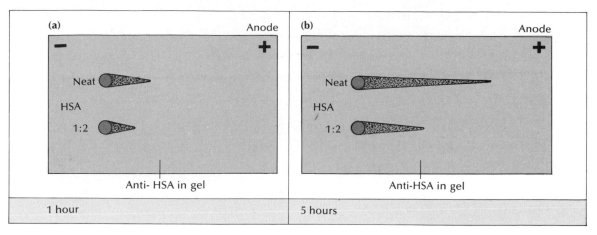

Fig. 6.21 Electrophoresis in antibody-containing media. Precipitates are formed (slide (**a**)) which re-dissolve in antigen excess until equivalence is reached at which point a stationary precipitate forms (slide (**b**)).

stationary. Rocket shapes of precipitation are usually formed and the area under the rockets is proportional to the concentration of antigen (see Figs 6.21 and 6.22).

Materials and equipment
2% agar in barbitone buffer (Section 6.5.1)
Human serum albumin, HSA (Appendix II)
Anti-HSA (Appendix II)
Phosphate-buffered saline, PBS (Appendix I)
Agar pre-coated slides (Section 6.5)
Levelling table
Gel punch
56° water bath
Electrophoresis tank and power pack

Method
1 Melt agar in a microwave oven and allow to cool to 56°.
2 Add antiserum to test tube and dilute for use (as a guide, use 0.1 ml of antiserum and add 0.9 ml PBS).

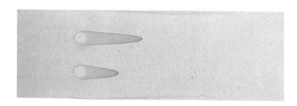

Fig. 6.22 Electrophoresis of human serum albumin (HSA) into agar containing anti-HSA. At equilibrium the height of the precipitation arc is proportional to the antigen concentration.

3 Mix and warm to 56°.

4 Add 2 ml agar to the diluted antiserum and mix.

5 Pour onto pre-coated slides on the levelling table.

6 Punch wells.

7 Fill the wells with antigen solutions—in the range 50–500 µg ml^{-1} should be suitable.

8 Electrophorese at about 8 mA slide^{-1}, 5–10 V cm^{-1}.

9 Run for at least 2 h.

10 The peaks may be measured immediately, but this is easier after staining (Section 6.6.1).

11 Plot the height of the peaks against the antigen concentration if a full standard curve has been determined.

If the slide was run until the precipitin arcs became stationary, the relationship of peak height to antigen concentration is linear.

Technical note

The assay cannot be used directly to quantitate IgG as both the antigen and antibody would be moving in the same direction in the electrophoretic field. However, the electrophoretic mobility of the IgG antigen may be altered by carbamylation.

6.10.1 Carbamylation of IgG

Materials

IgG samples

2 M KCNO (freshly prepared)

Method

1 Mix equal volumes of IgG sample and 2 M KCNO.

2 Incubate at 45° for 30 min.

3 Cool mixture to 10–15° and dilute appropriately with electrophoresis buffer.

6.11 Two-dimensional or crossed immunoelectrophoresis

This development combines the benefits of an electrophoretic separation of antigens with their quantitation by electrophoresis into an antibody-containing gel. The technique was originally introduced for the analysis of serum proteins but it has now been used in many systems. One application that is of particular interest is the analysis of C3 activation. The active and inactive forms of C3 share many antigenic determinants and so are detected simultaneously in simple immunodiffusion assays. However, C3 in its inactive state has a β_{1C} electrophoretic mobility which changes to a β_{1A} mobility after activation. It is therefore possible to show the appearance of activated C3 and the disappearance of inactive C3. The two forms of C3 are first separated by electrophoresis in agarose, and then form rockets of immune precipitates by a second electrophoretic step, at right angles to the first, into a gel containing anti-C3.

Materials and equipment

Barbitone buffer (Appendix I) containing 0.01 M ethylene diamine tetra-acetic acid, EDTA, disodium salt

Agarose

Anti-C3 serum (Appendix II)

Serum samples for C3 quantitation

Glass microscope slide (not pre-coated)

8 × 8 cm glass plate (pre-coated as in Section 6.5.2) (Appendix II)

Electrophoresis tank and power pack

Method

FIRST DIMENSION

1 Prepare a 2% agarose solution in the barbitone buffer containing EDTA (Section 6.5.1).

2 Layer 3 ml of agarose solution onto the microscope slide and allow to set. Use a levelled surface.

3 Cut a 1 mm well in the centre of the slide, remove the agarose plug, and fill the well with the serum sample.

4 Apply a potential difference of 150 V (constant voltage setting on power pack) for 2–3 h.

5 Cut and remove a 5 mm wide longitudinal strip of agarose from the centre portion of the slide, along its complete length. It must, of course, include the sample.

SECOND DIMENSION

1 Prepare 12 ml of a 1 : 50 to 1 : 100 dilution of anti-C3 in 2% agarose solution at 56° (as in Section 6.6); the precise dilution of the antiserum to be used must be determined empirically.

2 Place the agarose strip at one end of the square glass plate (pre-coated) and cover the whole slide with 12 ml of agarose containing anti-C3.

3 Place the plate in the electrophoresis tank. The cathode must be at the end of the plate with the agarose strip, i.e. the electric field will cause the separated complement components to enter the antibody-containing gel at right angles to the first electrophoresis. Electrophorese at 40–50 V overnight (if cooling apparatus is available a higher voltage may be used for a shorter time.)

4 Wash and stain the precipitin arcs (Section 6.6.1).

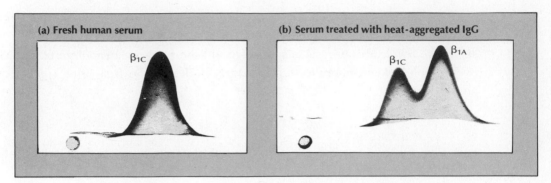

Fig. 6.23 Quantitation of C3 activation. Although the inactive and active forms of C3 share many antigenic determinants, the activation of C3 is accompanied by a change in electrophoretic mobility from β_{1C} to β_{1A}. It is therefore possible to quantitate C3 activation by combining electrophoresis in one dimension with 'rocket' immunoelectrophoresis in the second dimension.

Activation of C3: C1q, C1r, and C1s are linked, probably through calcium, to form a tri-molecular complex. The binding of C1q to the Fc of the immune complex (in this case we have substituted heat-aggregated IgG) initiates the esterase activity of the C1s component which activates C4 and C2. (The complement components were numbered before their order in the activation sequence was known.) The resulting C1.4.2. complex has 'C3 convertase' activity and so splits C3 (β_{1c} mobility) to C3a and C3b (β_{1A} mobility).

The two rocket arcs of C3a and C3b are fused because of shared antigenic determinants.

Fresh serum should give a pattern similar to Fig. 6.23a, while aged serum or serum with immune complexes should give a pattern more like Fig. 6.23b.

6.12 Antibody heretogeneity detected by isoelectric focusing

A mixture of proteins may be resolved into fractions of differing charge by their differential migration in an electric field (Section 6.9.1); however, the resolving power of this system is insufficient to detect minor charge differences. If the electric field is applied across a continuous pH gradient, the proteins will move to, and concentrate at their isoelectric point, i.e. the pH at which their net charge is zero. Unlike ordinary electrophoresis at a single pH, the protein is concentrated to a very narrow band while the electric current is applied.

The product of a single lymphocyte clone, for example a myeloma or hybridoma protein, may be resolved into two to five bands, each differing by a single unit of charge, because of post-synthetic changes in the molecule (Fig. 6.24).

The pH gradient is established using a mixture of carrier ampholytes. These molecules have a 'backbone' on which varying numbers of NH_3^+ and COO^- groups are attached. Under an electric field the ampholyte molecules migrate to their various isoelectric points and produce an ascending pH gradient from the anode to the cathode. Different mixtures of ampholytes are available commercially for various ranges of pH gradient (see Appendix II).

Although the technique described here is applied to the fractionation and identification of antibody molecules, a precisely similar technique can be applied to the analysis of any proteins where charge micro-heterogeneity exists. Further, the technique may be used for the small- or large-scale preparation of ultrapure proteins. In the former case, the pH gradient is stabilised by a Sephadex gel, whereas in the latter, it is formed in a sucrose gradient (Section 8.6).

Well-designed apparatus is now available from several commercial sources. An important feature is the presence of a cooling plate to prevent heating effects in the gel. Gels may be bought ready made, and this is certainly an advantage if only a small number are being run. It is, however, quite possible to pour ones own plates either using proprietary apparatus or alternatively making a mould as in Fig. 6.25.

Materials and equipment

Samples for analysis; for example, IgG isolated by ion-exchange chromatography (Section 8.5) or hybridoma antibody (Chapter 12)

Stock solutions for gel:

(a) N,N,N',N'-tetramethylene diamine (5% v/v)

(b) Acrylamide, 100 g, and N,N'-bismethylacrylamide 3 g dissolved in 300 ml with water

(c) Riboflavin, 2 mg in 100 ml water

Stock subbing solutions:

(a) Ilford No. 1 gelatine powder (5% w/v)

(b) Potassium chromium sulphate (1% w/v)

Ampholine, pH range for example 3–10 (Appendix II)

Ethylene diamine (5% v/v)

Phosphoric acid (5% v/v)

Staining and de-staining solutions as in Section 2.10.1.

Glass plates, 7.5 × 15 cm (as in Fig. 6.25) (Appendix II)

Electrophoresis tank with cooling plate

Power pack (500 V)

Whatman 3 MM filter paper (Appendix II)

6.12.1   Preparation of the gel

The gel may be prepared by chemical polymerisation using ammonium persulphate, but photopolymerisation with riboflavin is preferable as this avoids the risk of artifacts resulting from the action of persulphate on the sample.

For a 7.5 × 15 cm gel about 10 ml of solution is required.

1   Mix 0.05 ml stock solution (a) with 1.5 ml solution (b), plus 0.5 ml of 40% Ampholine carrier ampholytes and make up to 10 ml with water.

2   De-gas the mixture with a vacuum pump until bubbling ceases.

3   Add 1 ml of solution (c). Briefly gas solution with CO_2 until pH is 6.5. This is required because of the instability of riboflavin at a higher pH.

4   Cast the gel immediately.

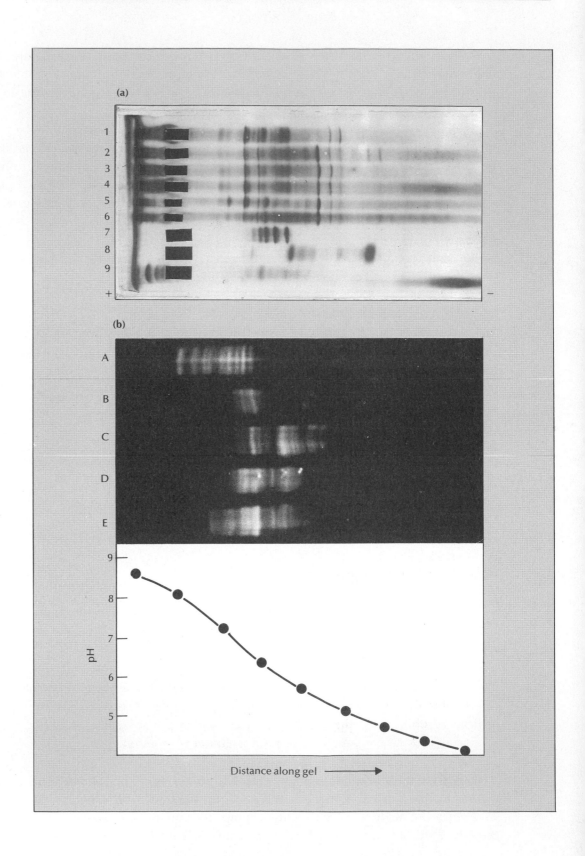

(a)

(b)

pH

Distance along gel

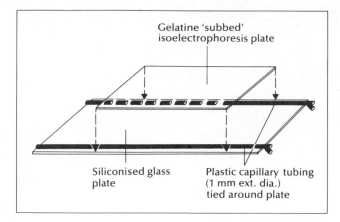

Fig. 6.25 Mould for casting thin-layer polyacrylamide gels. Run the 'gel solution' between the glass plates and, after photopolymerization, remove the siliconized plate with a scalpel blade.

6.12.2   Casting the gel

1 Dip the electrofocusing plate in the 0.1% gelatine 'subbing' solution containing 0.01% potassium chromium sulphate and air dry. If the electrofocusing tank being used does not require that the gel be inverted or you wish to separate the gel from its glass plate after running, do not sub the plate.

2 Siliconise the second plate (Section 1.16) and attach the polyethylene capillary tubing.

3 Assemble the mould as in Fig. 6.25.

Fig. 6.24 (*Facing page*) **(a) Serum isoelectric spectra: thin-layer polyacrylamide gel electrofocusing (5% gel, pH range 5–10)**. Samples were loaded on to filter-paper strips of various size depending upon the loading volume. After focusing, the plate was stained with Coomassie brilliant blue dye. *Samples 1–6*: serum samples from individual mice challenged with an antigen of very few determinants. Under these conditions, it is possible to limit the number of different lymphocyte clones stimulated and therefore an analysis of the resulting antibody is possible in terms of its isolectric spectrum. The migration of two antibodies from two different mice to the same position in the same pH gradient may be used as a criterion of clonal identity. This has been used, for example, to determine the frequency with which a single clone repeats within a population of mice.

It should be noted that in this case we are comparing proteins alone as no method has been used to demonstrate antibody activity in any of the observed bands (cf. section on identification of antibody, Section 6.12.6).

Samples 7–9 are myeloma proteins isolated by DEAE-cellulose chromatography. Each sample was eluted as a single peak.

Sample 7: IgG2a myeloma. The five bands probably result from a single clone of plasma cells. The spectrum of pI values could result from post-synthetic enzymic changes after secretion into the serum, or from differences in the glycosylation of the myeloma. Even though every molecule of immunoglobulin from a single clone has the same amino acid sequence the pattern of glycosylation is likely to be heterogeneous.

Sample 8: IgG2b myeloma. This preparation has at least three major contaminants.

Sample 9: IgA myeloma, partially purified. This protein is more basic and so has migrated towards the anode. To resolve this sample satisfactorily it would be necessary to use a lower pH range.

(b) Isoelectric spectrum of anti-DNP antibodies from CBA/J mice. Sera from X-irradiated CBA/J mice receiving column fractionated spleen cells (as in Section 9.10) were focused (Section 6.12) and then treated with ^{125}I-labelled DNP–HOP–lysine. Antigen-binding bands were detected by autoradiography with X-ray film.

4 Pipette 10 ml of the gel mixture into the mould and expose to UV light for 2–3 h to polymerise the gel. (This should be done in a humid atmosphere.)

5 Prise away the siliconised plate and store the gel in a humid box at 4° until use. (Cast gels may be stored in this way for 2–3 weeks. The small amount of expressed acrylic acid is an excellent bacteriostat.)

6.12.3 Sample application

1 Pipette about 10 µl of sample (10–20 mg ml^{-1}) onto a 10 × 5 mm square of Whatman 3 MM paper.

2 Place the paper on the gel surface towards the anodal end. Leave the paper in place during the electrofocusing. Several samples may be placed on the gel at the same time (as in Fig. 6.24a).

6.12.4 Electrofocusing

The precise details will depend on the design and sophistication of the apparatus. Apply the current. The maximum power per plate must not exceed 500 mW to avoid excessive heating and distortion of the gel. As the pH gradient is established the current will fall and so the voltage may be increased. An integrating power supply will do this automatically once the maximum power level has been set.

The following table will provide a guide if the voltages are to be set manually (use constant voltage setting on power pack):

Time (h)	Voltage (V)	Corresponding current (mA)
0 – 4	150	3
4 to overnight	250–300	1.5–2
last 3 h	500	<1

A higher power may be used if an efficient cooling plate is available.

6.12.5 Examination of the gel

MEASUREMENT OF THE PH GRADIENT

Ideally the pH along the gel should be measured directly using a flat membrane electrode or, if rainbow markers (Appendix II) have been used, with a ruler. If neither of these techniques are possible the ampholytes must be eluted from the gel:

1 Remove 5 mm discs of gel with a sharp cork borer at close intervals along the plate (away from the sample tracks).

2 Disperse each disc in 1 ml freshly distilled water for 2 h.

3 Measure the pH with a micro-electrode.

STAINING THE PROTEIN BANDS

Many protein stains are unsuitable as they bind to the ampholytes as well as the proteins. The following procedure is suitable without ampholyte removal:

1 Immerse the gel in the Coomassie brilliant blue staining solution for 30 min (see Section 2.10.1).
2 Differentiate in the de-staining solution until the background is clear.

INTERPRETATION OF RESULTS

The major difficulty with this technique is the embarrassing number of protein bands resolved, even with so-called 'purified' proteins. The IgG from normal serum will give so many lines that any real interpretation is impossible, except to give some idea of the heterogeneity of immunoglobulins.

Hybridoma protein should be more restricted. If the previous isolation steps have been thorough, only four or five bands should be seen. When monoclonal proteins are isolated directly from the cells a single predominant molecular species may be seen. After contact with serum for just 1 h, post-synthetic modifications occur producing the multiple bands resolved by isoelectric focusing. However, even when first secreted, heterogeneity may exist as the oligosaccharide chains can differ in their sugar sequences, even within the products of one clone of cells.

6.12.6 Identification of antibody

In contrast to SDS-PAGE (Section 2.10 and 8.4), proteins separated by isoelectric focusing are not exposed to any harmful detergents or reducing agents and should retain most of their antibody activity. It is possible to detect individual species of antibody reacting with a particular hapten by autoradiography following radio-labelled hapten binding. When sera are focused on the same plate it is possible to identify common clonal products between individual sera (Fig. 6.24). Because of their size, IgM molecules are not included in conventional polyacrylamide gels and so cannot be analysed by the system described. This is not, however, a problem if agarose is used instead of polyacrylamide or during preparative isoelectric focusing using a sucrose density gradient. The tendency for these large molecules to precipitate at their isoelectric point may be overcome by using 6 M urea in the medium.

6.13 Secondary interactions: agglutination

Particulate antigens may be cross-linked by antibody to give visible agglutination in a manner analogous to the formation of precipitates with soluble antigens. The agglutination reaction has principally been exploited using red cells as the particles and, as might be expected, the reaction is of vital importance in blood grouping. Other particles such as latex and bentonite suspensions have also proved useful. Antisera may be compared semi-quantitatively by determining the end points of their respective titration curves. The sera are diluted until they no longer give a visible reaction with antigen by agglutination. This is a measure of the relative antigen-binding capacity of a serum and can only be used to compare antisera when they are tested at the same time and with the same antigen.

Conversely, the concentration of an antigen in solution may be determined by the degree of inhibition of a standard, homologous agglutination system.

6.14 Haemagglutination

The simplest form of this test involves the agglutination of erythrocytes (as antigens) by increasing dilutions of anti-erythrocyte sera.

Materials and equipment
Anti-sheep erythrocyte sera, anti-SRBC (Appendix II and Section 6.14.1)
Normal serum, as control
SRBC in phosphate-buffered saline, PBS, 2 % v/v (Appendix II)
0.1 M 2-mercaptoethanol in PBS
Micro-haemagglutination trays (V-shaped) (Appendix II)
Diluting loops or tulips (25 µl) (Appendix II)
Standard dropping pipettes (25 µl) Appendix II) or multi-channel automatic pipette
    (Appendix II)
Sealer strip (Appendix II)

PREPARATION IN ADVANCE
Aged sera may be used directly but fresh sera must first be incubated at 56° for 30 min to inactivate complement.

Method
For each antiserum and control serum prepare two rows of dilutions as follows:
1 Add 25 µl of PBS to all the test wells with the dropping or multi-channel pipette. (Hold the dropping pipette vertically to deliver precisely 25 µl.)
2 Flame the diluting loops to incandescence in a Bunsen flame and quench in distilled water.
3 Blot the tips of the loops on absorbent paper. (Do not dry around the outside.)
4 Touch the meniscus of the test serum with the tip of the loop. (This will collect exactly 25 µl of serum provided the loop is not immersed in the serum.)
5 Put the loop in the first well of the tray. Repeat for a second row of the same serum.
6 Rotate the loops in the wells, take care not to grind away at the plastic surface, lift out cleanly and rotate in the next well. Repeat to the end of the plate.
7 Add 25 µl of PBS to each well of the left-hand row of each replicate pair of dilutions.
8 Add 25 µl of 0.1 M 2-mercaptoethanol in PBS to each well of the right-hand

dilutions. (This reagent is toxic and so this and all subsequent steps *must* be carried out in a fume cupboard.)

9 Add 25 µl of SRBC suspension to all the wells used, and 25 µl to an empty well, as control. (Add 50 µl of PBS to this control well.)

10 Cover the tray with a sealer strip and mix the contents of the wells by gentle shaking.

11 Leave the tray at room temperature for 1 h.

Assessment of results

Read the plate either on a white surface or using a magnifying mirror (Appendix II). A typical pattern of agglutination is shown in Fig. 6.26. Positive agglutination is seen when the cells form a continuous carpet on the base of the cup. If no agglutination has occurred the cells fall as a tight button to the bottom of the V-shaped cup. If round-bottomed wells are used the non-agglutinated cells form a ring around the bottom. The 2-mercaptoethanol in each right-hand row of the duplicate dilutions

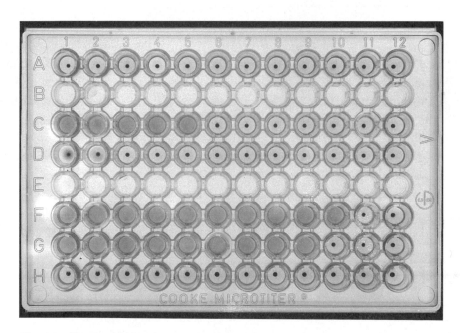

Fig. 6.26 Haemagglutination test on primary and secondary response antisera. Doubling dilutions left to right along the plate starting at 1:2, antigen:sheep erythrocytes.

Well A: normal mouse serum, pre-immunization bleed.

Well C: mouse serum from an animal 5 days after one intraperitoneal injection of 10^8 sheep erythrocytes.

Well D: as for C but with 1 drop of 2-mercaptoethanol (0.1 M).

Well F: mouse serum from an animal 7 days after third injection of 10^8 sheep erythrocytes (previous injections given at 0, 10 and 29 days).

Well G: as for F but with 1 drop of 0.1 M 2-mercaptoethanol.

Well H: sheep erythrocytes alone.

   (Note in wells not receiving 2-mercaptoethanol, 1 drop of saline was added to equalize the dilution effect.)

reduces the disulphide bonds holding together the subunits of the IgM pentamer so that it is no longer able to agglutinate the cells. The titre of the 2-mercaptoethanol-resistant antibody is roughly equivalent to that of the IgG in the serum, and so the greater titre obtained without 2-mercaptoethanol is due to the IgM. A more exact estimate of the IgG and IgM agglutination titres may be determined using indirect haemagglutination with specific anti-class sera.

Technical notes

1 Many antisera or normal human sera contain spontaneous anti-SRBC antibodies (heterophile antibodies). These are usually of low titre ($< 1:10$).

2 The final concentration of SRBC in the trays may be varied from 0.5 to 1.5%. If the cells are valuable, for example RBC coupled with a soluble antigen, a lower concentration may be used for reasons of economy.

3 The haemagglutination test detects IgM antibodies preferentially not only because of the multi-valency of this antibody, but also because of the relatively large size of IgM. Hence, as erythrocytes are further apart when agglutinated by IgM compared with IgG, the repulsive force which is due to the cell's ζ potential is less.

4 You should not see any spontaneous agglutination of red cells in the control well. This is seldom a problem with fresh cells as they have a high negative ζ potential which causes the cells to repel each other. When erythrocytes are coupled to soluble antigens, however, the surface charge is often reduced and so spontaneous agglutination may occur. This is discussed in Section 6.14.3, Technical notes.

5 Greater sensitivity may be obtained with U-shaped wells if the cells are allowed to sediment in the normal way and the plate then tilted to an angle of 45 degrees. Unagglutinated cells stream to the edge, whereas cross-linked cells are fixed in place by antibody.

6 Agglutinated and unagglutinated erythrocytes have different light-scattering properties, this may be quantitated using an ELISA reader (Section 10.6).

6.14.1 Primary versus secondary antibody response

In the primary response there is an early production of IgM antibody which soon declines and is replaced by IgG. In contrast, IgG production is greatly accelerated in the secondary response (Fig. 6.26), the peak titre is attained rapidly and declines slowly. There appears to be no accelerated IgM production, the kinetics are essentially that of the primary response.

The differences between these two responses can be conveniently demonstrated using haemagglutination, comparing the total and 2-mercaptoethanol-resistant antibody titres of sera taken from mice immunised with sheep erythrocytes (SRBC) as follows:

(a) 2×10^8 SRBC given i.p., bleed 3–4 days later.

(b) 2×10^8 SRBC given i.p. on day 0 and day 7, bleed 7 days later.

6.14.2 Agglutination of antigen-coated erythrocytes

Erythrocytes may be coupled to soluble antigens by various methods and agglutinated by antisera to the coupled antigens.

(a) Spontaneous uptake. Erythrocytes will adsorb polysaccharides to their surface during incubation. Although this is a non-covalent binding, there is very little leaching off of the antigen during the assay.

(b) Coupling to chemically modified erythrocytes.

6.14.3 Tanned erythrocytes

This procedure is suitable for many protein antigens; in the method below human serum albumin is used.

Materials
Sheep erythrocytes, SRBC, in Alsever's solution (Appendix II)
Phosphate−saline buffer (Appendix I)
Borate−succinate buffer (Appendix I)
Saline (Appendix I)
Tannic acid
Human serum albumin, HSA (Appendix II)
40% aqueous formaldehyde

Method
1 Wash SRBC three times with 40 volumes of saline by centrifugation (300 g for 10 min).
2 Adjust SRBC suspension to 40% v/v in phosphate−saline buffer, pH 7.5.
3 Add 2.5 mg of tannic acid to 50 ml of phosphate−saline buffer and mix with 50 ml of 4% SRBC suspension.
4 Incubate at 37° for 15 min.
5 Spin down cells very gently (100 g for 20 min). If the cells are pelleted too quickly they will agglutinate.
6 Divide the cells into two aliquots, and wash each with 50 ml phosphate−saline buffer by centrifugation (100 g for 20 min). One aliquot will be used for antigen coating and the other as control cells.
7 Re-suspend 1 aliquot of cells in 50 ml phosphate−saline buffer and add 50 ml of HSA solution (2 mg ml^{-1} initial concentration).
8 Incubate at 37° for 30 min.
9 Wash in phosphate−saline buffer by gentle centrifugation and re-suspend in 100 ml of borate−succinate buffer.
10 Re-suspend the second aliquot of cells in 100 ml of borate−succinate buffer. The control cells are not coated and are used both to absorb the test antisera and as control cells in the assay.

11 Add 10 ml of 40% formalin to both cell suspensons while stirring. The formalin must be added dropwise during 20–30 min.

12 Leave overnight at 4° and add a further 10 ml of formalin to both suspensions.

13 Leave the cells to settle (24 h) and pour off the supernatant.

14 Add a large volume of borate–succinate buffer and re-suspend the cells by vigorous shaking.

15 Allow cells to settle (24 h) and wash again by sedimentation in borate–succinate buffer.

16 Adjust both cell suspensions to 1% v/v and add 0.2% formalin (final concentration) as a preservative.

The cells can be stored at 4° for up to 2 years.

Assay procedure

Materials and equipment

As for Section 6.14, but use antigen (HSA)-coated erythrocytes (SRBC) and control erythrocytes as prepared above together with appropriate antiserum.

Method

1 Titrate the antiserum as described in Section 6.14, but use an initial dilution of 1 : 5 (100 μl of buffer to the first well) (*omit* the 2-mercaptoethanol from the left-hand row and the 25 μl of buffer from the right-hand row).

2 Add 25 μl of the 1% suspension of HSA-coated SRBC to the right-hand row of dilutions.

3 Add 25 μl of 1% control (uncoated but tanned) SRBC to the left-hand row of dilutions.

4 Place 25 μl of coated and uncoated cells in two separate empty wells to test for spontaneous agglutination. (Add 25 μl of buffer to each of these control wells.)

5 Gently shake and leave to stand for 1 h.

Again, positive agglutination is seen when the cells form a continuous carpet on the base of the cup.

Technical notes

1 If agglutination occurs with control cells the antiserum must be absorbed to remove heterophile antibodies as follows:
   a Add 0.1 ml of serum to 1 ml of packed control cells.
   b Incubate at 37° for 10 min and spin off the erythrocytes.
   c Repeat the agglutination assay and re-absorb if necessary.

2 If the coated or control cells agglutinate spontaneously, add 1% normal serum to the buffers used in the assay.

Antigens may also be coupled to erythrocytes using bisdiazotised benzidine, glutaraldehyde and chromic chloride. The basic principles are similar to those described above and the exact technical details may be found in the references cited at the end of this chapter. Other particles such as bentonite or latex may be used as antigen carriers for agglutination tests. They have the advantage of not being antigenic but have a more limited range of applications than the antigen-coated erythrocyte assay described above.

6.14.4 Indirect agglutination

IgG antibodies are less efficient at agglutinating red cells. Addition of 25 µl of 1% bovine serum albumin to each well can sometimes enhance the agglutination. Otherwise the addition of a second antibody can be used. The red cells should be gently centrifuged down, the supernatant removed, and the red cells gently re-suspended in 50 µl of suitably diluted anti-IgG.

6.14.5 Latex agglutination

Latex beads provide a convenient carrier for antigens in agglutination tests. They have not yet achieved the popularity of erythrocytes, perhaps because it is not so easy to perform quantitative assays in micro-titre plates with these beads. However, sophisticated equipment has been developed to quantitate the degree of agglutination of the latex beads very accurately. This apparatus has led to a whole new field of immunoassay known as particle-counting immunoassay which has a sensitivity approaching that of radioimmunoassay. It is, however, simple to set up basic slide agglutination tests without any expensive equipment.

Coating the beads with antigen is not difficult especially when using IgG or albumin as these antigens adsorb readily to polystyrene latex. However, many proteins, including immunoglobulin isotypes other than IgG, bind less well and require covalent coupling with carbodiimide.

Latex coating

Materials
Latex suspension, 10% w/v (Appendix II)
Antigen; for example, IgG
0.27 M and 0.054 M glycine–saline buffer, pH 8.2 (Appendix I)

Method
1   Wash 800 µl latex suspension twice by adding 40 ml 0.054 M glycine–saline; mix and centrifuge at 12 500 g for 15 min.

2 Re-suspend the latex in 20 ml 0.054 M glycine–saline and add 300 µl of a 10 mg ml^{-1} solution of antigen.

3 Mix the suspension for 30 min at room temperature.

4 Wash the latex two times by adding 40 ml 0.054 M glycine–saline; mix and centrifuge the latex 12 500 g for 15 min.

5 Re-suspend the latex in 20 ml 0.27 M glycine–saline containing 0.1% of an irrelevant protein to block any remaining protein-binding sites and store at 4°.

Slide agglutination

Materials
Antigen-coated latex (as above)
Specific antiserum
0.27 M glycine–saline buffer, pH 8.2 (Appendix I)

Method
1 Prepare doubling dilutions of the test antiserum.
2 Mix 25 µl of each antiserum dilution with 25 µl coated latex on a glass slide.
3 Rock gently for 2 min and read agglutination visually, illuminating the slide from the side, against a dark background.

Technical note
It is advisable to dilute the sera for use, as a prozone effect (where no agglutination is seen at the highest concentrations of serum) can easily occur.

Applications
Several commercial latex agglutination tests are available, one of the most widely used being that for the detection of autoantibodies in rheumatoid arthritis. Patients with rheumatoid arthritis often develop antibodies to 'self IgG'. This anti-globulin antibody, known as rheumatoid factor, is readily detected by its ability to agglutinate latex particles coated with IgG.

6.14.6 Blood grouping

A simple slide agglutination test may be used for demonstrating blood grouping.

Materials
Standard Group A serum or monoclonal antibody (Appendix II)
Standard Group B serum or monoclonal antibody (Appendix II)
Human erythrocytes

Method
1 Adjust the erythrocyte suspension to approximately 4% v/v and place 2 separate drops on a glass slide.

2 Add 1 drop of group A serum to the first drop of erythrocytes, and 1 drop of group B serum to the second.

3 Rock the slide and observe the agglutination over 5 min.

To avoid a transfusion reaction it is necessary to cross-match the donor and recipient blood. One drop of recipient serum is mixed with donor cells and vice versa. If no agglutination occurs in either combination, the donor and recipient are compatible. Slide agglutination has now been largely replaced by a tube agglutination test which, among other advantages, offers greater sensitivity.

AGGLUTINATION REACTIONS

Blood group	Standard antiserum*		Saline
	Anti-A (group B serum)	Anti-B (group A serum)	
O	−	−	−
A	+	−	−
B	−	+	−
AB	+	+	−

* A full typing reaction would normally include anti-AB serum from an O donor to detect the rare A samples not agglutinated with anti-A.

The only other blood-group antigens for which donor and recipient must be routinely typed is the rhesus or Rh system; the most important antigen of which is the Rh_0 or D antigen. Red cells are typed as positive or negative using an anti-D(Rh_0) serum.

Rhesus incompatibility

If a Rh_0 positive child is borne to a Rh_0-negative mother there is a danger of sensitisation to the D antigen following the escape of fetal cells into the maternal circulation at parturition. Two classes of antibody have been detected in this situation: one which is able to induce agglutination of D-positive erythrocytes and later shown to be IgM. The second type of antibody could not induce agglutination and was originally referred to as incomplete antibody (a misnomer as will be seen later). This second antibody belongs to the IgG class. Clinically the IgG anti-D antibody is of much greater importance as this class alone is able to cross the placenta. Thus during a second pregnancy with a Rh_0 positive fetus, anti-D antibody may enter the fetal circulation and bring about the destruction of fetal erythrocytes by the processes described in Section 5.8.4.

Anti-D antibodies may be detected using rabbit anti-human immunoglobulin antibodies which cross-link IgG anti-D in the presence of a serum−BSA mixture (the latter mixture is used to reduce the red cell surface charge and so facilitate agglutination).

6.15

Immunoglobulin idiotypes

When an animal is immunised with a monoclonal immunoglobulin from another species it responds by making antibodies against many different parts of the foreign molecule: anti-Fc, anti-Fab, anti-light chain and anti-heavy chain. Antibodies are produced against the constant region and also against the variable region. These antibodies directed against the variable region form the anti-idiotype antibodies. If the resultant antiserum is absorbed with pooled serum from a normal donor all the antibodies against constant region determinants will be absorbed out, but those directed against the variable region will remain. The antiserum will now constitute a specific anti-idiotypic serum. Anti-idiotypic antibodies may also be prepared using hybridoma technology. In this case no absorption will be necessary as each anti-idiotype will be specifically directed against a unique variable region determinant. Anti-idiotypes may also be induced against polyclonal antibodies directed against a specific antigen.

6.15.1

Production of anti-idiotypes

The production of anti-idiotype antibodies does not differ in principle from the production of any other type of antibody. The following protocol works well in our experience for the production of monoclonal anti-idiotype antibodies.

Method

1 Concentrate and purify the monoclonal antibody. In the case of tissue culture supernatants, purification by ammonium sulphate precipitation will probably be sufficient (Section 8.1), whereas separation from polyclonal immunoglobulin will be necessary with ascitic fluid (Section 12.8).
2 Give a total of three subcutaneous injections of 50 μg of purified monoclonal antibody to BALB/c mice, with an interval of 2 weeks between each injection. For the first injection the antibody should be combined with Freund's complete adjuvant (Section 1.7.1), for the second use incomplete Freund's adjuvant and in the third the antibody should be adsorbed onto alum (Section 1.8).
3 Give each mouse a final intravenous boost with 20–50 μg antibody 3 days prior to removing the spleens for fusion.
4 Fuse the spleen cell suspensions with the hybridoma parent by conventional hybridoma technology (Chapter 12).
5 Screen each hybridoma supernatant against idiotype and normal immunoglobulin of the same subclass, using radio or enzyme immunoassay (Section 10.4 or 10.5).

16.15.2

Idiotypic networks

A major stimulus to work on idiotypes has been the network hypothesis of Jerne in which it was proposed that lymphocytes formed a network through interactions

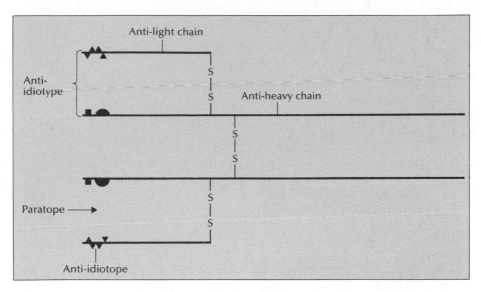

Fig. 6.27 Anti-idiotypes and idiotopes. All regions of the immunoglobulin molecule
are potentially immunogenic. Antibodies raised against constant region
determinants of the light or heavy chains will cross-react with other immunoglobulins
from the same species. Antibodies may also be produced against the variable region.
Polyclonal antisera will bind a range of determinants — anti-idiotype sera, whereas
individual monoclonal antibodies will recognize individual idiotopes.

between idiotypes and anti-idiotypes on different lymphocytes. The physiological
significance of such a network is still the subject of discussion, but manipulation of
the immune response by anti-idiotypes has been shown to be a potent means of
both enhancing and suppressing immune responses.

6.16 Summary and conclusions

The rate of association between antibody and antigen is very rapid and largely
dependent on the rates of diffusion of the molecules towards each other. The
dissociation rate is usually much slower and varies for different antibodies. It is this
difference in dissociation rate which contributes to the variations in equilibrium
constant—antibody affinity. This concept of antibody affinity applies only to
homogeneous systems with monovalent hapten and single antibody-combining sites.
More often, in the real world, multi-valent antigens are binding to antibodies
possessing from two to 10 combining sites. This multi-valent reaction leads to the
formation of complexes of variable size depending on the ratio of antibody : antigen.
The quantitative precipitin curve demonstrates the full range of complexes from
antibody to antigen excess.

The concept of the formation of complexes of variable size, some of which are
soluble, is of importance not only for the interpretation of the patterns of precipitation
in gels, but also for understanding the different *in vivo* pathological processes which
may occur with changes in complex size. The presence of high concentrations of

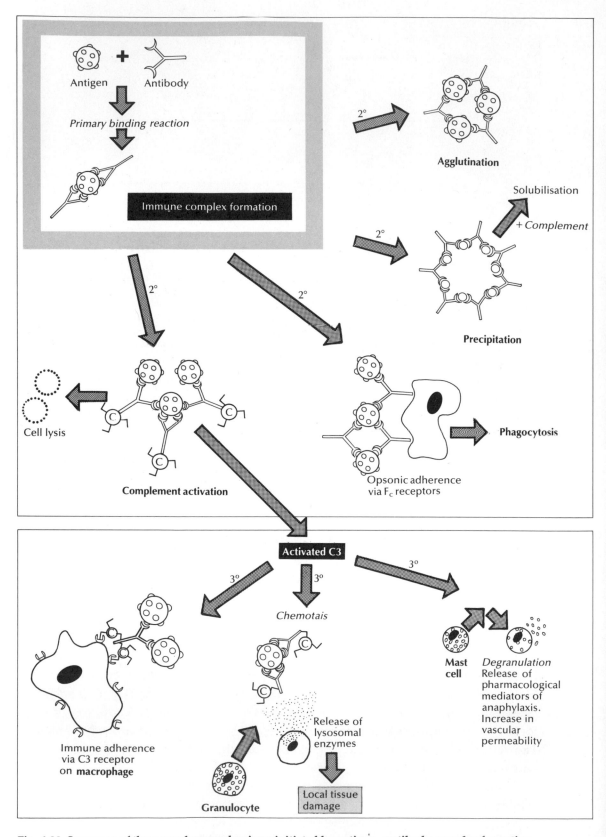

Fig. 6.28 Summary of the secondary mechanisms initiated by antigen–antibody complex formation.

soluble complexes may give rise to immune complex-mediated hypersensitivity (Sections 5.8.5 and 14.6) with all the associated immunopathological complications.

Once complex formation commences, further secondary effector functions may be activated (Fig. 6.28). These are dependent upon the Fc region; even for effective precipitation an intact Fc region is necessary. To understand all the implications of an antigen−antibody interaction it is necessary to consider the following:

(a)   Amounts of antibody and antigen.
(b)   Affinity of the combination.
(c)   Antibody class and sometimes subclass.
(d)   Associated biological activity of antibody, antigen and complex.

6.17

Further reading

Axelsen NH (1983) Handbook of precipitation in gel techniques. *Scand. J. Immunol.* **17**, Suppl. 10.

Dunhar BS (1987) *Two-dimensional Electrophoresis and Immunological Techniques.* Plenum, London.

Marchalonis JJ and Warr GW (editors) (1982) *Antibody as a Tool: the Applications of Immunochemistry.* John Wiley and Sons, Chichester.

Mayer RJ and Walker JH (editors) (1987) *Immunochemical Methods in Cell and Molecular Biology.* Academic Press, New York.

Ouchterlony O and Nilsson LA (1986) Immunodiffusion and immunoelectrophoresis. In *Handbook of Experimental Immunology*, Weir DM (editor), volume 1, 4th edition. Blackwell Scientific Publications, Oxford.

Steward MW (1986) Introduction to methods used to study the affinity and kinetics of antibody/antigen reactions. In *Handbook of Experimental Immunolgy*, Weir DM (editor), volume 1, 4th edition. Blackwell Scientific Publications, Oxford.

Vunakis HV and Langonc JJ (editors) (1986 onwards) Immunochemical Techniques. In the *Methods in Enzymology* series, volumes 70, 73, 74, 84, 92 and 93. Academic Press, New York.

7 Complement

Antigen−antibody interaction can result in a visible expression of complex formation such as precipitation or agglutination. These complexes can, in turn, activate several accessory systems such as complement fixation and phagocytosis. The complement pathway is a multi-component system of at least 20 different serum proteins which are present in normal serum in an inactive state. In the absence of other information, the importance of the complement components could be inferred from their high concentration in plasma; about 3 mg ml^{-1} of total complement protein. For convenience, the complement system may be considered in three parts: (a) the classical pathway, which is activated by immune complexes, (b) the alternative pathway which is activated directly by certain microorganisms or fed by activated components from the classical pathway (both the classical and alternative pathway have the cleavage of C3, the major component of complement, as their principle activity); and (c) the lytic, membrane-attack pathway, which is a common route from the earlier pathways to cell lysis.

The complement system is a triggered enzyme cascade in which each component activates several molecules of the next component. This amplification of the original signal, therefore, can result in a potent cytotoxic activity. The other effector functions of complement are triggered before the assembly of the full membrane attack complex and, in many situations, they are probably more important than cell lysis in protection of the host. These secondary effector functions include:

(a) Adherence, via receptors for activated C3b on many cell types; for example, primate erythrocytes, neutrophils, basophils, lymphocytes and dendritic cells.

(b) Anaphylotoxin activity, mediated by C3a and C5a causing the release of mediators and enzymes from cells such as basophils and mast cells.

(c) Chemotaxis, by C3a and $\overline{C567}$.

7.1 Total haemolytic complement

The lysis of antibody-coated erythrocytes has long been used as a means of estimating the complement activity of a serum. As complement is added to antibody-coated erythrocytes an increasing proportion of the cells are lysed as shown in Fig. 7.1. As the curve approaches 100% lysis asymptotically, it is difficult to determine the total lytic unit of complement (CH_{100}) and so one normally defines the 50% lysis point (CH_{50}).

The von Krogh equation for the sigmoid dose−response curve of complement-mediated cytolysis was derived empirically and, in its basic form, may be written as:

$$x = k \left\{ \frac{y}{100 - y} \right\}^{1/n}$$

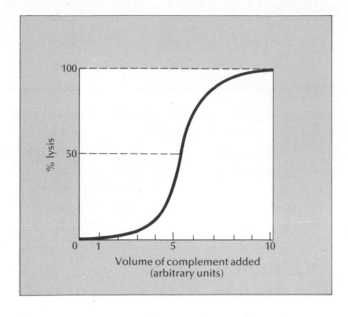

Fig. 7.1 Lysis of sheep erythrocytes (SRBC), sensitized by horse anti-SRBC, in the presence of human complement. The curve of complement-mediated lysis approaches the 100% lysis value asymptotically and so accurate determinations of serum complement levels are made on the 50% lysis point as shown in the graph.

where:

x = amount of complement (ml of undiluted serum),
y = proportion of cells lysed,
k = 50% unit of complement,
n is a constant.

The CH_{50} unit is determined under standardised conditions which depend upon:
(a)   Erythrocyte and antibody concentration.
(b)   Buffering conditions of the medium.
(c)   Temperature.
Hence, the definition of the CH_{50} unit is arbitrary and depends wholly on the conditions used. The assay may be performed in tubes, without reference to a standard or in agar with reference to a standard serum.

7.1.1   ## Standardization of erythrocytes

Materials and equipment
Barbitone-buffered saline for complement tests (Appendix I) (this contains essential calcium and magnesium ions)
Sheep erythrocytes, SRBC, in Alsever's solution (Appendix II)
0.04% ammonia solution
Serum, this should be fresh , or guinea-pig serum preserved specially for complement fixation assays (Appendix II)
Horse haemolytic serum (source of anti-erythrocyte antibody) (Appendix II)
Spectrophotometer

Method

1 Dilute the barbitone-buffered saline to working strength. Check for fungal or bacterial contamination, as these are anti-complementary.
2 Wash 4 ml of the erythrocyte suspension (supplied at *c.* 25% v/v in Alsever's solution) three times in barbitone-buffered saline (200 g for 3 min).
3 Re-suspend the washed erythrocytes in 15 ml of barbitone-buffered saline (use a measuring cylinder).
4 Mix 1 ml of erythrocytes with 25 ml of ammonia solution to lyse the cells and read the absorbance at 541 nm. For a 6% SRBC suspension, in a 1 cm cuvette, the absorbance should be 0.48−0.50. Adjust the suspension as required.
5 Mix 15 ml barbitone-buffered saline, 0.1 ml of horse haemolytic serum and 15 ml of 6% SRBC. Strictly, the anti-erythrocyte serum should be titred until the highest dilution still giving full complement fixation is reached; however, for most purposes it is sufficient to use a 1 : 150 dilution.
6 Incubate at 37° for 15 min.

This method is for the preparation of 30 ml of 3% v/v sheep erythrocytes, use the sensitised cells within 24 h.

7.1.2 Estimation of CH_{50} tube assay

Method

1 Set up the tubes as in the Protocol and remember to use fresh or specially preserved serum as the complement source.
2 Incubate at 37° for 60 min.
3 Place the tubes on ice and add 2 ml of buffer to each tube.
4 Centrifuge at 200 g for 10 min at 4°.
5 Remove a sample of each supernatant (tubes 1−7) and read their absorbance at 541 nm.

Protocol

	Tube numbers						
	1	2	3	4	5	6	7
Buffer (ml)	1.10	1.05	1.00	0.90	0.80	1.20	1.20 ml of ammonia solution
Guinea-pig serum (ml) initial dil. 1 : 30	0.10	0.15	0.20	0.30	0.40	0.00	
Sensitised erythrocytes (ml) suspension	0.3 ————————————————————————→						

Calculation of results
1 Assuming that tube 7 represents total lysis, calculate the % lysis for each tube.
2 Plot the % lysis against the complement concentration (ml of undiluted serum). This will yield a sigmoid curve as in Fig. 7.1.

This dose–response curve follows the von Krogh equation given earlier. However, this equation may be logarithmically transformed so that the data fall on a straight line:

$$\log x = \log k + 1/n \log \left\{ \frac{y}{100 - y} \right\}$$

where terms defined as previously (Section 7.1).

3 Plot $\log x$ against $\log [y/(100-y)]$ for each dilution of complement used. The straight line has a slope of $1/n$ (the exact value depends on experimental conditions, but it should be within 20% of 0.2). The abscissa intercept of the line, where $\log [y/(100-y)] = 0$, is the log dilution resulting in 50% lysis. The complement level of a serum is normally expressed as the number of CH_{50} units ml^{-1} of serum.

Technical notes
1 Complement components are highly labile and so fresh serum must be prepared by clotting the blood at 4°. Preserved guinea-pig serum is available commercially, in which the complement components are stabilised by lyophilisation of serum in a hypertonic salt solution.
2 The whole assay may be made more sensitive, and use less reagents if the red cells are radiolabelled with ^{51}Cr (Section 7.5.2) for the radioisotopic variant of this assay.

7.1.3 Estimation of CH_{100} by assay in agar

The amount of complement in a serum may be determined accurately using the tube assay above; however, a much simpler assay, which is analogous to single radial immunodiffusion, may be used on a routine basis with reference to a standard serum. Antibody-sensitised red cells are incorporated into molten agarose and the mixture allowed to set. Wells are cut in the agarose and filled with either the sera under test or dilutions of a standard serum. The complement diffuses into the agarose and reacts with and binds to the antibody-coated red cells. Circles of lysis appear, the size of which depend upon the complement content of the serum.

Materials and equipment
All reagents should be made up in barbitone buffer for complement fixation (Appendix I)
Sensitised red cells (Section 7.1.1, made up to 10% v/v)
Agarose, 2% w/v in barbitone buffer

Glass plates (microscope slides are suitable for a small number of estimations)
Gel cutter (Appendix II)

Method
1 Warm 1.5 ml of the barbitone buffer to 56° in a water bath.
2 Cool 1.2 ml of molten 2% agarose to 56° and add to the barbitone buffer.
3 Mix and cool to 45° in a water bath.
4 Add 0.2 ml of sensitised red-cell suspension and mix gently.
5 Place the glass plate on a level surface, use a spirit level to check.
6 Pour the mixture quickly onto the plate to form a smooth, even surface.
7 When set, place the plate in a box containing moist filter paper and chill to 4° for a few minutes to harden the agarose.
8 Cut two rows of five wells, approximately 3 mm across using an Ouchterlony gel cutter and remove the agarose plugs with a Pasteur pipette attached to a Venturi pump.
9 Dispense 8 μl samples of the sera under test into separate wells. Similarly, add four doubling dilutions of a standard serum to a series of wells. (For accurate research studies, a larger plate can be used to permit replicate determinations.)
10 Incubate the plate in a moist box, overnight at 4°.
11 Warm the plate, still in the box, to 37° for 2 h, to allow cell lysis to occur.
12 Measure two diameters at right angles across each well and calculate their mean.
13 Plot the value of the areas (πr^2) of the standard serum dilutions (linear scale) against the log dilution. Determine the concentration of the unknown sera as a percentage of the standard by extrapolation from the standard curve.

Technical note
This technique is eminently suitable for detecting complement deficiencies both in total and in individual components of complement. Qualitative assay reagents may be prepared in which just one component is missing from the lytic pathway of complement. These reagents are incorporated in agarose and will only lyse the indicator erythrocytes if the missing component is present in the test serum added to the well.

7.2 Detection of antibody or antigen by complement fixation

An antibody, antigen or antigen–antibody complex may be detected by estimating either complement consumption or fixation. As mentioned earlier, because of the amplifying cascade sequence of complement, a small amount of antigen–antibody complex will cause massive complement fixation or consumption (depending upon whether you assay the complex or the supernatant for complement components). Accordingly, the complement fixation reaction is a very sensitive technique for measuring small amounts (<1 μg) of antigen or antibody. However, it has the disadvantage that it detects only certain antibody classes. In the human, for example, IgG1, IgG2 (weakly), IgG3 and IgM activate the classical pathway, whereas IgG4, IgA and IgE cannot. There may, however, be some activation by these three latter classes via the alternative pathway. In many instances complement fixation has been replaced by other techniques, such as ELISA and RIA, but it is still used in many microbiological assays. It does have the advantage of showing that the reaction being measured is capable of activating a biological effector function.

7.2.1 Quantitative complement fixation assay

It is possible to standardise complement activity using antibody-sensitised erythrocytes (Section 7.1.1).

If instead of defining the CH_{50} as before, we define the minimum amount of complement required to lyse all of a standard volume of sensitised red cells (minimum haemolytic dose, MHD) we have an extremely good indicator system for complement consumption tests.

Hence in the complement fixation assay a soluble antigen is allowed to react with

(a)

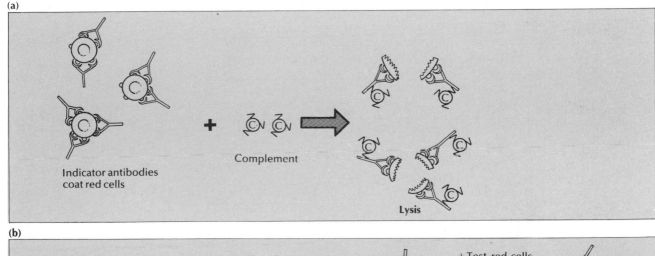

(b)

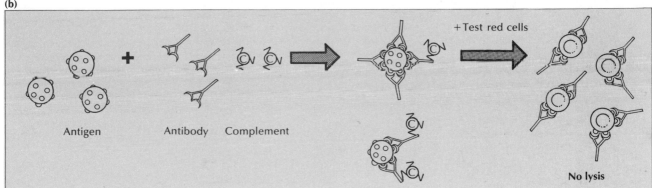

Fig. 7.2 Complement fixation test to detect either antigen or antibody. A detection system of antibody-coated red cells is set up. On the addition of complement the red cells will be lysed (**a**). To test for antibody the mixture of antigen plus test sample is incubated with complement. Indicator antibody-coated red cells are then added to test for free complement. If antibody is present in the test sample, the complement will have been bound by the immune complexes and *no lysis* of red cells will occur. If no antibody is present in the test sample no complexes will be formed and the complement will not be consumed and so will be free to bind to the antibody-coated red cells and lysis will occur (**b**).

antibody and so fix complement. When the indicator system of sensitised erythrocytes is added, the degree of lysis observed will be proportional to the amount of complement remaining in the supernatant.

This principle has been widely used in clinical screening procedures, notably in the Wasserman complement fixation test for anti-treponemal antibodies in syphilis. The principles of interpretation of this test may be easily appreciated by reference to Fig. 7.2.

The assay is made semi-quantitative by titrating the test serum to determine the lowest dilution that still gives positive complement fixation.

Materials and equipment

Human serum albumin, HSA (1 mg ml^{-1}) (Appendix II)

Anti-HSA (Section 1.9 or Appendix II)

Sensitised erythrocytes (Section 7.1)

Barbitone-buffered saline for complement fixation (contains magnesium and calcium ions, use this for all dilutions) (Appendix I)

Complement source; for example, guinea-pig serum (fresh or preserved, see Appendix II)

Micro-titre apparatus (Appendix II)

Micro-titre trays — U-shaped wells (Appendix II)

Protocol **A**

	Tube number						
	1	2	3	4	5	6	7
Barbitone-buffered saline (ml)	0.1	0.2	0.3	0.4	0.5	0.6	0.7
Guinea-pig serum (ml 1 : 10 initial dil.)	0.1 ⟶						
Final C dilution	1 : 20	1 : 30	1 : 40	1 : 50	1 : 60	1 : 70	1 : 80

There should not be any complement fixation in either the antigen or antiserum controls, i.e. haemolysis should be complete.

7.2.2 Estimation of MHD of complement

1 Re-constitute the guinea-pig serum if required.
2 Adjust to 1 : 10 dilution.
3 Set up the complement dilutions as in the Protocol A.
4 Take 0.1 ml of each complement dilution and add 0.2 ml buffer plus 0.1 ml of sensitised erythrocytes.
5 Incubate for 30 min at 37° and centrifuge at 100 g for 15 min.

The titre of the first tube in the curve to show a button of erythrocytes is then taken as the MHD. In the assay 2 MHD units are used.

Protocol **B**

	Tube number						
	2	3	4	5	6	7	8
Barbitone-buffered saline (ml)	1.0						
HSA (ml, initial conc. mg ml^{-1})	1.0						
		mix	*mix*	etc.			
		1.0 ml	1.0 ml				
Final HSA dilution	1:2	1:4	1:8	1:16	1:32	1:64	1:128

ANTIBODY AND ANTIGEN ASSAY

The test is set up as shown in Fig. 7.3. The antiserum is diluted out down the plate (columns) and the antigen is diluted out across the plate (rows).

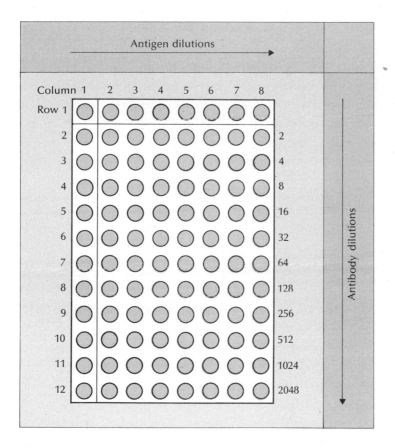

Fig. 7.3 Micro-titre plate for quantitative complement fixation assay.
Row 1 contains antigen dilutions only and is a control for anti-complementary activity of the antigen.
Column 1 contains antibody alone, again this is a control for anti-complementary activity.

1 Put 1 drop (25 µl) of buffer in each well. (Hold the dropping pipette vertically.)
2 Dilute out the antiserum in the eight columns as for haemagglutination (Section 6.14), but start at row 2. Row 1 is used as an antigen control (see Fig. 7.3).
3 Set up antigen dilutions in tubes as in the Protocol B.
4 Add 1 drop of antigen to each well in columns 2–8, tube number should correspond to column number (see Fig. 7.3). Leave column 1 free of antigen — this is the antiserum control.
5 Add 2 MHD units of complement to each well.
6 Mix by shaking and incubate at 37° for 30 min.
7 Add 1 drop of sensitised cells to all wells.
8 Mix by shaking and incubate at 37° for 30 min.
9 Shake and stand at 4° for 60 min.

Examine the wells for the presence of unlysed erythrocytes; indicating previous complement fixation. The end-point titre of this test is usually taken as the first well showing approximately 50% lysis of indicator cells.

Technical notes
1 Because IgM has a higher haemolytic efficiency (cf. Section 7.1), this antibody class is preferentially detected.
2 In the chequer-board design given above, both the antigen and antiserum concentration were varied. For routine use, once the optimum level of either antigen or antibody has been established, a single concentration is usually used for the detection of unknown concentrations of antigen or antibody.
3 The final step of settling the indicator cells at 4° for 60 min may be considerably shortened by gently centrifuging the trays in special micro-titre plate holders (Appendix II).
4 If any component is anti-complementary the test must be repeated with fresh reagents.

7.3 Assay of complement components with specific antibodies

Most complement components occur in sufficiently large amounts in serum for accurate quantitation by a precipitin reaction in gel (Section 6.6). A problem with the detection of complement components as antigens is that some antisera do not distinguish between active and inactive complement fragments. However, fragment-specific antisera can be obtained and these can give useful information about the state of complement activation *in vivo*. In addition some components change their electrophoretic mobility on activation, a qualitative change that may be used to advantage in two-dimensional crossed immunoelectrophoresis to monitor the activation of C3 (Section 6.11).

7.4 Estimation of immune complexes using C1q

Immune complexes are pharmacologically very active when formed in the body. Normally, they are very quickly removed by cells of the mononuclear phagocyte system and so little, if any, harm results. Under certain circumstances; however, complexes tend to persist in the circulation and may eventually fix complement, leading to the release of anaphylotoxins and chemotactic factors. The anaphylotoxins mediate histamine release and consequently produce increased vascular permeability. Neutrophils are attracted to the site of complement fixation and release their proteolytic enzymes while engulfing the complexes, thus causing local tissue damage. Immune complexes containing C3 are readily bound by the CR1 receptor on primate erythrocytes leading to erythrocyte clearance in the liver.

C1q is frequently used for the detection of circulating complexes. The simple binding of C1q to immune complexes may be determined, but this has the disadvantage that some molecules, such as DNA, also bind C1q. Utilisation of a solid-phase immunoradiometric C1q assay has the advantage that the complexes are identified by two, rather than one, marker molecules. In the assay described below, human C1q is bound to the surface of plastic tubes and patients' sera added. Complexes adsorbed to the C1q are then revealed with radiolabelled anti-human IgG.

7.4.1 Preparation of human C1q

Materials and equipment
Fresh human serum
C1q buffers 1 to 6 (Appendix I)
Dialysis tubing (Appendix II)
Refrigerated centrifuge capable of 10 000 g

Method
Important: the samples and buffers must be kept at 4° at all times during this preparation.

1 Dialyse 127 ml fresh human serum against 1 litre of buffer 1 for 4 h.
2 Transfer the dialysis bag to a second 1 litre of buffer 1 and dialyse for a further 11 h.
3 Centrifuge the sample at 10 000 g for 15 min at 4°.
4 Discard the supernatant and re-suspend the precipitate in buffer 1.
5 Centrifuge at 10 000 g for 15 min at 4°.
6 Discard the supernatant, loosen the precipitate with a glass rod and add 32 ml of buffer 2. Dissolve the precipitate by mixing on a slow roller for 10 min.
7 Centrifuge at 5000 g for 5 min at 4° to remove undissolved material.
8 Dialyse the supernatant against 4 litres of buffer 3 for 4 h.
9 Centrifuge at 10 000 g for 15 min.
10 Discard the supernatant and re-suspend the precipitate in buffer 3.

11 Centrifuge at 10 000 *g* for 15 min at 4°.

12 Discard the supernatant and re-dissolve the precipitate in 32 ml of buffer 4 as in step 6.

13 Centrifuge at 5000 *g* for 5 min at 4° to remove undissolved material.

14 Dialyse the supernatant against 4 litres of buffer 5 for 5 h.

15 Centrifuge at 10 000 *g* for 15 min at 4°.

16 Discard supernatant and re-suspend precipitate in buffer 5.

17 Centrifuge at 10 000 *g* for 15 min at 4°.

18 Discard the supernatant and re-dissolve the precipitate in 16 ml of buffer 6.

19 Measure the absorbance at 280 nm and calculate the C1q concentration. (The absorbance of C1q at 280 nm in a 1 cm cell is 1.0 for a 1156 µg ml^{-1} solution.)

20 Aliquot the C1q and store at −70° for use.

Technical notes

1 Animal, rather than human, C1q may be used. This has the advantage that any slight residual contamination with immunoglobulin will not be detected if specific anti-human immunoglobulin antibodies are used in the assay.

2 Do not extend the time for re-solution of the precipitates. Although more protein will go into solution, the eventual product is less pure.

3 The degree of purity may be determined by immunoelectrophoresis (Section 6.9) against anti-human serum and anti-C1q or by SDS polyacrylamide gel electrophoresis (Section 2.10).

4 Anti-C1q antibodies have been reported in some SLE patients. This could produce false positive results in some situations.

7.4.2 ## Immune complex assay

Materials and equipment

Human C1q (prepared as above)

Test sera

Gelatin (Appendix II)

Antibody against human IgG, immunoadsorbent purified and radiolabelled (Sections 9.6 and 2.5).

Phosphate-buffered saline, PBS (Appendix I)

Tween 20

0.2 M ethylene diamine tetra-acetic acid, EDTA, disodium salt, pH 7.5

γ spectrometer

Polystyrene tubes (LP3) (Appendix II)

Method

1 Dilute the human C1q to 10 µg ml^{-1} in PBS.

2 Place 1 ml volumes of C1q solution in polystyrene tubes and leave for 3 days at 4°.

3 Empty tubes and wash three times with PBS.

4 Fill the tubes with 0.01 % w/v gelatin solution in PBS to block any free protein-binding sites on the tubes, and incubate at room temperature for 2 h.

5 While the tubes are being blocked, mix 50 μl of each test serum with 100 μl EDTA solution and incubate at 37° for 30 min. Transfer the samples to an ice bath.

6 Empty the C1q tubes and wash three times with PBS.

7 Place duplicate 50 μl samples into C1q-coated tubes, together with 950 μl of PBS containing 0.05% v/v Tween 20 (PBS–Tween).

8 Coated tubes containing 1 ml PBS–Tween (background controls) should be prepared in the same way as the sample tubes.

9 Incubate the tubes at 37° for 1 h and at 4° for 30 min.

10 Remove free serum proteins by washing three times with cold PBS.

11 Detect the bound complexes by adding 1 μg radiolabelled anti-IgG antibody in 1 ml PBS–Tween to each tube and incubate at 37° for 1 h and then at 4° for 30 min.

12 Remove free radiolabelled reagent by washing three times with cold PBS.

13 Count the tubes in a γ spectrometer.

The amount of radiolabelled antibody bound is a measure of the concentration of immune complexes in the patient's serum. Generally sera from normal subjects bind less than 20 ng of radiolabelled antibody, while patients may bind as much as 200 ng.

Technical notes

1 Enzyme-labelled antibodies (Section 2.3) may be used for the detection of complexes bound to the C1q.

2 The use of antibody can be avoided altogether by using labelled protein A. Staphylococcal protein A binds specifically to IgG, especially subclasses IgG1, IgG2 and IgG4. It is difficult to label by conventional techniques but this can easily be done by the method below. Protein G, which binds to a much wider range of IgG molecules, can also be used.

Materials and equipment
Staphylococcus aureus protein A (5 mg ml^{-1} in water) (Appendix II)
0.12 M carbonate–bicarbonate buffer, pH 9.0 (Appendix I)
Dioxane containing 10 mg ml^{-1} hydroxyphenol succinimide
Phosphate-buffered saline, PBS (Appendix I)

Method

1 Add 0.8 ml carbonate–bicarbonate buffer and 10 μl hydroxyphenol solution to 0.2 ml protein A solution (5 mg ml^{-1}, initial concentration).

2 Incubate at room temperature for 25–30 min with occasional mixing.

3 Dialyse overnight against 1 litre of PBS.

4 Iodinate as in Section 2.5.

3 A positive control should be included in all assays for immune complexes. International reference preparations are available from the World Health Organisation,

Division of Immunology, but a simple 'in house' standard can be prepared from heat-aggregated IgG, as below.

Materials and equipment
Human IgG (Section 8.5.2)
Phosphate-buffered saline, PBS (Appendix I)
Water bath at 63°
Ice

Method
1 Prepare 1 ml of a 27 mg ml^{-1} solution of IgG in PBS.
2 Place in a glass test tube and incubate at 63° for 10 min. This aggregates approximately 10% of the IgG.
3 Cool immediately in ice.
4 Make dilutions, from 100 to 1000 µg ml^{-1} in normal serum.
5 Include these dilutions in each immune complex assay.

7.5

Complement-mediated cytolysis

This technique is probably one of the *in vitro* equivalents of cytotoxic hypersensitivity (Section 5.4); antisera directed against cell-surface antigens are used to kill cells carrying these antigens with the aid of complement. We will describe two techniques that differ in the means by which cell death is assayed.

7.5.1

Dye exclusion test

This test is an extension of the method used to estimate cell viability described in Section 3.4.

Materials
Anti-lymphocyte serum, ALS (Section 3.8.1).
Rabbit anti-mouse immunoglobulin (Section 1.7.2).
Guinea-pig serum (complement) (Appendix II)
Nigrosin dye (Appendix II)
Inbred mice, 4–6 weeks old

Method
1 Absorb the complement with mouse spleen and erythrocytes; approximately 0.1 ml packed cells ml^{-1} of serum, for 30 min at 4°.
2 Centrifuge the absorbed complement. Use immediately or store at −20°.
3 Prepare thymus and lymph-node suspensions from mouse donors. Estimate viability and adjust to 5×10^7 viable lymphocytes ml^{-1} (Section 1.16 for removal of dead cells).
4 Prepare cell and serum mixtures according to the following Protocol, and incubate at 37° for 30 min.

Protocol

	Tube number					
	1	2	3	4	5	6
ALS or NRS final dilution	1:20	1:40	1:80	1:160	1:320	1:640
Lymph-node cells (5×10^7 ml^{-1})	0.1 ml ————————————————————————→					
Absorbed guinea-pig serum (1:5 initial dilution)	0.1 ml ————————————————————————→					

Repeat this Protocol using thymus cells with the same dilution of ALS and NRS.

ASSAY 1 (see Protocol above)

Cells: lymph node.

Antisera: ALS and pre-immunisation serum (normal rabbit serum, NRS). Titrate NRS only to 1:40.

ASSAY 2 (see Protocol below)

Cells: lymph node.

Antisera: anti-immunoglobulin (if assays 1 and 2 are performed simultaneously a second NRS control is not required).

5 After incubation stand the tubes in ice to prevent further complement fixation and cell lysis.

6 Count the number of viable cells in each suspension as described in Section 3.4.2.

7 Calculate the number of viable cells ml^{-1} and from this the percentage lysis for each tube according to the following equation:

$$\% \text{ lysis} = C_N - C_A \times 100/C_O$$

where:

C_N = number of live cells in NRS,

C_A = number of live cells in ALS or anti-Ig,

C_O = original number live cells.

Protocol

	Tube number				
	1	2	3	4	5
Anti-immunoglobulin dilution	1:10	1:20	1:40	1:80	1:160
Lymph-node cells (5×10^7 ml^{-1})	0.1 ml ————————————————————→				
Absorbed guinea-pig serum (1:5 initial dilution)	0.1 ml ————————————————————→				

Repeat this Protocol using thymus cells with the same dilutions of anti-immunoglobulin.

8 Plot a graph of % lysis against antiserum dilution for each tissue and antiserum.

Interpretation of results

1 You should find that ALS kills all nucleated cells in the thymus and the lymph-node suspension to a high dilution of antiserum. This lack of T-cell specificity is, of course, to be expected as lymphocytes share many surface antigens.

2 The percentage of cells killed by the anti-immunoglobulin serum should coincide with the expected % of B cells in the tissue used (Fig. 1.3, p. 23).

3 If the killing of thymocytes by anti-immunoglobulin or NRS exceeds 5%, there are probably anti-species antibodies present, not related to the original immunising procedure. In this case it is necessary to absorb *all* sera with liver membranes (see Section 2.1.7, p. 39).

Technical notes

1 The sensitivity of this assay depends upon a high initial cell viability. Frequently 20–30% dead cells are encountered in lymph-node suspensions. Dead cells may be removed as described in Section 1.16.

2 The guinea-pig serum complement source must be absorbed with spleen and red cells before use as it is sometimes itself cytotoxic. It was discovered that an agarose absorption may also be used to remove anti-mouse antibodies. Use 100 mg of agarose ml^{-1} of serum, absorb for 60 min at 4°.

In this assay it is advisable to count the number of viable cells after lysis rather than the number of dead cells, especially if centrifugation steps are included after killing. Dead cells are often broken up and lost during centrifugation.

7.5.2 ## ^{51}Cr-labelled cell lysis

Estimating cell death by dye exclusion, although simple, is rather time consuming and so not many assay points can be performed simultaneously. If the cells are labelled with ^{51}Cr it is possible to estimate cell death by the amount of isotope released. In this case it is an advantage to centrifuge the cells after killing to enhance cell dissolution and isotope release.

Materials and equipment
Sodium ^{51}chromate (Appendix II)
Inbred mice, 4–6 weeks old
γ spectrometer

Method

1 Prepare thymus and lymph-node suspensions in tissue culture medium containing HEPES (20 mM) and 5% foetal bovine serum (Section 1.15).

2   Adjust to 5×10^7 lymphocytes ml^{-1} and add 37×10^5 Bq of sodium ^{51}chromate to 1 ml of each cell suspension.

3   Incubate at 37° for 40 min.

4   Wash cells twice with medium and allow to stand on ice for 30 min.

5   Wash cells three times with medium and re-suspend to 5×10^6 lymphocytes ml^{-1}.

6   Mix 0.1 ml of each cell suspension with antibody and complement (see Protocols, Section 7.5.1) and incubate at 37° for 30 min.

6   After incubation adjust final volume to 0.5 ml, mix well and centrifuge (150 g for 10 min at 4°).

7   Remove 0.1 ml of supernatant and determine its radioactive content (amount of released isotope) in γ spectrometer.

Many investigators determine the maximum (100% ^{51}Cr release) by lysing an aliquot of cells, either by freezing and thawing or with 10% Saponin. Under the labelling conditions described this is usually $10\,000-14\,000$ c.p.m. (for 5×10^6 cells). For some applications, however, this is not a realistic value. This technique may be used, for example, for quantitative absorption experiments by which the relative amount of cell-surface antigen on different cell types may be compared. A fixed number of cells is used to absorb a fixed concentration of antiserum and the original and absorbed antisera are then assayed on ^{51}Cr-labelled cells. In this case it is advisable to determine the dilutions of original antiserum giving a plateau release value, and to use this as the 100% ^{51}Cr release. Alternatively, one may work more sensitively with the dilution of antiserum required to give 50% of this maximum release (cf. Section 7.1). The Technical notes given in Section 7.5.1 also apply to this technique.

7.6   Summary and conclusions

The innate immune system provides an important means of defence against micro-organisms. Complement and phagocytosis form two major parts of this activity. Whereas phagocytosis is a cell-based defence mechanism, complement is a collection of more than 20 different molecular components which act in a cascade fashion to provide enormous amplification of a small initial signal. The adaptive immune system has been able to feed into this pathway via antibody and C1q.

Many complement components are very labile and so studies involving complement must be carried out on fresh or fresh-frozen biological samples. In fresh serum the presence of activation products of the complement system is an indication of inflammation somewhere in the body.

Total complement activity may be easily quantitated, and if a deficiency is found, assays for individual components may be performed to see if a single component in the cascade is limiting. Although complement fixation assays provide a sensitive means of detecting antigen or antibody, because of the marked amplification achieved, care must be taken with the reagents as they can be anti-complementary and so yield anomalous data.

7.7 **Further reading**

Harrison RA and Lachman PJ (1986) Complement technology. In *Handbook of Experimental Immunology*, DM Weir (editor), Volume 1, 4th edition. Blackwell Scientific Publications, Oxford.

Whaley K (editor) (1985) *Methods in Complement for Clinical Immunologists*. Churchill Livingstone, Edinburgh.

Whaley K (editor) (1987) *Complement in Health and Disease*. MTP Press, Lancaster.

8 Isolation and Structure of Immunoglobulins

The immunoglobulin classes differ from each other and from the other serum proteins by their solubility in aqueous solution, molecular size, electrostatic density and isoelectric point. These characteristics can be used to isolate immunoglobulins and to fractionate them into classes. Recently, it has been found that certain immunoglobulin classes are bound by particular proteins such as protamine for IgM, protein A for IgG and Jacalin for IgA. This has led to the development of affinity techniques for the isolation of immunoglobulin isotypes.

8.1

Salt fractionation

The relative solubility of proteins in pure water, ethanol or in various salt solutions has been used for over 100 years as a basic fractionation technique. Serum may be separated into its euglobulin (insoluble) and pseudoglobulin (soluble) fractions by dialysis against distilled water. Although this is often used as the first step in the purification of IgM, the euglobulin fraction is always contaminated with some IgG. In addition, the method gives a low yield but it can be of use when a source rich in IgM, such as Waldenstrom macroglobulinaemia serum, is available.

As the salt concentration of the medium is raised there is an interference with the interaction of water molecules with the charged polar groups on protein molecules, thus rendering them less hydrophilic. This allows a greater hydrophobic interaction between protein molecules and they eventually become insoluble. The salt concentration at which each protein precipitates is different, but between closely related molecules such as immunoglobulins the difference is not sufficiently great to give a precipitate with high-grade purity. However, as many unwanted serum proteins, for example albumin, will remain in solution when immunoglobulins are precipitated, salt-induced differential precipitation is often a useful first step in many isolation procedures. Besides its use for purification, salting out is useful for concentration of immunoglobulins from dilute solution. Ammonium sulphate precipitation is a widely used laboratory technique for the preparation of a crude immunoglobulin fraction from whole serum, although on a commercial scale cold ethanol (Cohn fractionation) is more usual. The use of ammonium, rather than sodium sulphate, as the precipitating salt offers the advantage of a high solubility which is only minimally dependent on temperature, it varies by only about 3% between 0° and 25°. Sodium sulphate is five times as soluble at 25° as at 0°. Although relatively 'pure' IgG may be rapidly prepared by precipitation at a 33.3% saturation of ammonium sulphate, if a higher yield at lower purity is required, 50.0% saturation may be used. Smaller fragments of the molecule require higher salt concentrations for precipitation.

8.1.1 Rapid concentration of immunoglobulins

After column chromatography, samples are often recovered in dilute solution in large volumes of buffer. It is important to concentrate these rapidly as denaturation occurs in dilute solution. Ammonium sulphate precipitation is useful for this, using the solid salt to limit the total working volume of solution (nomogram, front inside cover). The method below is suitable for light chains (Section 8.7) and Fab regions (Section 8.8), and is also applicable for preparing Bence-Jones proteins from the urine of patients with multiple myeloma.

Materials

Material for concentration; for example, Fab or light chains from column chromatography, urine from patient with multiple myeloma, or urine from a mouse with a transplanted mineral oil-induced plasmacytoma or hybridoma
Solid ammonium sulphate
Phosphate-buffered saline, PBS (Appendix I)

Method
Steps 1–2 are only for urine samples, otherwise start at 3.

1 Dialyse the urine against cold, running tap water for 24 h to remove inorganic salts and urea.
2 Filter or centrifuge to remove any insoluble material.
3 Adjust to pH 5.5 (salt precipitation is most effective at the isoelectric point of the protein required).
4 Add solid ammonium sulphate to 75% saturation. At 25°, 575 g solid ammonium sulphate is required for 1000 ml of solution (see also nomogram, front inside cover). Add the salt slowly with stirring, otherwise it will form lumps bound up with protein which are very difficult to dissolve.
5 When all the salt has been added, stir for 1 h at room temperature to equilibrate.
6 Centrifuge at 1000 g for 15 min and discard the supernatant. (Take care to wash any salt off the rotor head or corrosion will occur.)
7 Re-dissolve the precipitate in PBS.

Technical note

Ammonium sulphate precipitation is often used to prepare crude γ-globulin fractions from whole serum (Section 1.3). For many applications this may provide protein of sufficient purity, but even if highly purified material is required, salt precipitation may provide a useful first step in the isolation procedure.

8.2 Size fractionation

Serum proteins may be isolated and fractionated on the basis of their molecular size using gel filtration.

Principles of molecular sieving

Using porous gels of cross-linked dextran (Sephadex), agarose (Sepharose or Biogel-A), polyacrylamide (Biogel-P) or mixtures of agarose and acrylamide (Sephacryl) proteins may be separated on the basis of their molecular dimensions. An equilibrium is maintained between the liquid phase around the gel particles and the gel phase. Depending upon the pore size of the gel, molecules may diffuse from the liquid phase into the gel phase. The rate at which a molecule moves down a column of the gel depends upon the number of beads that are entered. Because the solute molecules maintain a concentration equilibrium between the gel and liquid phases the sample moves down the column as a band. Large proteins, above the exclusion limit of the gel, will not enter the beads and so move with the advancing solute front while small molecules enter the beads and must traverse this space as well as the volume around the beads. All sizes of excluded proteins appear in the effluent simultaneously and so will not be separated. Molecular weight is not the only factor governing the entry of molecules into the gel; molecular shape and degree of hydration are also important. Proteins and polysaccharides have very different exclusion limits in terms of molecular weight. However, within a related group of molecules, for example immunoglobulins, the molecules will leave the column in order of decreasing size (Fig. 8.1). Some molecules such as nucleotides have a tendency to bind to dextran columns and this will alter their behaviour during separation.

Many gels are available for exclusion chromatography, each differing in their chemical composition, physical form and pore size. The following basic requirements should be considered in selecting a gel for separation of any protein mixture.

8.2.2 ## Basic requirements for gel filtration chromatography

(a)   Correct pore size. The proteins must be able to diffuse into the gel for molecular sieving to occur. The exclusion limits of the different grades and types of gel are shown in Fig. 8.2.

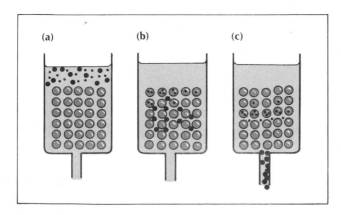

(a)   (b)   (c)

Fig. 8.1 Principles of molecular size sorting on a gel bead column. When a mixture of proteins is applied to a gel filtration column (a) the smaller molecules, within the fractionation range of the gel, diffuse into the gel beads and are retarded. Larger molecules are excluded, as they are unable to enter the bead pores, and move with the advancing solute front (b), leaving the column first with the void volume, smaller molecules leaving later in the eluted volume (c).

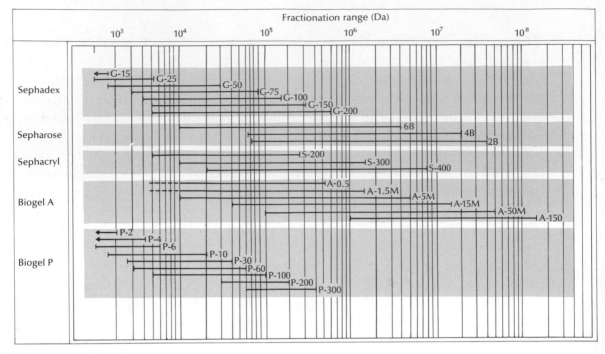

Fig. 8.2 Effective fractionation ranges for gel filtration media.

G-15—G-200, Sephadex dextran gels: available in a range of bead sizes. The finest beads give better resolution but at the expense of slower flow rates.

2B—6B, Sepharose beaded agarose gels: suitable for fractionation in the higher molecular weight ranges. Cross-linked, CL, agarose gels have similar fractionation ranges with increased thermal and chemical stability.

S-200—S-400, Sephacryl acrylamide—agarose combination gel: for high stability and increased resolution.

A-0.5—A-150, Biogel A: agarose gels extending into high molecular weight fractionation ranges.

P-2—P-30, Biogel P: polyacrylamide gels for high resolution, narrow range fractionation.

(b)   Chemical nature. The gel must be inert, any charged groups on the gel or affinity for the material to be separated will complicate size separation.

(c)   Bead size. The gel must be finely dispersed to allow rapid diffusion and effective separation, but this must be balanced against optimum flow rate as very fine particles tend to slow the flow of solute molecules. The presentation of the gel in bead form gives good flow characteristics.

Sephadex (Appendix II). This is the most widely used material for gel filtration. It is prepared by cross-linking alkaline dextran with epichlorohydrin and is swollen in phosphate-buffered saline or water for use.

Sepharose and Biogel-A (Appendix II). These gels consist of small spheres of agarose, a linear polysaccharide of D-galactose and 3,6-anhydro-L-galactose. It contains no ionizable groups but has the unfortunate characteristic of liquefying at elevated temperatures or in the presence of solutes capable of breaking hydrogen bonds, for example urea. This latter problem has been overcome by the introduction of cross-linked CL-Sepharose. Unlike Sephadex it can be used to separate very large molecules, even in the range of viruses.

Biogel-P (Appendix II). This gel is a copolymer of acrylamide and methylene bisacrylamide. Its fractional range corresponds roughly to that of agarose gels, but, as it is a plastic, it has the enormous advantage of not being susceptible to attack by microorganisms.

Sephacryl. This gel exhibits a combination of properties as each bead consists of a mixture of agarose and acrylamide. It is a rigid gel capable of good resolution at comparatively high flow rates, S-300 is especially useful for fractionating large serum proteins including immune complexes.

Fast preparative liquid chromatography (FPLC). A complete system for the reproducible preparation of proteins has now been introduced using pre-prepared columns with high resolving power.

High-performance liquid chromatography (HPLC). This form of column uses high resolving gels on silica supports. The characteristics of the columns necessitate the use of high pressures leading to its alternative name of *high-pressure liquid chromatography*.

8.2.3   ## Parameters of gel filtration (see also Section 1.5)

Large molecules, above the exclusion limit, cannot enter the gel pores and remain in the solute around the beads, i.e. in the *void volume*, V_0. Small buffer molecules are able to pass into the gel freely and so enter the *included volume*, V_i, as well as the space around the beads. They therefore traverse the volume $V_i + V_0 = V_t$, the *total solvent volume*. Molecules of intermediate size may enter the gel, but less freely than buffer molecules, and so they are eluted from the column at an intermediate volume between V_0 and V_t, known as the elution volume V_e.

8.2.4   ## Applications of gel chromatography

De-salting or rapid buffer exchange. Sephadex G-25 excludes all molecules over 5000 molecular weight. Its use in de-salting and buffer exchange of protein solutions has been described in detail in Section 1.5.

Protein fractionation. From the previous section it is obvious that a major use of gel chromatography is the isolation and purification of molecules of different molecular size. It is possible, however, to separate molecules of the same size if they have different affinities for the gel material.

Molecular weight determination of proteins. Although an estimate of molecular weight and shape of a native molecule may be obtained from its elution volume from a calibrated column, more accurate determinations of relative apparent molecular weight may be obtained from SDS-PAGE (Section 2.10).

8.2.5   Basic column technique

Figure 8.3 shows a suitable basic arrangement of equipment for gel filtration.

Equipment

Columns. Many different types of column are available each with their own advantages and disadvantages. Many manufacturers now supply a wide range of apparatus, from simple manual columns to fully integrated systems (Appendix II).

Pump. Peristaltic pumps provide an even flow rate with little solvent turbulence. Alternatively, a simple reservoir such as a Marriotte flask can be used. It is important to maintain a constant pressure on the column.

Monitoring and collection of fractions. A fraction collector and flow through UV analyser connected to a chart recorder are necessary (Appendix II).

8.2.6   Fractionation of serum on G-200 Sephadex or S-200 Sephacryl

Sephadex G-200 excludes proteins over 800 000 molecular weight and so is extremely useful for the isolation of IgM. Sephacryl S-200, which is pre-swollen, is also useful for fractionation in this molecular weight range. The same principles apply to the use of other gels fractionating in different size ranges.

Materials and equipment
Sephadex G-200 or Sephacryl S-200 (Appendix II)
Phosphate-buffered saline, PBS (Appendix I)
Column chromatography equipment (Fig. 8.3, Section 8.2.5, Appendix II)
Serum

Method
Start at step 1 for Sephadex, Step 3 for Sephacryl.

1 Heat 17 g (dry weight) Sephadex G-200 in about 750 ml PBS in a boiling water bath for 5 h. This will provide enough swollen gel for a 100 × 2.5 cm column. Swelling of the gel in boiling water is more rapid than at room temperature and expels the air from the gel.
2 Cool the gel to the operating temperature. Generally room temperature is suitable but with labile materials 4° should be used. The gel must be poured and the column run at the same temperature. As gases are more soluble at lower temperature, bubbles will form in a column poured at 4° and run at room temperature.
3 De-gas the gel under a vacuum. Air bubbles in the gel will distort the protein bands during the run.
4 Pour the gel into the column along a glass rod to avoid air bubbles. Take great

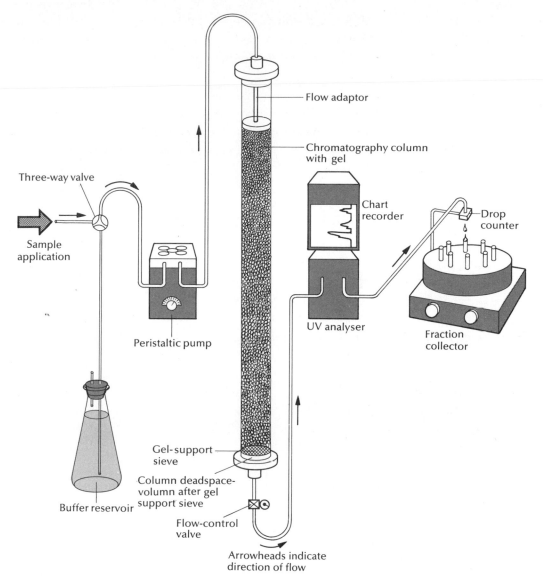

Fig. 8.3 Equipment for column chromatography. The equipment shown above allows efficient chromatographic separation of protein mixtures. It is an advantage to have an insulating jacket around the column to protect it from draughts and temperature changes. If the column is equipped with flow adaptors at either end, this will allow the column to be inverted and run in the opposite direction, or to be run with the buffer flow in the ascending direction which will lessen the chances of the column packing down.

care that the column is vertical. All the gel must be poured into the column at one time. Use an extension tube or reservoir (Appendix II). Leave the column outlet open during packing. A column of 100×2.5 cm generally takes about 5 h to settle.

5 Once the gel has settled fit the flow adapter.

6 Pack the column by running through at least two column volumes of buffer. The flow rate should be about 20 ml h^{-1} (faster flow rates are possible with Sephacryl). After packing lower the flow adapter if necessary.

If the column tends to pack down after several runs you are probably running the column too fast. If a flow adapter is used, packing after extended use may be avoided by using descending and ascending flow chromatography alternatively.

7   When the column is not in use add thiomersal to a concentration of 0.005% to stop microbial growth. This must be completely flushed out of the column before adding a sample as it absorbs at the same wavelength as protein. Alternatively columns may be run with buffer containing sodium azide 0.01 M. Azide gives less absorption at 280 nm.

SAMPLE APPLICATION

The gel surface must not be disturbed during sample application as this would cause distortion of the bands. The simplest procedure is to feed the sample through the pump and then through the flow adapter, but this will cause some mixing and dilution of the sample in the dead space of the pump tubing.

If an adapter is not available place a nylon net or a layer of G-25 Sephadex (about 5 mm) on top of the gel to protect the surface. Add a little sucrose to the sample to increase its density and layer it gently onto the gel surface below the free buffer with a long Pasteur pipette or a syringe with capillary tubing.

1   Apply a sample volume of up to 8 ml of serum.
2   Run the column at 20 ml h^{-1}.
3   Collect samples of 2–5 ml.

Distribution of serum proteins in eluted volume

Three major peaks should be eluted. On fractionating mouse serum the peaks shown in Fig. 8.4 were obtained.

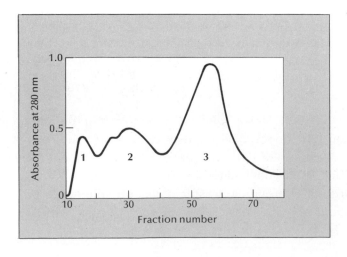

Fig. 8.4 Elution profile of serum proteins from a column of G-200 Sephadex. A 5 ml sample of mouse serum was applied to a column of bed volume 100 × 2.5 cm, and the proteins eluted with phosphate buffered saline.

PEAK 1

The first peak contains the macroglobulins, IgM and α-macroglobulin, plus some lipoproteins. Also on some occasions large haemoglobin—haptoglobin complexes are present. These are easily distinguishable by their reddish-brown colour. Some IgA may be found towards the end of the elution of this peak.

PEAK 2

Most of the IgG is in this peak, together with IgA in the first fractions.

PEAK 3

This contains mainly albumin and other small globulins.

Occasionally the first two peaks are not resolved satisfactorily. This is due to weak non-covalent interactions between the IgG molecules causing them to aggregate and so contaminate the first peak. In these cases, run the column in 0.1 M acetate buffer, pH 5.0. Lowering the pH increases the positive charges on the IgG molecules increasing the repulsive forces between them, so preventing aggregation.

Examination of fractions

After concentration the fractions may be examined, either with reference to their molecular weight, by SDS-polyacrylamide gel electrophoresis (Section 8.4) or immunologically by immunoelectrophoresis (Section 6.9.2). Fractionated mouse serum analysed by immunoelectrophoresis is shown in Fig. 8.5.

8.2.7 ## High-pressure liquid chromatography (HPLC)

High-pressure or high-performance size exclusion columns have been developed which have increased the HPLC molecular weight fractionation range sufficiently to

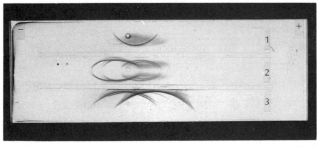

Fig. 8.5 Immunoelectrophoretic analysis of protein peaks eluted from G-200 Sephadex. Sample wells 1—3 contain the eluted peaks 1—3 from Fig. 8.4. The electrophoresed proteins were visualised by precipitation with a rabbit anti-mouse immunoglobulin serum. It can be seen that the peaks contain mixtures of immunoglobulins of similar molecular size except ror peak 1 where IgM is easily separated from the other immunoglobulins. It must be remembered that this peak will still be contaminated with non-immunoglobulin proteins, such as α_2-macroglobulin, not revealed by the anti-immunoglobulin serum.

deal with immunoglobulins. These columns are particularly useful for analysing the products of enzymic digestion and for monitoring the purity of fractions from gel exclusion columns. For example, they are capable of resolving F(ab')$_2$ from whole IgG and they are very fast; typically 30 min instead of the hours needed on a conventional gel column. The columns are generally small with sensitive detection systems capable of detecting 1–5 µg of protein, making them more suitable for analytical than preparative purposes.

8.3 Ultracentrifugation

The techniques of analytical and preparative ultracentrifugation have been widely applied in immunochemistry, both for molecular weight determinations and isolation procedures.

Preparative ultracentrifugation in sucrose density gradients is particularly useful for the isolation of chicken IgM. Chicken IgM cannot be easily isolated by gel filtration as the IgG forms soluble aggregates very readily and so appears within the excluded fraction of Sephadex G-200 as a major contaminant of the IgM. However, the difference in size between the IgG dimers and the IgM is still sufficiently great to allow good resolution in the ultracentrifuge.

A detailed treatment of the basic techniques available, for example rate separation and isopycnic separation, both with and without a density gradient, is beyond the range of this book. (See McCall and Potter, 1973).

8.4 SDS polyacrylamide gel electrophoresis (SDS-PAGE) for analysis of immunoglobulin proteins

In electrophoresis the migration of proteins is dependent upon the charge, size and shape of the molecules. However, in the presence of sodium dodecyl sulphate (SDS), proteins bind the SDS, all become negatively charged and have similar charge: weight ratios. When SDS-coated proteins are placed in an electric field, their spatial separation will depend only upon their size and shape. By varying the concentration of the polyacrylamide gel, used as the medium for the electrophoretic separation, different resolution ranges of molecular weight may be obtained. Proteins may be fractionated in the native state, but more information is usually obtained if the disulphide bonds are first reduced, allowing separation of the individual peptide chains. After heating to 100° in the presence of reducing agents and SDS, the proteins unfold and bind about 1.4 g SDS g^{-1} protein. The strong negative charge on the proteins thus means that their electrophoretic mobility will be inversely proportional to the logarithm of their molecular weight. There are exceptions to this behaviour: (a) heavily glycosylated proteins bind less SDS than unglycosylated molecules of similar molecular weight; (b) some proteins, such as J chains, do not unfold completely and retain some of their native configuration.

In practical terms, a stacking gel is cast on the top of the separating gel, this has both a lower percentage polyacrylamide concentration (typically, between 3 and 5%) and is prepared using a buffer with a slightly different composition. The different mobilities of chloride and glycine and the slow rate of entry into the separating gel relative to the rate of progression through the stacking gel are exploited to concentrate the proteins in a narrow band at the interface between the stacking and separating gels. This allows the loading of variable volumes of sample.

Originally the technique was performed in gel tubes but these have almost entirely been replaced by flat gel slabs. The basic technique described in Section 2.10 may be applied to the analysis of immunoglobulin molecules and their fragments to good effect. However, a large improvement in resolution can be obtained by running a two-dimensional gel (Section 8.4.2) in which the proteins are first separated in one direction in the absence of reducing agents and then electrophoresed in a second direction, at right angles to the first, under reducing conditions. This allows the determination of the molecular weight of a protein in its multi-chain structure and also the composition and weight of its individual chains. The introduction of gradient gels with an increasing concentration of polyacrylamide from the cathode (top) to the anode (bottom) has greatly increased the useful fractionation range of a single gel.

8.4.1 Gradient gels

Homogeneous polyacrylamide gels are widely used, partly because of the ease of pouring these gels, but gradient gels give increased resolution. Gradients of varying ranges may be prepared, for example from 4 to 30%. Proteins continue to move within the gel until they effectively reach their pore size in the sieving gradient.

8.4.2 Two-dimensional SDS-PAGE

Increased information may be obtained about a protein by running a two-dimensional electrophoresis. This may be performed in two ways to give three separate sets of information about a protein. A conventional SDS-PAGE may be run in one direction in non-reducing conditions, then following incubation of the gel with reducing agent, the proteins may be run into a second reducing SDS-PAGE. From this analysis the molecular weight of the native protein may be calculated and also if the protein is made up of several polypeptide chains, this will be revealed in the second dimension. Alternatively the first dimension may be run as an isoelectric focusing gel, to give information on the isoelectric point and the second dimension can be run as an SDS-PAGE to reveal the molecular weight.

8.4.3 Blotting onto nitrocellulose

The analytical power of the SDS-PAGE technique has been greatly enhanced by the use of immunological techniques to augment simple protein staining. However, reactions of antibody or lectins with protein in acrylamide gels are inefficient because of the slow diffusion kinetics and associated high backgrounds. Analysis of the fractionated components is much easier if they are transferred from the polyacrylamide gel and absorbed onto the surface of a nitrocellulose membrane.

Transfer onto nitrocellulose after electrophoretic separation was first developed by Ed Southern for the analysis of DNA. Later RNA blots were introduced and aptly named Northern blots. Following this tradition, transfer of electrophoretically separated proteins onto nitrocellulose has become known as Western blotting.

In Western blotting a sheet of nitrocellulose is placed against the gel surface and a current applied across the gel (at right angles to its face), thus causing the proteins to move out of the gel and onto the nitrocellulose where they bind firmly by non-covalent forces. Two variants of the basic apparatus are available to accomplish this electrophoretic transfer, the so-called wet and semi-dry blotters. In wet blotters the gels are immersed in large volumes of buffer whereas semi-dry blotters use only filter-paper pads moistened with buffer.

The technique is described in detail in Section 2.11.

8.5 Ion-exchange chromatography

Ion-exchange chromatography is an extremely useful method for the separation of proteins and the isolation of immunoglobulins. Proteins are bound electrostatically onto an ion-exchange matrix bearing an opposite charge. The degree to which a protein binds depends upon its charge density. Proteins are then eluted differentially by:

(a) Increasing the ionic strength of the medium. As the concentration of buffer ions is increased they compete with the proteins for the charged groups upon the ion-exchanger.

(b) Alteration of the pH. As the pH of the buffer approaches the isoelectric point of each protein, the net charge becomes zero and so the protein no longer binds to the ion-exchanger.

Both cation, for example carboxymethyl (CM) cellulose, and anion exchangers such as diethylaminoethyl (DEAE) cellulose, are available but the latter is used more widely for the fractionation of serum proteins. Cellulose remains the favoured support for the diethylaminoethyl group. Various forms are available to suit particular applications, and high-pressure liquid chromatography columns are available for analytical work.

8.5.1 Batch preparation of rabbit IgG with DEAE cellulose

DEAE cellulose can be used in columns or in batches. The batch technique is useful when large volumes of serum must be processed under standardised conditions. The

DEAE cellulose is equilibrated under conditions of pH and ionic strength which allow all the serum proteins to bind except IgG. The serum must be pre-equilibrated to the same pH and ionic strength as the DEAE cellulose and is then simply stirred with the cellulose prior to recovering the supernatant containing IgG. This method, although suitable for rabbit IgG, is not nearly as efficient for human IgG and so a gradient separation will be described for the latter.

Materials
Diethylaminoethyl (DEAE) cellulose — DE52 Whatman (Appendix II)
0.01 M phosphate buffer, pH 8.0 (Appendix I)
1.0 M HCl

Method
1 Place 100 g DE52 in a 1 litre flask and add 550 ml 0.01 M phosphate buffer, pH 8.0.
2 Titrate the mixture back to pH 8.0 by adding 1.0 M HCl.
3 Leave the slurry to settle for 30 min, then remove the supernatant with any fines it may contain. Re-suspend the cellulose in enough phosphate buffer to fill the flask.
4 Repeat this cycle of settling, decantation and re-suspension two times.
5 Pour the slurry into a Buchner funnel containing two layers of Whatman No. 1 filter paper. Suck the cellulose 'dry' for 30 sec to leave a damp cake of cellulose.

Preparation of IgG

The degree of purity of the IgG is governed by the ratio of ion-exchanger to serum, Fig. 8.6 illustrates the problems involved. For high purity more cellulose is added but this leads to losses of IgG through binding to the ion-exchanger. The precise proportions used depend upon the required purity of the IgG. Reasonable purity (about 96%) and good yield (about 70%) are obtained using 5 g (wet weight) cellulose for every ml of serum.

1 Weigh the cellulose into a beaker; for every 10 ml serum use 50 g wet weight of cellulose. Mix 10 ml serum with 30 ml distilled water, to lower its ionic strength, and add to the cellulose at 4°.
2 To equilibrate stir thoroughly every 10 min for 1 h at 4°.
3 Pour the slurry onto a Buchner funnel and suck through the supernatant; this contains the required IgG. Rinse the cellulose with 3 volumes of 20 ml of 0.01 M phosphate buffer, pH 8.0.

Collect and combine all the filtrates.

Examination of IgG preparation

1 If a determination of yield is required, then the IgG content in the original serum and the filtrate may be measured immunologically; for example, using either rate nephelometry (Section 6.8) or radial immunodiffusion (Section 6.6).

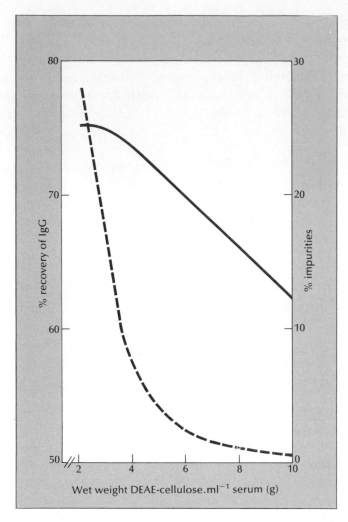

Fig. 8.6 Relationship of purity and yield of IgG to the amount of ion-exchanger used per ml of serum. This illustrates a universal rule of all protein purifications that the higher one tries to make the yield the lower will be the purity.
——— curve of percentage recovery of IgG.
----- curve of percentage of impurities.
(After Reif, 1969, *Immunochemistry* 6:723.)

2 The purity of the preparation may be determined by comparing the IgG content (measured above) of the filtrate with its total protein content (determined by UV spectrometry, Section 1.4 and Appendix III)

3 Use SDS-PAGE (Section 2.10) or immunoelectrophoresis (Section 6.9) against anti-whole rabbit serum to identify the main contaminants of the IgG.

8.5.2 Preparation of IgG with an ionic strength gradient

For maximum yield and purity a column technique using gradient elution is preferred for the preparation of IgG of any species. For human and mouse IgG gradient elution is essential. Initially, buffering conditions are adjusted such that virtually all the serum proteins bind to the ion-exchanger. The proteins are then eluted sequentially by gradually increasing the ionic strength of the buffer running through the column.

Materials and equipment
Serum sample
Diethylaminoethyl (DEAE) cellulose DE52 Whatman (Appendix II)

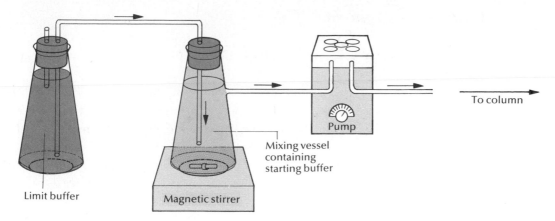

Fig. 8.7 Simple apparatus for the production of an exponential gradient. When the buffer concentration in the limit vessel is greater than the initial concentration in the mixing vessel a convex gradient is produced. Sophisticated pumps are now supplied for FPLC and HPLC systems, with microprocessor controllers, which allow the programming of an almost limitless range of gradients.

Arrows indicate direction of flow.

Column and fraction collection apparatus (as in Section 8.2.5, Fig. 8.2 and Appendix II)

Gradient device (commercially available, Appendix II or constructed as in Fig. 8.7)

Conductivity meter (Appendix II)

Phosphate buffers, pH 8.0, 0.005 M and 0.3 M (Appendix I)

Equilibration of ion-exchanger

1 Place the ion-exchanger in a beaker — use 2–5 g (wet weight) DE52 for every 1 ml of serum.

2 Add the basic component of the phosphate buffer (0.5 M disodium hydrogen phosphate) until the pH reaches 8.0.

3 Add 0.005 M phosphate buffer, pH 8.0. There should be 6 ml buffer for every 1 g of wet ion-exchanger.

4 Disperse the cellulose and pour into a measuring cylinder and allow to settle (settling time [min]= 2 × height of the slurry [cm]). Remove the supernatant which contains cellulose 'fines'; these may block the column.

5 Add a volume of 0.005 M buffer equal to half the volume of settled cellulose and re-suspend.

6 Pour the slurry into the column with the flow-control valve open. (A short wide column is preferable; for example, 25 × 3.3 cm.)

7 Pack the column by pumping 0.005 M, pH 8.0, phosphate buffer through at 45 ml h^{-1} for each cm^2 internal cross-section.

8 Monitor the buffer effluent with a conductivity meter. When the ionic strength of the effluent is the same as that of the original buffer, the ion-exchanger is equilibrated. If a meter is not available, pass 2–3 litres of buffer through the column.

Running the column

1 Dialyse the sample against the starting buffer (0.005 M, pH 8.0 phosphate buffer) (Section 1.5).
2 Centrifuge the sample. (Some protein will precipitate at this low ionic strength.)
3 Apply the serum to the column and pump through the starting buffer (about 60–100 ml h^{-1}). Monitor the effluent for protein. Most of the proteins should bind to the ion-exchanger.
4 Elute the proteins with a gradient of increasing ionic strength (see below). Collect fractions of approximately 5 ml.

Technical note

If a high concentration of protein is detected in the column effluent prior to the application of the ionic strength gradient either: (a) the ion-exchanger or serum was not fully equilibrated; or (b) the absorbing capacity of the cellulose has been exceeded.

Ionic strength gradient

Gradients of varying shapes are used for different purposes. A great variety of commercial gradient-forming equipment is available, ranging from relatively simple devices which are essentially two chambers joined together (similar to Fig. 8.9) to the very sophisticated electronic systems in which the rate of advance of the gradient is controlled by a monitor for protein in the column effluent. In the latter system a discontinuous gradient can be formed automatically and greatly increases the resolution of ion-exchange chromatography (see Fig. 8.8 for illustration of this point).

A continuous exponential gradient may be produced as shown in Fig. 8.7. The limit buffer enters the mixing vessel at the same rate as the buffer is pumped onto the column. The gradient is established according to the following equation:

$$C_m = C_1 - (C_1 - C_0)e^{-v/v_m}$$

where:

C_m = concentration in mixing vessel,
C_1 = concentration in limit vessel,
C_0 = initial concentration in mixing vessel,
v = volume removed from mixing vessel,
v_m = volume of the mixing vessel.

For ease of calculation this equation may be re-written as:

$$2.303 \cdot \log \frac{C_1 - C_m}{C_1 - C_0} = \frac{-v}{v_m}.$$

When $C_1 > C_0$ the gradient is convex; when $C_1 < C_0$ the gradient is concave. (Latter used for density gradient formation not ion-exchange chromatography; the highest ionic strength buffer will emerge first and elute everything off the column.)

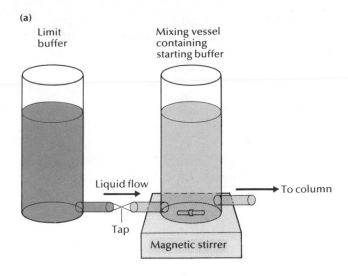

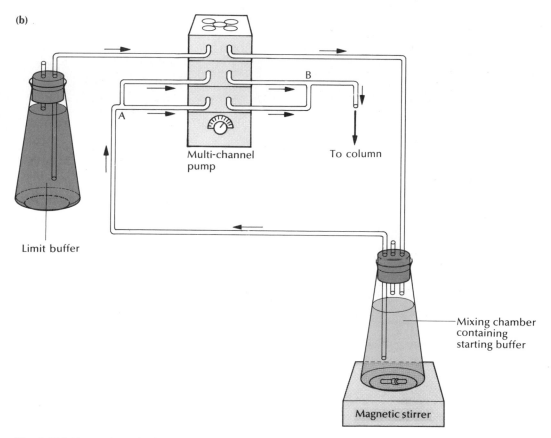

Fig. 8.8(a) Formation of a linear gradient using an open mixing vessel. The effective volume of the mixing chamber reduces as the gradient is formed.
(b) The production of a linear gradient by means of a multi-channel pump. Tubing from B to the column must be of sufficient internal diameter to take twice the flow rate in the rest of the system.
Arrows indicate direction of flow. A and B are 'h'-type functions.

Linear gradients may be established using an open mixing vessel (Fig. 8.8a) or by means of a multi-channel pump as shown in Fig. 8.8b. In this case the equation for the gradient is:

$$C_m = C_0 + (C_1 - C_0) \frac{v}{2v_0}$$

where:

v_0 = initial volume of buffer in the mixing vessel.
Other symbols as in equation for exponential gradient.

Distribution of serum proteins

Assuming that the ion-exchanger has not been over-loaded with protein the first peak should contain only IgG (Fig. 8.9). This is the only pure protein that can be isolated under these conditions of pH and buffer molarity, the remaining peaks contain several proteins. Beta-lipoproteins, haptoglobin and α_2-macroglobulin will contaminate the IgA and IgM fractions.

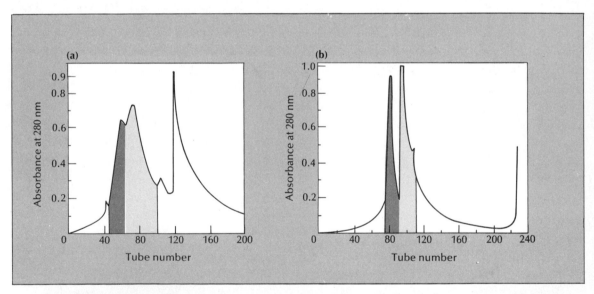

Fig. 8.9 Elution profile of serum proteins from a DEAE-cellulose column using a gradient of increasing ionic strength. Tubes contain 5 ml aliquots.
(a) A sample of 30 ml mouse serum, equilibrated with 0.005 M phosphate buffer, pH 8.0, was applied to a column of DEAE-cellulose (bed volume 25 × 3.3 cm) equilibrated in the same buffer. Elution was by means of a convex gradient, limit buffer 0.18 M phosphate buffer, pH 8.0, volume of mixing vessel 110 ml. The first two major peaks (tinted) are difficult to resolve as the ionic strength of the buffer increases before the first protein has been fully released from the cellulose.
(b) Using a sophisticated controller, the gradient can be held stationary as soon as a peak is detected, allowing isolation of the first protein. As soon as the absorbance of the eluate falls to a pre-set lower limit the ionic strength gradient is re-started to elute the second component. The striking increase in resolution is readily apparent. The first peak contains IgG1 and the second the other IgG subclasses.

Regeneration of the ion-exchanger

1 Remove the ion-exchanger from the column by washing out with distilled water.
2 Add 0.1 M HCl (0.5–1 × bed volume of cellulose).
3 Place on Buchner funnel and rinse through with distilled water.
4 Add 0.1 M NaOH (volume equivalent to the HCl used) and then rinse through with distilled water.
5 Wash through with full strength buffer and then re-equilibrate with low ionic strength buffer.

Technical note
To store cellulose ion-exchangers add chlorhexidine to a concentration of 0.002% for anion-exchangers and sodium azide to 0.02% for cation-exchangers.

<table><tr><td>8.5.3</td><td></td></tr></table>

Mass production and mini-column ion-exchange chromatography

The conditions for running ion-exchange columns are far less critical than for gel filtration, therefore it is possible to set up large numbers of mini-columns in cheap apparatus such as disposable syringe barrels. The conditions are sufficiently reproducible that fixed volumes of cellulose, serum and buffer give reproducible preparations of IgG and are technically so simple that up to 20 syringe columns in a rack with gravity flow may be run simultaneously. The following procedure will rapidly give very pure IgG.

Materials and equipment
Serum (human)
Saturated ammonium sulphate
Phosphate buffers 0.02 M and 0.2 M, pH 7.2 (Appendix I)
1 M potassium chloride in 0.02 M phosphate buffer, pH 7.2
Disposable syringe (10 ml)
Diethylaminoethyl (DEAE) cellulose DE52 (Appendix II)
Glass or nylon wool, or sintered plastic disc (Appendix II)

Method
1 Add 1 ml saturated ammonium sulphate dropwise to 2 ml human serum to give a 33% saturation. Stir for 30 min. Precipitating the serum with ammonium sulphate eliminates much of the material which would otherwise bind to the ion-exchanger and reduce its capacity.
2 Spin the precipitate at 1000 g for 15 min and re-suspend the pellet in 40 % saturated ammonium sulphate.
3 Stir for 10 min and then spin at 1000 g for 15 min.
4 Re-suspend the pellet in 0.02 M phosphate buffer, pH 7.2.
5 Dialyse the sample against 0.02 M buffer overnight.

6 Block the outlet of a disposable syringe with a little glass or nylon wool or a sintered plastic disc.

7 Place 3 g (wet weight) of DEAE-cellulose in the syringe and wash through with 5 ml of 0.02 M phosphate buffer containing 1 M KCl.

8 Wash the column with 20 ml 0.02 M phosphate buffer (without KCl).

9 Add the dialysed protein sample to the cellulose.

10 Elute the IgG with 15 ml of 0.02 M phosphate buffer and collect 3 ml fractions.

11 Determine the absorbance at 280 nm of the fractions and pool those containing protein. These contain the IgG.

12 Calculate the yield of IgG using the extinction coefficient given in Appendix III.

13 Elute the bound protein from the column with 0.02 M phosphate buffer containing 1 M KCl and regenerate the column. The DE52 may then be regenerated as in step 8 above.

Technical note

Greater through-put efficiency may be achieved by combining the protein dialysis and ion-exchange media in the same column. Layer Sephadex G-25 on top of the DE52 cellulose and equilibrate both as above. Filtration of the protein sample through the Sephadex G-25 will allow sample equilibration by buffer-exchange prior to interaction with the DE52 cellulose. Using this procedure many samples of highly purified IgG may be prepared during one working day.

8.5.4 QAE-Sephadex isolation of IgG

Quaternary aminoethyl (QAE) Sephadex is a strongly basic anion-exchanger which is particularly suitable for the column separation of proteins using pH gradient elution as the swelling of QAE-Sephadex is not affected by changes in pH. It offers the distinct advantage that IgG may be prepared using a volatile buffer and freeze dried without prior salt removal. It is advisable to remove β-lipoproteins from the serum before chromatography, otherwise they may break through and contaminate the IgG.

Materials and equipment
Human serum
Aerosil (Appendix II)
Diamino ethane−acetic acid buffer, ionic strength 0.1, pH 7.0 (Appendix I)
Acetic acid−sodium acetate buffer, ionic strength 0.1, pH 4.0 (Appendix I)
Quarternary aminoethyl (QAE) Sephadex A-50 (Appendix II)
Column and fraction collection apparatus (as in Section 8.2 and Appendix II)
1.0 M sodium hydroxide
Aquacide (Appendix II)
Dialysis tubing (Appendix II)
Centrifuge capable of 12 000 *g*

Method

1 Swell QAE-Sephadex A-50 in the diamino ethane−acetic acid buffer. A bed volume of 20 ml of swollen gel is required per 10 ml serum.

2   Pack the gel into a suitable chromatography column and equilibrate with the diamino ethane—acetic acid buffer.

3   Remove β-lipoprotein from the serum by adding 0.2 g Aerosil to 10 ml serum and stir at room temperature for 4 h.

4   Centrifuge the serum at $12\,000\,g$ for 30 min and remove the lipid layer.

5   Equilibrate the serum with the diamino ethane—acetic acid buffer by dialysis or column buffer exchange (Section 1.5).

6   Dilute the equilibrated serum with an equal volume of diamino ethane—acetic acid buffer. (If column buffer exchange was used the sample will have already been diluted by passing through the column.)

7   Apply the sample to the column at a flow rate of 8 ml $cm^{-2}\,h^{-1}$ and continue the elution with the diamino ethane—acetic acid buffer. IgG will come straight through the column while other proteins will be retained.

8   Elute the other proteins with the acetate buffer, pH 4.0.

9   Regenerate the column by running through two bed volumes of diamino ethane—acetic acid buffer.

10 Concentrate the IgG in the first peak to 1/10 volume as quickly as possible; for example, using dialysis tubing and Aquacide.

11 The concentrated sample may now be freeze dried without removing salt as the buffer is volatile.

Technical notes

1   It is important to concentrate the sample prior to lyophilisation otherwise an insoluble precipitate may form.

2   The yield of IgG should be about 70% of the serum IgG.

8.6   Preparative isoelectric focusing

A mixture of proteins may be resolved into fractions of differing charge by their differential migration in an electric field (Section 6.12). If this electric field is applied across a continuous pH gradient, then the proteins will move to, and concentrate at their isoelectric point, i.e. the pH at which their net charge is zero. Unlike ordinary electrophoresis at a single pH, the protein is concentrated to a very narrow band while the electric current is applied.

In isoelectric focusing a protein purified to apparent homogeneity by molecular sieving and ion-exchange chromatography may be resolved into several fractions. Indeed, the product of a single lymphocyte clone, for example a myeloma or hybridoma protein, may be resolved into two to five bands because of post-synthetic changes in the molecule (see Fig. 6.24). The major post-synthetic change involves the hydrolysis of amide residues to carboxyl groups by serum enzymes, thus gaining one negative charge for each deamidation.

PRODUCTION OF STABLE pH GRADIENT

The pH gradient is established using a mixture of carrier ampholytes. These molecules have a 'backbone' on which varying numbers of NH_3^+ and COO^- groups are attached. In an electric field the ampholyte molecules migrate to their various isoelectric points and produce an ascending pH gradient from the anode to the cathode. Different mixtures of ampholytes are available commercially for various ranges of pH gradient (see Appendix II).

PREPARATIVE FRACTIONATION

On a large preparative scale the pH gradient can be established in a column and stabilised by a sucrose density gradient. Because the pH gradient is not completely continuous, pronounced heating effects are produced which necessitates complex cooling circuits in the column. For general, low-resolution fractionation, a pH gradient of 3.0–10.0 is used, whereas for high resolution, a narrower pH gradient of 5.0–8.0 or 7.0–10.0 is preferable.

After focusing, the fractions are recovered by running the sucrose out of the bottom of the column through a UV analyser cell. This must be done immediately the electric field has been turned off to prevent diffusion of the bands.

Small-scale preparative isoelectric focusing may be carried out as described for the analytical system (Section 6.12) but using thin-layer Sephadex, rather than poly-acrylamide gels which are then sliced and mixed with buffer to elute the protein. It is possible to obtain sufficient ultrapure material by this route for the immunisation of experimental animals.

8.7 | Reduction of IgG to heavy and light chains

The heavy and light chains of IgG are covalently linked together by disulphide bonds. These bonds may be broken by reduction. As well as interchain disulphide bonds there are also intrachain disulphide links. Although the latter are less easy to break, a balance has to be found between breaking enough interchain bonds to permit chain separation but at the same time limiting the number of intrachain bonds broken so that biological activity is retained. The reduced heavy and light chains are still held together by non-covalent forces but can be dissociated by fractionation in an acid medium.

Materials and equipment
IgG
0.15 M Tris–HCl buffer, pH 8.2 (Appendix I)
2-mercaptoethanol
Iodoacetamide
1 M propionic or acetic acid
Trimethylamine
Nitrogen cylinder
Aquacide (or other means of concentration) (Appendix II)
G-100 Sephadex column, equilibrated with 1 M propionic or acetic acid at 4°
Dialysis tubing

Method

1 Dialyse the IgG against Tris—HCl buffer (Section 1.5) and adjust the protein concentration to 30 mg ml^{-1}.

2 De-gas the IgG solution with a vacuum pump and then bubble in nitrogen.

3 Add 2-mercaptoethanol to a final concentration of 0.75 M. *2-mercaptoethanol is toxic and so this procedure must be carried out in a fume cupboard.* (The solution is de-gassed and the reduction carried out in the presence of nitrogen as 2-mercaptoethanol is oxidised by atmospheric oxygen. Alternatively, reduction may be carried out with 0.02 M dithiothreitol which is less susceptible to oxidation. *Again this agent is dangerous and will cause a severe headache if inhaled*.)

4 Incubate at room temperature for 1 h.

5 Cool the mixture in ice water and add iodoacetamide to a final concentration of 0.75 M. This prevents re-association of the reduced interchain S—S bonds by alkylating the liberated sulphydryl groups.

6 Maintain the pH at 8.0 by the dropwise addition of trimethylamine.

7 Concentrate the sample; for example, by placing in dialysis tubing and covering with Aquacide.

8 Apply the sample to the G-100 Sephadex column equilibrated with 1 M propionic or acetic acid at 4° (see Section 8.2.5) and collect fractions of 5 ml.

A typical elution profile is shown in Fig. 8.10.

9 Concentrate and return the fractions to neutrality.

Technical note

A similar procedure may be followed for the reduction of the other immunoglobulin classes

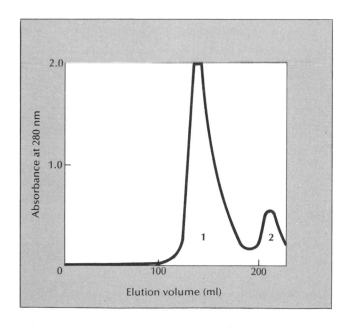

Fig. 8.10 Elution profile of reduced and alkylated IgG from a Sephadex G-100 column. Following reduction of the interchain disulphide bonds the heavy and light chains still hold together through non-covalent forces. They are separated by gel filtration in an acid dissociating buffer. The intra-chain S—S bonds in each domain are more resistant to reduction and are more readily broken by treating with reducing agents in the presence of 8 M urea or 5 M guanidine which allow the IgG to unfold.

ANALYSIS OF THE FRACTIONS

The success of the reduction can be assessed by SDS-PAGE in non-reducing conditions (Section 2.10). Alternatively, the samples can be examined immunologically by immunodiffusion against specific anti-light chain and anti-Fc antisera.

8.8 Cleavage of IgG by proteolytic enzymes

In the pre-antibiotic era a major use of immunoglobulins was in immunotherapy. Immunoglobulins from animals immunised with antigens such as tetanus and diphtheria toxin were used to passively immunise patients suffering from diseases caused by these toxins. Unfortunately these foreign immunoglobulins were themselves immunogenic and could often provoke a type III hypersensitivity serum sickness. To try to reduce the immunogenicity of these foreign immunoglobulins, they were treated with a range of proteolytic enzymes including pepsin and papain. These enzymes were known to cleave the antibodies into active and inactive fragments. In 1958 Porter exploited these observations in his Nobel prize-winning studies on antibody structure.

Many enzymes have now been introduced for the production of immunoglobulin fragments, but papain and pepsin are still the two most commonly used in the immunology laboratory. For many years immunologists have studied immunoglobulins either from humans or from experimental animals such as the rabbit, where reasonably large amounts of antiserum could be produced. Thus most of the accumulated wisdom on enzymic fragmentation applies to human and rabbit immunoglobulin. In addition, digestion conditions have been determined using biochemically heterogeneous polyclonal antibodies and so relate only to the average properties of the mixture. With the advent of the hybridoma technique for producing monoclonal immunoglobulins from mice it has become necessary to produce similar fragments from mouse immunoglobulins. Two problems thus present themselves: (a) far less is known about the fragmentation of mouse immunoglobulins in general; and (b) each monoclonal antibody is unique and requires its own digestion conditions. In this section the general principles learned from the digestion of human and rabbit immunoglobulins will be described, followed by some guidance on the determination of optimum digestion conditions for novel monoclonal mouse immunoglobulins (Section 2.10).

8.8.1 Papain digestion

Papain is an enzyme that contains active site cysteine. It splits the IgG molecule to the N-terminal side of the disulphide bonds linking the two heavy chains, thus giving rise to two Fab fragments and one Fc fragment.

Rabbit IgG

Materials and equipment
IgG (Rabbit)

Papain (Appendix II)
Cysteine
Ethylene diamine tetra-acetic acid, EDTA, disodium salt
Carboxymethyl cellulose (CM-cellulose)
Sodium acetate buffers, 0.01 and 0.9 M, pH 5.5 (Appendix I)
Phosphate-buffered saline, PBS (Appendix I)
Chromatography column
Fraction collector

Method

1   Adjust the concentration of the IgG to 20 mg ml^{-1} in PBS.
2   Add cysteine to a final concentration of 0.02 M.
3   Add EDTA to a final concentration of 0.002 M.
4   Add 1 mg papain for every 100 mg IgG used.
5   Incubate at 37° for 4 h.
6   Dialyse the digest against 0.01 M sodium acetate buffer, pH 5.5.

When the cysteine and EDTA are removed by dialysis, the enzyme is inactivated. More controlled termination of the reaction can be obtained by adding iodoacetamide to a final concentration of 0.1 mg ml^{-1}.

7   Apply the dialysate to a CM-cellulose column. This column should be prepared as for DEAE-cellulose (Section 8.5.2) but should be pre-equilibrated with 0.01 M, sodium acetate buffer, pH 5.5.
8   Allow 200 ml of 0.01 M sodium acetate buffer, pH 5.5, to run through the column.
9   Apply a gradient of increasing ionic strength (starting buffer 0.01 M sodium acetate, pH 5.5; limit buffer 0.9 M sodium acetate, pH 5.5), as in Section 8.5.2.
10 Collect and concentrate each peak. The first two peaks contain Fab, while the third smaller peak contains the Fc.
11 Dialyse against PBS. Crystals of the Fc fragment may form at this stage.

Human IgG

In contrast to rabbit, human IgG subclasses differ in their sensitivity to papain, in the order: IgG3 > IgG1 > IgG4 > IgG2. Thus, any one set of conditions will have a tendency to over-digest some subclasses while under-digesting others. Excessive digestion results in the further fragmentation of the Fc portion.

The same digestion conditions may be used here as described for rabbit IgG; however, the fractionation of the products of digestion is more complex. Although it is possible to obtain pure fragments by a two-stage ion-exchange separation, the first on CM-cellulose followed by re-fractionation on DEAE-cellulose, in practice it is easier to take advantage of the ability of staphylococcal protein A to bind to IgG Fc regions. Protein A has no affinity for the Fab region. As IgG3 does not bind to protein A, the IgG preparation should be selected for protein A-binding species before digestion (Section 9.1). Some of the IgG invariably remains undegraded after digestion so it is necessary to remove this on a gel filtration column before use of the protein A column.

Materials and equipment
Sephadex G-150 (Appendix II)
Chromatography column and fraction-collection apparatus (as in Section 8.2.5, Fig. 8.2 and Appendix II)
Aquacide (or other means of concentrating samples) (Appendix II)
Protein A—Sepharose CL-4B (Appendix II)
Phosphate-buffered saline, PBS (Appendix I)
1.0 M sodium hydroxide
0.1 M glycine—HCl buffer, pH 2.8 (Appendix I)

Method
1 Prepare a G-150 Sephadex column and equilibrate with PBS (Section 8.2.5).
2 Pass the dialysed digest through the column and collect fractions.
3 Any undigested IgG will come through in the breakthrough volume. The Fab and Fc will come later in one peak.
4 Concentrate the Fab/Fc peak to the pre-gel filtration volume; for example, by placing in a dialysis bag and covering with Aquacide.
5 Prepare a protein A—Sepharose CL-4B column as in Section 9.2.
6 Apply the Fab/Fc peak to this column and wash through with PBS. The capacity of the column for binding Fc is 8 mg ml^{-1} of swollen gel.
7 Collect the Fab which comes straight through the column.
8 Elute the bound Fc with glycine—HCl buffer pH 2.8.
9 Titrate the pH of the purified Fc to near neutrality with NaOH and then dialyse against PBS.
10 Regenerate the column by running through 2 column volumes of PBS. Store the column at 4°.

Examination of fragments

The fragments can be analysed by SDS-PAGE (both under reducing and non-reducing conditions) to determine the molecular weights of the fragments (Fig. 12.2). Then blot the fragments onto nitrocellulose and confirm their immunological identities with specific antisera. Alternatively they may be more simply examined by immuno-electrophoresis (illustrated for mouse fragments in Figs 8.11 and 8.12) although this will have less sensitivity for detecting contaminants.

8.8.2 ## Pepsin digestion

Pepsin digestion of IgG yields a fragment with two-thirds the molecular weight of the original molecule but with intact, divalent antigen-binding activity. This is the

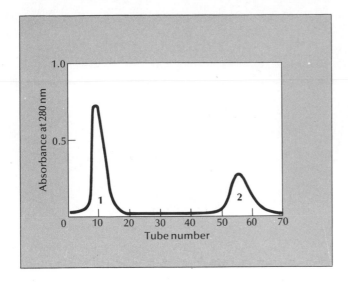

Fig. 8.11 Elution profile of papain digest of mouse IgG from DEAE-cellulose. After digestion with papain the sample was equilibrated in 0.005 M phosphate buffer, pH 8.0 and applied to a DEAE-cellulose column equilibrated in the same buffer. The column was eluted with a linear gradient, limit buffer 0.2 M phosphate, pH 8.0.

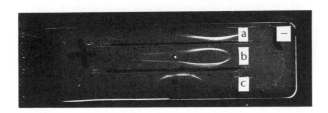

Fig. 8.12 Immunoelectrophoresis of fractions from DEAE-cellulose chromatography of papain digest of mouse IgG
Sample (a): peak 1, DEAE-cellulose, Fab fragments.
Sample (b): original IgG.
Sample (c): peak 2, DEAE-cellulose, Fc fragments.
    The proteins were visualised by precipitation with rabbit anti-mouse whole IgG. (Photograph of unstained preparation.)

F(ab')$_2$ fragment. The other one-third of the IgG molecule is digested into a smaller pFc' fragment corresponding to the CH$_3$ domains held together non-covalently, while the CH$_2$ domains are digested away to small peptides.

Materials and equipment
IgG (rabbit or human)
Pepsin (Appendix II)
0.1 M sodium acetate
Phosphate-buffered saline, PBS (Appendix I)
Acetic acid, glacial
Sephadex G-150 or G-100 column equilibrated with PBS

Method
1   Adjust the IgG solution to 20 mg ml^{-1} and dialyse 10 ml against 0.1 M sodium acetate for 3 h.
2   Adjust the dialysate to pH 4.5 with acetic acid.
3   Add 2 mg pepsin for each 100 mg of IgG used.

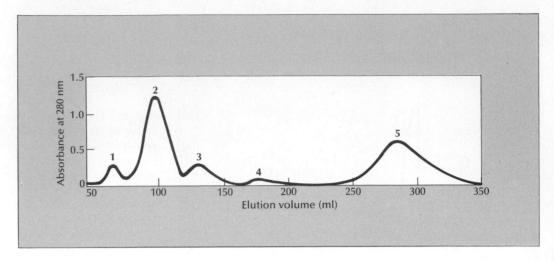

Fig. 8.13 Elution profile of a pepsin digest of IgG on Sephadex G-100. A 2 ml sample of digest (20 mg ml^{-1}) was applied to a column of Sephadex G-100 (bed volume 90 × 2.5 cm) equilibrated with phosphate-buffered saline.

4 Incubate at 37° overnight.
5 Adjust the supernatant to pH 7.4. This inactivates the enzyme.
6 Centrifuge and discard any precipitate that may form.

Analysis and isolation of fragments

Apply the digest to the Sephadex column equilibrated with PBS, monitor the eluate and collect fractions. Generally this will give fragments of sufficient purity but re-

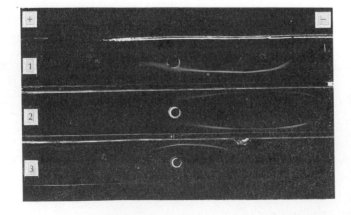

Fig. 8.14 Immunoelectrophoresis of Sephadex G-100 fractions of IgG pepsin digest. The fractions from the separation in Fig. 8.13 were examined by immuno-electrophoresis. The samples were visualised after electrophoresis. By precipitation with rabbit anti-human immunoglobulin.
Well 1: human IgG before digestion.
Well 2: Sephadex G-100 fraction 2 — F (ab')$_2$.
Well 3: Sephadex G-100 fraction 4 — pFc'.

cycling on a G-200 Sephadex column will get rid of any remaining contamination. A typical elution profile on G-100 is shown in Fig. 8.13. Peak 1 contains some undigested IgG; the amount will vary from preparation to preparation and may only show as a slight bulge on the leading edge of the second peak. Peak 2 contains the F(ab')$_2$. Peak 4 contains pFc', the small CH$_3$ fragment, while the remaining material is composed of small peptides (Fig. 8.13).

8.9 Enzymic digestion of IgA and IgM

Enzymic fragmentation of IgA and IgM is possible but is not nearly so well established. Pepsin digestion is effective but needs to be monitored continually. Short digestion times can yield small amounts of F(ab')$_2$ from IgM but longer digestion proceeds to a Fab-like fragment. IgA is also a suitable substrate for pepsin digestion but, from work with myeloma proteins, there appears to be considerable variation in sensitivity between different IgA preparations.

8.10 Summary and conclusions

Many techniques are now available for isolating immunoglobulin molecules. For example, using a combination of ion-exchange chromatography and gel filtration it is easy to obtain immunoglobulins of reasonable purity directly from serum samples. With a combination of techniques, for example isoelectric focusing of ion-exchange purified material, even single homogeneous immunoglobulins may be isolated. Although very high sample purity may be obtained, it is important to remember that the degree of protein denaturation increases with the number of manipulations. Thus, many properties may be attributed to the final purified sample that are simple artifacts introduced by denaturation during preparation. Aggregate formation is a particular problem, as properties such as complement fixation and macrophage binding will be activated even with small soluble aggregates. Endotoxin contamination is also a potential problem. Immunochemical separations are rarely carried out under sterile conditions so growth of bacteria is frequent. You will certainly not be the first person to have discovered the properties of endotoxin rather than your purified immunoglobulin.

When planning the fractionation and isolation of immunoglobulin fragments it is important to work out a logical pathway based on the structure of the molecule (Fig. 8.15). This is especially important with monoclonal antibodies where individual susceptibilities to particular enzymes will favour one fractionation route rather than another. In this chapter physico-chemical techniques have been discussed but is often advantageous to combine affinity methods (Chapter 9) with these procedures for optimum purification.

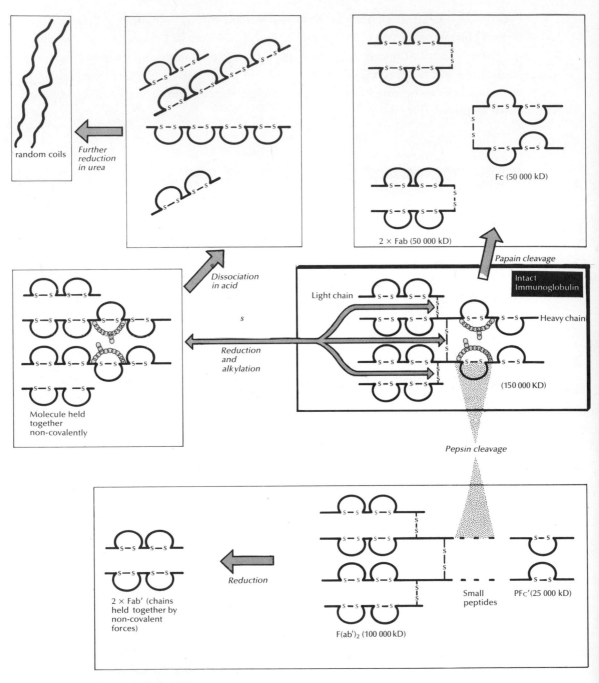

Fig. 8.15 Summary of the structure of human IgG and its reduction and enzymic cleavage products.
The IgG molecule is composed of four polypeptide chains covalently joined through S—S bonds.
These bonds may be split by reduction and alkylation and then dissociated under acid pH. The
individual chains also possess intrachain disulphide bonds and these may be split by further
reduction after unfolding the chains in 8 M urea.

Throughout most of the molecule the chains are also held together by non-covalent protein–
protein interactions but in the first half of the Fc region, close to the hinge region, carbohydrate
chains attached to the asparagine 297 residues interupt the structure and hold the heavy chains
apart. This more open structure is accessible to proteolytic enzymes and the IgG may be split with a
number of enzymes including papain and pepsin. Papain leads to the formation of three fragments
with similar molecular weight (2 × Fab plus Fc), while pepsin gives the divalent F (ab')$_2$ and a small
C-terminal fragment pFc'.

8.11

Further reading

Andrews AT (1986) *Electrophoresis: Theory, Techniques, and Biochemical and Clinical applications*, 2nd edition. Oxford University Press, Oxford.

Catty D (1988) *Antibodies: a Practical Approach*, Volume 1. IRL Press, Oxford.

Hames BD and Glover DM (1988) *Molecular Immunology*. IRL Press, Oxford.

Hames BD and Richwood D (editors) (1981) *Gel Electrophoresis of Proteins: a Practical Approach*. IRL Press, Oxford.

Hancock WS (editor) (1984) *CRC Handbook of HPLC for the Separation of Amino Acids, Peptides and Proteins*, Volume II. CRC Press.

McCall JS and Potter BJ (1973) *Ultracentrifugation*. Macmillan, London.

Parham P (1986) Preparation and purification of active fragments from mouse monoclonal antibodies. In *Handbook of Experimental Immunology*, Weir DM (editor), Volume 1, 4th edition. Blackwell Scientific Publications, Oxford.

Scopes RK (1987) *Protein Purification: Principles and Practice*, 2nd edition. Springer-Verlag, Berlin.

Stanworth DR and Turner MW (1986) Immunochemical analysis of human and rabbit immunoglobulins and their subunits. In *Handbook of Experimental Immunology*, Weir DM (editor) Volume 1, 4th edition. Blackwell Scientific Publications, Oxford.

Towbin H and Gordon J (1984) Immunoblotting and dot immunobinding — current status and outlook. *J. Immunol. Methods* **73** 313.

9 Affinity Techniques for Molecules and Cells

MOLECULES

The series of techniques described in this chapter combine the two most sought-after attributes in any purification procedure: large gains in purity in single-step procedures and technical simplicity. In affinity chromatography (technique summarised in Fig. 9.1), the former is achieved by the selection of an affinity ligand that shows strong, selective and reversible binding to the molecule being purified (in operational terms, the ligand's substrate), whereas the latter is facilitated by the use of an insoluble (and, preferably, chemically inert) affinity matrix thus permitting rapid partitioning of the ligand and its substrate.

In 1967 Axén, Porath and Ernbach introduced a general technique for affinity chromatography in which molecules containing primary amino groups could be

Fig. 9.1 (*Facing page*) **Affinity chromatographic separation of substrate molecules**.
(a) *Preparation of the affinity matrix*. Although we have chosen to illustrate cyanogen bromide activation of Sepharose, there are an enormous range of different solid supports and derivatisation reactions available (see references at end of chapter). The solid support should be chemically and biologically inert (before and after derivatisation); it should have a large surface area and a physical form (for example, beaded) that will permit a high flow rate; its physical and chemical stability should not be affected by the conditions used for desorption (treatment with free ligand, chaotropic agents, agents which disrupt hydrogen bonding detergents, etc. or changes in pH and ionic strength). The derivatisation reaction should result in an uncharged covalent bond between the ligand and solid support which is stable both during desorption and long-term storage. It should not inactivate ligand! Sometimes the ligand is sterically hindered by the support, resulting in a low adsorptive capacity (the theoretical upper limit of the affinity matrix may be calculated from the amount of ligand bound and the stoichiometry of the ligand—substrate interaction). This can be frequently overcome by the use of a 'spacer arm' between the support and ligand (see references at end of chapter).
(b) *Capture of the substrate molecules*. Practical considerations are very important at this stage; for example, the mixture containing the substrate should be in complete solution (this can be a particular problem with detergent solubilised cells — Section 9.7), the insolublised ligand and substrate should have sufficient time to interact (do not run the columns too fast and re-cycle the column effluent several times) and the final washing of the column should be exhaustive to ensure that no unbound or weakly bound material is trapped in the interstices of the column.
(c) *Desorption of the purified substrate*. The details of the desorption process are considered in Section 9.6.4. It is only rarely possible to desorb the substrate purely by competition with free ligand. Consider, for example, a relatively simple system such as the purification of anti-dinitrophenyl (anti-DNP) antibodies on a DNP—bovine serum albumin affinity column. Even when using very small molecules for free ligand competition, such as DNP—lysine, it is impossible to achieve a sufficiently high local concentration of free ligand, in the environment of the affinity matrix and anti-DNP-binding site of the antibody, to be able to compete with the high-avidity multi-point interaction. Instead it is necessary to reduce or neutralise the forces of interaction, originally responsible for capturing the bound substrate. A reduction of the interactive forces will sometimes permit the final release of the bound substrate molecules by free ligand competition; this brings an additional specific desorption step to the whole technique and so gives greater purity of product.

The simultaneous desorption of substrate and regeneration of the matrix is a particularly appealing feature of affinity chromatography; the column need only be returned to the adsorptive conditions to start the whole process again.

coupled to insoluble polysaccharide matrices activated by cyanogen bromide. This route of derivatisation is still the most widely employed today, even though the matrix so formed has the disadvantage of charged isourea groups, leading to a bioselective matrix with ion-exchange properties, and unstable covalent bonds between the matrix and ligand, which are susceptible to nucleophilic attack.

Support matrix — beaded agarose gels. Commercial agarose beads consist of linear chains of agarobiose units in which the ionic charge of the repeating 1,3-linked β-D-galactopyranose and 2,4-linked 3,6-anhydro-α-galacto-pyranose moieties is removed by reduction with sodium borohydride under alkaline conditions. As there are no natural covalent bonds between the linear polysaccharides, these are introduced by treatment with epi-chlorohydrin; improving the mechanical and chemical properties of the gel, thus permitting higher flow rates without compression of the gel bed and leading to improved stability at higher temperatures and in the presence of denaturing or chaotropic agents, etc. (Sepharose CL-4B [Appendix II] is a commercially available gel with these physical and chemical properties.)

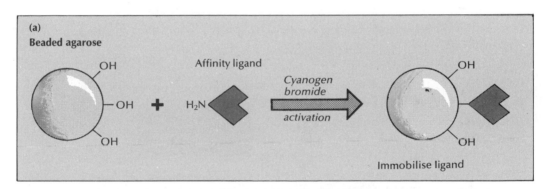

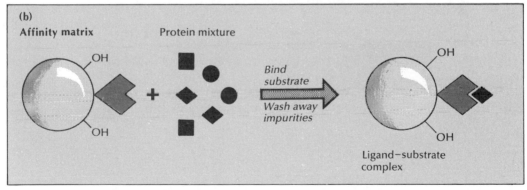

Matrix derivatisation — cyanogen bromide activation. Cyanogen bromide reacts with the vicinal diols of agarose (also dextran [Section 9.10.1] and cellulose) to produce an activated matrix which will react with ligands (or spacer arms) containing unprotonated primary amines as summarised in Fig. 9.2. The isourea group which is positively charged at physiological pH and can act as an ion-exchange matrix with negatively charged proteins (Section 8.5).

CELLS

The purification of molecules from cells (Section 9.7), and even of viable, functionally enriched cells, use the same general principles — and many of the same techniques — described above. However, cell-derived molecules tend to be highly hydrophobic and so require the presence of a detergent throughout the procedure, to maintain

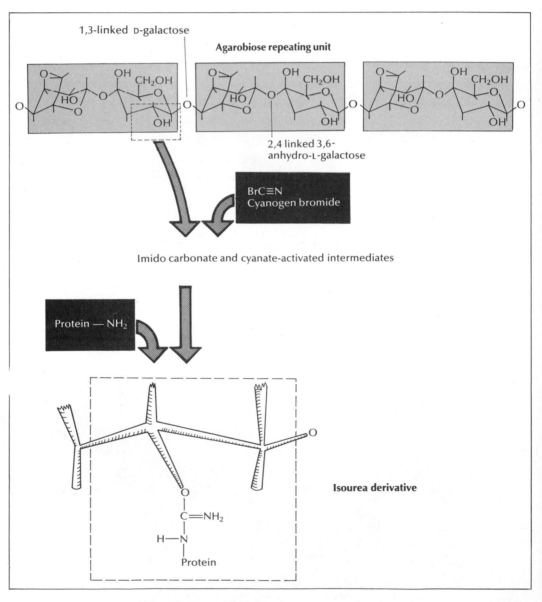

Fig. 9.2 Cyanogen bromide activation of agarose.

solubility. Living cells bring their own problems; not only because the affinity columns need to be run in physiological buffers at 4°, to maintain viability and reduce non-specific interaction between the matrix and cell, but also because, in the case of lymphocytes, contact between the ligand (in particular, antigen) and cell changes the nature of the latter irrevocably. Thus, even the sophisticated positive selection made possible by the development of electronically programmable flow cytometers (Section 9.11) still yield a population of lymphocytes that are no longer truly virginal cells.

9.1 Preparation of immunoglobulin isotypes by affinity chromatography

Affinity chromatography may be used to purify immunoglobulin isotypes as an alternative to the physical chemical methods described in Chapter 8. The most obvious way to use affinity adsorption would be to prepare an insoluble antibody specific for the required isotype. However, this requires that the purified isotype first be available to prepare the antibody for immunosorption! Fortunately, it is possible to take advantage of the affinity that immunoglobulins have for a range of other molecules. For instance, IgG binds strongly to protein A, a cell-wall protein derived from *Staphylococcus aureus*, while IgM binds to protamine and IgA1 binds to the lectin Jacalin.

9.2 Preparation of IgG on protein A—agarose

The IgG binding properties of protein A make affinity chromatography with protein A—Agarose immunoadsorbents a very simple method for preparing IgG. However, IgG subclasses show differential binding; for example, human IgG subclasses 1, 2 and 4 bind to protein A but IgG 3 does not.

Materials
Human serum
Protein A—agarose; for example protein A—Sepharose CL-4B (Appendix II)
Phosphate-buffered saline, PBS (Appendix I)
0.1 M glycine—HCl, pH 2.8 (Appendix I)
1 M sodium hydroxide or solid Tris (hydroxymethyl) aminoethane

Method
1   Swell 1.5 g protein A—Sepharose CL-4B in 10 ml PBS for 1 h at room temperature and then pack it into a small chromatography column. Store and use this column at 4°.
2   Dilute 10 ml human serum with an equal volume of PBS.
3   Filter the serum through the column at a flow rate of 30 ml h^{-1}.
4   Wash through unbound proteins with PBS until no more protein leaves the column (monitor the protein with a UV flow cell).

5 Elute the bound IgG with glycine–HCl buffer, pH 2.8.

6 Titrate the pH of the purified IgG solution to near neutrality with NaOH or solid Tris, and dialyse against PBS.

7 Regenerate the column by washing with 2 column bed volumes of PBS. Store the column at 4°.

Technical notes

1 The protein A content of the swollen gel is 2 mg ml^{-1} and the binding capacity for human IgG is approximately 25 mg ml^{-1} of packed gel.

2 Small quantities of some types of IgM will bind to protein A. You should be aware of this possibility and monitor the IgG preparations if absolute purity is required. Remove the IgM by gel filtration (Section 8.2).

3 Protein G is also useful for preparing IgG. It has a slightly different range of subclass specificities and is particularly good for preparing rat IgG.

9.3 Isolation of IgG subclasses using protein A–agarose

Although in both human and mouse, the IgG subclasses differ markedly from each other in their biological properties, they are structurally very similar. This similarity has made it almost impossible to isolate single subclasses using physical chemical techniques. Fractionation of the IgG subclasses is, however, possible using protein A affinity chromatography and pH gradient elution.

9.3.1 Isolation of mouse subclasses

Mouse serum may be fractionated on protein A–agarose by allowing all the IgG to bind to the adsorbent and then eluting the separate subclasses with a stepped gradient of increasing acidity.

Materials and equipment
Mouse serum
Protein A–Sepharose CL-4B (Appendix II)
Phosphate-buffered saline, PBS (Appendix I)
0.1 M phosphate buffer, pH 8.0 (Appendix I)
0.1 M citrate buffers, pH 6.0, 5.5, 4.5, 3.5 (Appendix I)
1.0 M Tris–HCl buffers, pH 8.5, 9.0 (Appendix I)
Chromatography column or disposable syringe
Antisera to the mouse IgG subclasses (Appendix II)

Method

1 Swell 1.5 g protein A–Sepharose in 10 ml PBS for 1 h at room temperature and then pack it into a small chromatography column. Store and use this column at 4°.

2 Equilibrate the column with 0.1 M phosphate buffer, pH 8.0.

3 Add 2 ml of 0.1 M phosphate buffer, pH 8.0 to 4 ml mouse serum and adjust to pH 8.1 with 1 M Tris−HCl buffer, pH 9.0.

4 Apply the diluted serum to the column and wash through with 30 ml of 0.1 M phosphate buffer, pH 8.0 (flow rate 0.4−0.5 ml min^{-1} throughout).

5 Elute the IgG1 with 30 ml of 0.1 M citrate buffer, pH 6.0.

6 Wash the column with 25 ml of 0.1 M citrate buffer, pH 5.5.

7 To minimise the denaturation of the IgG2a and IgG2b antibodies, collect the eluates of steps 7 and 8 into tubes containing 1.0 M Tris−HCl buffer, pH 8.5.

8 Elute the IgG2a with 30 ml of 0.1 M citrate buffer, pH 4.5.

9 Elute the IgG2b with 25 ml of 0.1 M citrate buffer, pH 3.5.

10 Re-equilibrate the column to pH 8.0.

11 Determine the composition of each fraction with specific antisera preferably using immunoassay (Sections 10.4 or 10.5).

Figure 9.3 shows the purity of fractions obtained from a protein A fractionation of mouse serum. An enzyme linked immunosorbent assay has been used to examine the protein fractions dot blotted onto nitrocellulose (Section 2.11).

Technical note

IgG3 usually elutes with the IgG2a fraction. Immunoaffinity chromatography on subclass-specific antibody affinity columns is required to remove this contamination.

9.3.2 Isolation of human IgG subclasses

Protein A may be used to obtain fractions of human IgG which, although not completely pure, are certainly much enriched for individual subclasses. IgG3 does not bind to protein A, so if total IgG is filtered through a column of protein A−Sepharose, IgG1, IgG2 and IgG4 will bind to the adsorbent but IgG3 will come straight through. The IgG1 and IgG2 may then be differentially eluted from the adsorbent with a pH gradient of increasing acidity. Although IgG4 is a slight contaminant in the IgG2 fractions, this problem may be reduced by starting with IgG prepared using DEAE-cellulose ion-exchange chromatography (Section 8.5); this is relatively deficient in IgG4.

Materials and equipment

Protein A−Sepharose CL-4B (Appendix II)

Human IgG, DEAE-cellulose purified (Section 8.5.2) or human serum

0.15 M citrate−phosphate buffers, pH 7.0, 5.0, 4.5 (Appendix I)

0.1 M citric acid, pH 2.2

Antisera to human IgG subclasses (Appendix II)

Chromatography column or disposable syringe

UV flow cell

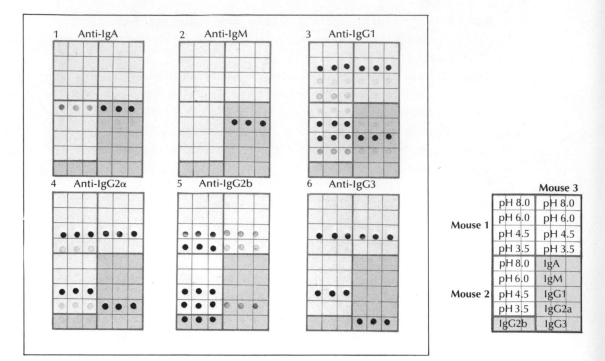

Fig. 9.3 Protein A fractionation of mouse IgG subclasses. Sera from MRL/lpr mice have been fractionated on protein A—agarose. The material coming straight through the column at pH 8.0 and fractions eluted at pH 6.0, 4.5 and 3.5 have been collected and dot blotted, in triplicate, on to six nitrocellulose membranes. Each membrane has been incubated with a biotinylated specific anti-class or subclass antibody. The blots were then incubated with Streptavidin labelled with peroxidase.

Blot 1, anti-IgA; Blot 2, anti-IgM; Blot 3, anti-IgG1; Blot 4, anti-IgG2a; Blot 5, anti-IgG2b; Blot 6, anti-IgG3. Grid key to each blot shown on right of main figure.

Commercially obtained, purified myeloma IgA, IgG1, IgG2a, IgG2b, IgG3 and HPLC-purified IgM were included on the blots as standards.

The blots show that it is possible to considerably enrich fractions for single subclasses from whole mouse serum. Some slight cross-reactivity is seen with the antibodies reacting with the myeloma proteins. Here there is the problem of determining whether the myeloma proteins or the antisera (all obtained commercially) are impure, or even possibly both. This experiment cautions the reader to not always take the manufacturers, publicity at face value.

Method

1 Swell 1 g protein A—Sepharose with 10 ml citrate—phosphate buffer pH 7.0.
2 Pack the swollen gel into a small chromatography column and equilibrate with citrate—phosphate buffer pH 7.0.
3 Load either 5 mg human IgG or 0.5 ml human serum (pre-mixed with 0.5 ml buffer pH 7.0) onto the column.
4 Wash the column through with pH 7.0 buffer. If purified IgG was used on the column, pure IgG3 will come out with the washing buffer. Otherwise, it will come out mixed with all the other non-IgG serum proteins.
5 Elute the IgG2 and IgG1 with a pH gradient of citrate—phosphate buffer. This is constructed by using a gradient maker of three equivolume chambers connected in series. The first chamber should contain 6 ml of 0.1 M citric acid, pH 2.2, the

middle chamber 6 ml of citrate−phosphate buffer, pH 4.5, and the final chamber, which is connected to the column, should contain 6 ml of citrate−phosphate buffer, pH 5.0.

6   Use a flow rate of 12 ml h^{-1} and monitor the eluate with a UV flow cell.

Two overlapping peaks will be obtained, the first being enriched for IgG2, the second for IgG1.

7   Each peak should be concentrated and re-cycled on the re-equilibrated protein A column to increase resolution.
8   To re-equilibrate the column, wash sequentially with 6 ml 0.1 M citric acid and 30 ml citrate−phosphate buffer, pH 7.0.
9   Check the purity of the IgG subclasses with specific antisera preferably using immunoassay (Section 10.4 *et seq.*).

Preparation of IgM on protamine sepharose

Protamine, covalently coupled to Sepharose, may be used to adsorb IgM from normal serum. After washing away free serum proteins, the IgM is eluted with sodium chloride. It is thought that the binding is mainly through electrostatic forces; the probable interaction being between negatively charged areas on the IgM molecule (where there are clusters of carbonyl groups) and suitable collections of positive groups on the protamine. Only the whole 19S IgM or the fragment composed of five Fc regions is able to bind; single IgM subunits have no affinity for protamine.

Materials and equipment
Normal serum
Protamine sulphate (Appendix II)
Sepharose CL-4B (Appendix II)
Cyanogen bromide (Appendix II) (*this chemical is very toxic and **must** be handled in a fume cupboard*)
2.0 M sodium hydroxide
0.08 M phosphate buffer, pH 7.4 (Appendix I) containing 1.1 M or 0.007 M sodium chloride
Tris-buffered saline (Appendix I)
0.1 M sodium bicarbonate buffer, pH 8.9 (Appendix I)
Sephacryl S-300, superfine (Appendix II)
Column and fraction collection apparatus (as in Section 8.2.5, Fig. 8.3 and Appendix II)

Preparation of immunoadsorbent

1   Pipette 14 ml of Sepharose (about 200 mg) into a 50 ml glass beaker and add 10 ml of distilled water.

All procedures must now be carried out in a fume cupboard:

2 Weigh a stoppered tube, add some solid cyanogen bromide, replace the stopper and re-weigh the tube.

3 Dissolve the cyanogen bromide in distilled water to a final concentration of 50 mg ml^{-1}.

4 Place the Sepharose beads on a magnetic stirrer and titrate the pH to 11.0−11.5 with 2.0 M sodium hydroxide.

5 Add 10 ml of the cyanogen bromide solution.

6 Maintain the pH at 11.0−11.5 by dropwise addition of sodium hydroxide for 5−10 min, until the pH becomes stable.

7 Wash the activated beads in a sintered glass funnel with 100 ml of water, and then 100 ml of 0.1 M sodium bicarbonate buffer, pH 8.9.

The rest of the procedure can now be completed outside the fume cupboard.

8 Wash the beads into a glass beaker with the bicarbonate buffer, allow them to settle and remove the supernatant.

9 Add 112 mg protamine sulphate in 22 ml 0.1 M bicarbonate buffer, pH 8.9.

10 Leave the beads stirring with the protamine overnight at 4° (most of the uptake occurs within the first 4 h and so this stage can be abbreviated).

11 Wash the beads on a sintered glass funnel with 10 ml PBS and collect the washings. (Use negative pressure and collect washings in a tube standing in a side arm flask.)

12 Wash the beads thoroughly with PBS to remove the rest of the unbound protamine.

13 A UV spectrophotometer reading of the washings will give the amount of unbound protein and so the approximate quantity of protein bound to the column can be calculated.

The immunoadsorbent is now ready. Store in PBS containing 0.1 M sodium azide.

Technical notes

1 In step 6, wash the gel with borate−saline buffer as soon as the pH becomes stable. The rate of inactivation by hydrolysis is highly pH dependent and increases sharply above pH 9.5.

2 For maximum uptake, the coupling pH should be above the pK$_a$ of the protein, but below pH 10.0.

3 Avoid buffers containing amines as they will compete with the amino function on the protein for the activated groups on the gel. Borate and bicarbonate buffers are the most useful (Appendix I); however, Tris buffers (Appendix I) may be used as the amino group on the Tris moiety is sterically hindered.

4 After coupling, it is possible to add 1.0 M glycine, pH 8.0 for 6 h at 4° if you wish to be completely sure that all the activated hydroxyls have been derivatised.

9.4.2 Use of immunoadsorbent

1 Wash the adsorbent with 0.08 M phosphate—saline buffer, pH 7.4, containing 0.077 M NaCl.
2 Add 28 ml normal serum mixed with 28 ml distilled water.
3 Stir slowly at 4° for 3 h.
4 Pour the gel slurry onto a sintered glass funnel and wash with diluted phosphate—saline buffer (1 volume 0.08 M phosphate containing 0.077 M NaCl plus 2 volumes distilled water). At this stage the gel may appear blue, due to adsorbed ceruloplasmin.
5 Pack the washed gel into a chromatography column and wash with further diluted phosphate—saline buffer.
6 Elute the IgM with 0.08 M phosphate buffer containing 1.1 M NaCl.
7 Concentrate the eluate to 2—4 ml (for example, by placing in a dialysis bag covered with Aquacide).

This preparation still contains proteins with molecular weights lower than IgM. These can be removed by gel filtration using either Sephacryl S-300 superfine, Ultrogel AcA22 or Sepharose 6B (as below; general principles Section 8.2.6).

9.4.3 Gel filtration

1 Take 200 ml of Sephacryl S-300 and dilute with 40 ml Tris-buffered saline.
2 De-gas the gel under vacuum.
3 Attach a gel reservoir to the column (100 × 1.6 cm) and pour the gel into the column along a glass rod to avoid air bubbles.
4 Pack and equilibrate the column with Tris-buffered saline. As Sephacryl has a rigid structure it may be packed using fast flow rates, optimally 30 ml cm^{-2} h^{-1}. This is equivalent to 1.0 ml min^{-1} in the 1.6 cm diameter column.
5 Fit a flow adapter to the column and apply the sample.
6 Run the column at a flow rate of less than 25 ml cm^{-2} h^{-1}. There is greater resolution at lower flow rates.

The IgM will be found in the first major peak. The descending arm of this peak may contain some IgA, while the other large peak contains ceruloplasmin.

Technical note
Although this technique has been optimised for human IgM it can also be used for the preparation of mouse IgM.

9.5 Preparation of human IgA1 on Jacalin—agarose

IgA is a comparatively difficult immunoglobulin to isolate by physico-chemical methods. Recently, the lectin Jacalin, obtained from the seeds of the Jackfruit,

Artocarpus integrifolia, was shown to bind human IgA1, but not IgA2. The binding is through O-glycosidically linked oligosaccharides containing galactosyl (β-1,3) *N*-acetylgalactosamine, in the presence or absence of sialic acid. For use in affinity chromatography the lectin is available conjugated to agarose. An immunoglobulin fraction prepared with ammonium sulphate (Section 8.1) must be applied to the column, as non-immunoglobulin serum proteins also bind to the lectin. Bound IgA1 is then eluted with melibiose or galactose.

Materials

Jacalin—agarose (Appendix II)

Jacalin storage buffer: HEPES 10 mM, pH 7.5, containing 150 mM sodium chloride, 100 mM calcium chloride, 20 mM galactose and 0.08% w/v sodium azide (Appendix I)

175 mM Tris—HCl buffer, pH 7.5 (Appendix I)

Immunoglobulin preparation; for example, 45% saturated ammonium sulphate precipitate of human serum (Section 8.1)

Melibiose 0.1 M or galactose 0.8 M in Tris—HCl buffer.

Method

1 Pour 2 ml of Jacalin—agarose gel into a small chromatography column (or 5 ml disposable syringe barrel with the outlet covered by glass or nylon wool).

2 Wash the gel thoroughly with 50 ml of Tris buffer to remove the sugars used to stabilise the lectin during storage.

3 Slowly add 5 ml of human immunoglobulin (10 mg ml^{-1}) in Tris—HCl buffer.

4 Wash the column through with 20 ml Tris—HCl buffer (or until the absorbance returns to base line, if you are using a flow-through UV monitor).

5 Elute the IgA with 5 ml 0.1 M melibiose or 0.8 M galactose (if using a UV monitor, elute until the protein peak has been collected).

6 Collect fractions of 1 ml and determine their protein content by spectrophotometry at 280 nm.

7 Pool the fractions containing protein and examine for IgA1 content and purity by SDS-PAGE (Section 2.10) and Western blotting (Section 2.11) with isotype-specific antisera, or alternatively by immunoelectrophoresis (Section 6.9.2) with antisera to IgA and whole human serum.

8 Regenerate the column by washing through with 20 ml storage buffer and store the Jacalin agarose gel at 4°.

Technical note

The binding capacity of the Jacalin—agarose gel will vary between batches but is typically 4.0 mg monomeric IgA ml^{-1} of gel.

9.6 Purification of antibodies

As we know from Chapter 6 an antibody reacts specifically with its own antigenic determinant to form an antigen—antibody complex.

If an animal is immunised with an antigen it will respond with antibodies all reacting with the antigen to some degree. Serum from this animal will have the usual range of immunoglobulins but those reacting with this antigen will be at a relatively higher concentration, compared to normal serum. In the same way, an animal receiving a transplantable plasmacytoma or hybridoma, will produce large amounts of the monoclonal immunoglobulin or antibody, but there will still be a significant background of normal serum proteins and immunoglobulins, even in ascitic fluid.

To study a particular antibody in detail it is of great advantage to be able to separate it from the surrounding, non-specific antibody molecules. The precipitated antigen—antibody complex seen in Chapter 6 has already done this for us! Unfortunately, the antibody in combination with its antigen has already completed the interesting reactions before we could follow them.

To obtain reactive purified antibody we must separate the complex and remove the antigen. The forces binding antibody to antigen are those involved in any protein—protein interaction:

(a) Coulombic.
(b) Dipole.
(c) Hydrogen bonding.
(d) Van der Waals'.
(e) Hydrophobic bonding.

All these forces depend upon the charge of the molecules taking part in the reaction; the net charge of the molecules in turn depends on the pH of the medium. If the pH of the medium is lowered sufficiently the protein molecules change conformation, gain H^+ ions, and so repel each other. We are now faced with the problem of physically removing the antigen or the antibody, because when the pH is returned to neutrality the complexes would re-form.

If the antigen is insoluble it can be easily separated from soluble antibody. There are many methods available for rendering either the antigen or antibody insoluble, some of which are described in the following sections.

9.6.1 Preparation of a protein immunoadsorbent

In this experiment antibodies to mouse immunoglobulin are purified but the identical method can be used for other proteins.

Materials and equipment
Sepharose 4B (Appendix II)
Cyanogen bromide (*this chemical is very toxic and **must** be handled in a fume cupboard*) (Appendix II)
2.0 M sodium hydroxide
Phosphate-buffered saline, PBS (Appendix I)
Borate—saline buffer, pH 8.3, ionic strength 0.1 (Appendix I)
Mouse immunoglobulin (Section 1.3.2)

Method

1 Pipette 14 ml of Sepharose (about 200 mg) into a 50 ml glass beaker and add 10 ml of distilled water.

All procedures must now be carried out in a fume cupboard.

2 Weigh a stoppered tube, add some solid cyanogen bromide, replace the stopper and re-weigh the tube.
3 Dissolve the cyanogen bromide in distilled water to a final concentration of 50 mg ml^{-1}.
4 Place the Sepharose beads on a magnetic stirrer and titrate the pH to 11.0–11.5 with 2.0 M sodium hydroxide.
5 Add 10 ml of the cyanogen bromide solution.
6 Maintain the pH at 11.0–11.5 by dropwise addition of sodium hydroxide for 5–10 min until the pH becomes stable.
7 Wash the activated beads on a sintered glass funnel with 100 ml of water, and then 100 ml of borate–saline buffer.
8 Wash the beads into a glass beaker, allow them to settle and remove the supernatant.
9 Add 100 mg of mouse immunoglobulin at 5–10 mg ml^{-1} (initial concentration).
10 Leave the beads stirring with the protein overnight at 4° (most of the uptake occurs within the first 4 h and so this stage can be abbreviated).
11 Wash the beads on a sintered glass funnel with 10 ml PBS and collect the washings. (Use negative pressure and collect washings in a tube standing in a side-arm flask).
12 Wash the beads thoroughly with PBS to remove the rest of the unbound immuno-globulin.
13 A UV spectrophotometer reading of the washings will give the amount of unbound protein and so the approximate quantity of protein bound to the column can be calculated.

The immunoadsorbent is now ready for use. Store in PBS containing azide (0.1 M).

Technical notes
1 In step 6, wash the gel with borate–saline buffer as soon as the pH becomes stable. The rate of inactivation by hydrolysis is highly pH dependent and increases sharply above pH 9.5.
2 For maximum uptake, the coupling pH should be above the pK_a of the protein, but below pH 10.0.
3 Avoid buffers containing amines; they will compete with the amino function on the protein for the activated groups on the gel. Borate and bicarbonate buffers are the most useful (Appendix I); however, Tris buffers (Appendix I) may be used as the amino group on the Tris moiety is sterically hindered.
4 After coupling, it is possible to add 1.0 M glycine, pH 8.0, for 6 h at 4° if you wish to be completely sure that all the activated hydroxyls have been derivatised.

9.6.2 Use of immunoadsorbent for antibody purification

Materials and equipment

Rabbit anti-mouse immunoglobulin (Section 1.7.2)
Immunoadsorbent-mouse Ig on Sepharose 4B (Section 9.6.1)
0.1 M glycine—HCl buffer, pH 2.5 (Appendix I)
Trichloroacetic acid, TCA, 10% aqueous solution
Tris—(hydroxymethyl) aminomethane
Phosphate-buffered saline, PBS (Appendix I)
Chromatography column (Appendix II)

Method

1 Pour the immunoadsorbent into the column and equilibrate with 20 ml PBS. Close the column.
2 Run 20 ml of antiserum through the column — do not use positive pressure, allow to run under gravity.
3 Wash the unbound protein from the column until the absorbance measured in a flow through UV cell is <0.1, otherwise wash with 200 ml PBS. Close the column.

We now have the antigen—antibody complex.

DISSOCIATION OF COMPLEX

1 Pipette out 20 0.5 ml aliquots of TCA into small glass tubes. (Use this to sample the effluent for protein elution if a flow-through UV cell is not available.)
2 Add glycine—HCl buffer to the top of the column and collect the effluent when protein is first detected.
3 Stop collecting the effluent when protein is no longer detectable.

The first stage of the elution is now complete and part of the antibody has been recovered. The acid elution buffer will, however, eventually denature the antibody so we must raise the pH.

4 Titrate the protein to pH 8.5 with solid Tris. Mix thoroughly and monitor with a pH meter or indicator papers.

We are now to alter the elution conditions to recover a second batch of antibody.

5 Add glycine—HCl plus 10% dioxane to the column. Monitor the effluent and collect the second batch of antibody (Fig. 9.4).
6 Adjust the pH to 8.5 with solid Tris.
7 Read the absorbance of each protein solution at 280 nm and calculate the recovered protein. (Remember to use the buffer plus dioxane as reference for the spectrophotometer.)
8 Concentrate the samples in dialysis tubing with either sucrose or polyethylene

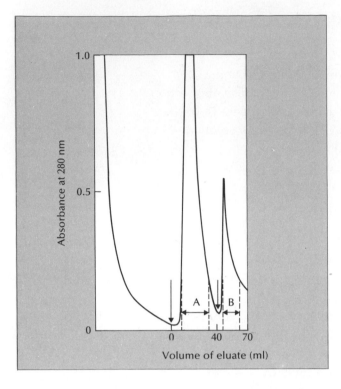

Fig. 9.4 Elution of antibody from an immunoadsorbent. The unbound protein was washed away with phosphate-buffered saline until the absorbance at 280 nm was below 0.1. A first population of antibody molecules was eluted with 0.1 M, pH 2.5 glycine−HCl buffer (first arrow). When elution was complete a second population of antibody was eluted off with the same buffer containing 10% dioxane (this second elution was started at the second arrow). To reduce the total sample volume only the volumes A and B were collected.

glycol 40 000 or by negative-pressure dialysis (Fig 9.5).

9 When the sample volume has been reduced to 3.0−5.0 ml, dialyse against 5 × 1 litre PBS.

10 Spin off the precipitate and determine the protein content of each sample.

This method of antibody purification is highly reproducible and so it is not necessary to calculate the antibody content of the sample routinely. However, a specimen calculation is given below.

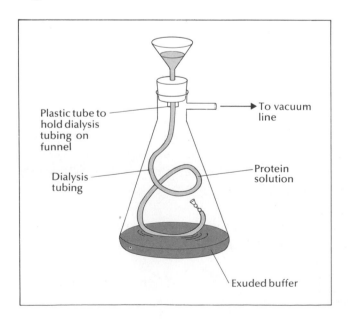

Fig. 9.5 Equipment for the rapid concentration of protein solutions by negative-pressure dialysis. It is advisable to test the system for leaks using phosphate-buffered saline before adding the protein solution to the dialysis tubing.

9.6.3   Calculation of recovery from immunoadsorbent

Total weight of immunoglobulin on column = 92.0 mg on 200 mg of Sepharose 4B.
Volume of antiserum for antibody purification = 10 ml.
Antibody content of serum calculated from Fig. 9.6, at equivalence condition as in Section 6.4.1.
Antibody content of serum = 5.2 mg ml^{-1}.

% yield of antibody protein from serum: immediately 81.5%; after concentration and dialysis 47.8%.

Eluates from immunoadsorbent
Total protein concentration in eluate:

Eluant	Immediately		After concentration and dialysis	
Glycine−HCL	36.4 mg	} 42.4 mg	23.0 mg	} 25.0 mg
Glycine−HCl + 10% dioxane	6.0 mg		2.0 mg	

Calculation of antibody content of eluate:

From Fig. 9.6: weight of antibody in 200 µg of eluted protein = 490 − 160
$$= \underline{230 \ \mu g.}$$

Hence, all the recovered protein has retained antibody activity. (In general, at least 90% of the recovered protein should be antibody.)

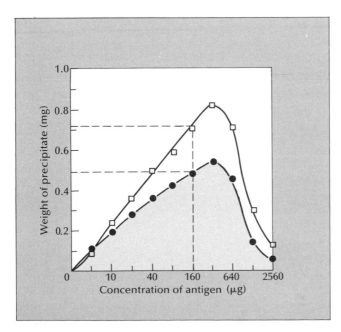

Fig. 9.6 Precipitin curves of anti-immunoglobulin serum and antibody.
□————□ 0.1 ml of original serum.
●————● 200 µg of purified antibody.

9.6.4   Elution conditions

Antibodies with high-affinity antigen-binding sites are the essential constituents of a 'strong' high-titred antiserum. However, when these antibodies are linked to Sepharose and used as solid-phase immunoadsorbents they give virtually irreversible binding to antigen. It is rarely possible, therefore, to isolate antigen or antibody by true affinity methods, simply because a sufficiently high concentration of free competitor cannot be obtained to compete effectively with the solid-phase reagents.

Most techniques for the release of material from antibody affinity columns rely on deforming agents to alter the shape of the reacting molecules and so lower their net binding affinity. Acid or alkaline buffers are usually sufficient to release an acceptable proportion of bound material, most of which will regain full activity when a near neutral pH is restored. The addition of dioxane to an acid buffer will increase yield from an affinity column (by reducing hydrophobic interactions) but with additional loss of recovered material due to irreversible denaturation.

Other, more effective eluting buffers may be used. These are more effective because they deform (and denature) to a greater extent. In order of increasing harshness they are:
(a)   3.5 M potassium thiocyanate in 0.1 M phosphate buffer, pH 6.6 (Appendix I).
(b)   8.0 M urea.
(c)   7.0 M guanidine hydrochloride.
Although these reagents will release bound protein more effectively, they may produce an unacceptably high proportion of denatured material.

When using anti-immunoglobulin affinity columns to isolate a particularly valuable antibody, for example a monoclonal antibody produced by a hybridoma cell line, it is good practice to saturate high-affinity anti-immunoglobulin sites by a cycle of pre-treatment with normal mouse immunoglobulin and acid elution (Section 12.9).

Technical notes
1   Under the conditions described, the Sepharose should bind 90−100 mg of mouse immunoglobulin. Approximately the same uptake can be expected with other common protein antigens, with the notable exception of bovine serum albumin where only 20−30 mg are bound.
2   Although the proportion of antibody in the final sample is fairly constant, the actual yield of antibody relative to the serum concentration varies with serum pool and species. The greatest loss of antibody occurs due to denaturation and precipitation after elution, concentration and dialysis.
3   In the experiment, the immunoadsorbent has been used below its maximal capacity; in general it should be able to deplete 1 ml of antiserum for each mg of antigen on the column.
4   Pre-activated Sepharose is available commercially (Appendix II); this avoids the use of cyanogen bromide. For large-scale preparations, however, it is relatively expensive.

Practical applications of immunoadsorbents

Besides their use for isolation of pure antibodies, immunoadsorbents are widely used to render antisera specific by depletion of cross-reacting antibodies (Section 2.1.8), and for quantitative adsorption.

Although the method described in Section 9.6.2 used an antigen immunoadsorbent to isolate antibody, it is possible to prepare antigen or immunoglobulin by the same procedure using an antibody immunoadsorbent column (Section 9.9.1) or a cellular immunoadsorbent column (Section 12.8.2).

9.7 ## Purification of cellular antigens

Much of our knowledge of the chemistry of the important antigens and receptors on cell surfaces has been gained by the purification of membrane molecules from detergent solubilised cells by immune affinity chromatography. The sheer specificity of the reversible binding reaction between antibody and its antigen permits impressive gains in purity in a single-step procedure. We describe below a general technique that can be applied to monoclonal antibodies (Chapter 12) or polyclonal sera, whether raised against a whole molecule or a partial sequence (Section 2.13.3).

Materials
Cells carrying the antigen of interest, solubilised in a non-ionic detergent (Section 2.8)
Monoclonal antibody, purified (Section 12.8) or IgG fraction (Section 8.5) coupled to Sepharose CL-4B (Section 9.6.1)
Irrelevant monoclonal antibody, purified (Section 12.8) or normal mouse IgG (Section 8.5) coupled to Sepharose CL-4B (Section 9.6.1)
0.05 M diethylamine—HCl buffer, pH 11.5 (Appendix I)
10 mM Tris—HCl buffer, pH 8.2 (Appendix I)
Sodium deoxycholate (Appendix II)
Bovine serum albumin, BSA
Glycine, solid
Absolute ethanol

Method
1 Before use, elute each column with 3 times its bed volume of diethylamine buffer.
2 Re-equilibrate with 3 times its bed volume of 10 mM Tris—HCl buffer, pH 8.2, containing 0.5% w/v sodium deoxycholate.
3 Saturate the non-specific protein-binding sites by treating each column with Tris—HCl buffer containing 1 mg ml^{-1} BSA, and wash through with Tris—HCl deoxycholate buffer.

4 Apply the detergent solubilised cells to the control column, collect the effluent and apply it immediately to the monoclonal antibody column.

5 Wash the monoclonal antibody column with 3 times its bed volume of Tris–HCl–deoxycholate buffer.

6 Elute the bound material by treating the monoclonal antibody column with 0.05 M diethylamine–HCl buffer, pH 11.5 containing 0.5% w/v deoxycholate.

7 Titrate the eluate back to pH 8.5 with solid glycine and dialyse against Tris–HCl–deoxycholate buffer.

8 If a further purification cycle is required the sample may be applied to the monoclonal antibody column after re-equilibration, as in steps 1–7.

9 Concentrate the final product by precipitation with ethanol; mix the effluent with 3 volumes of cold absolute ethanol and leave at $-20°$ overnight.

10 Recover the precipitate by high-speed centrifugation, re-dissolve in a minimum volume of 1% v/v non-ionic detergent (Section 2.8) and compare its purity with that of the starting material using SDS-PAGE (Section 2.10).

Technical notes
1 The detergent deoxycholate precipitates out of solution at high salt concentrations.
2 For maximum solubility after purification, the cell-derived proteins should be handled in slightly alkaline buffers.

9.8 Affinity chromatography of lymphoid cells

Cells can be isolated on the basis of any available molecule expressed on their surface membrane. These molecules can either be: (a) specific receptors, for example antigen receptors; or (b) antigens, for example immunoglobulin molecules (which are also receptors), histocompatibility or blood-group antigens, etc.

In the first, and simplest, system that we will describe, cells are adsorbed to the immunoadsorbent on the basis of their membrane content of immunoglobulin; however, these cells cannot be recovered and so we must work with the normal versus the depleted population. In the second system these cells may be recovered but in a slightly altered form; this is explained in Section 9.10.

9.9 B-cell depletion for T-cell enrichment

9.9.1 Anti-immunoglobulin columns

Materials and equipment
Degalan V$_{26}$ plastic beads (Appendix II)
0.1 M phosphate buffer, pH 6.4 (Appendix I)
Phosphate-buffered saline, PBS (Appendix I)
10 mg purified rabbit anti-mouse immunoglobulin antibodies (Section 9.6)

Method

1 Wash 5 g of Degalan beads with distilled water, and then equilibrate with 30 ml phosphate buffer. Remove all liquid with a pipette.
2 Add 10 mg purified antibody (initial concentration 5 mg ml^{-1}).
3 Incubate at 45° for 2 h, then at 4° overnight.
4 Recover unbound antibody and calculate amount adsorbed to beads as in Section 9.6.3.

CONTROL COLUMN

Many cells passing down a column of protein coated onto plastic beads will stick non-specifically because of the strong non-covalent intermolecular forces at the surface of the bead. Hence retention of the cells will not only be related to the antiserum on the column. As a control for non-specific retention of cells a column of an irrelevant antibody, for example anti-keyhole limpet haemocyanin, must be prepared and used in an identical manner to that described for the anti-immunoglobulin column.

CELL FRACTIONATION

Materials and equipment
Mouse spleen or lymph-node cells
Two 20 ml plastic syringe barrels
Sintered plastic discs for columns (Appendix II)
Tissue culture medium containing 5% fetal bovine serum and EDTA, 5 mM
Degalan beads coated with: (a) anti-Ig; and (b) an unrelated antibody.

Method

1 Pour the coated plastic beads into separate syringe barrels fitted with sintered plastic discs and equilibrate each with 30 ml of medium.
2 Seal off the column with a needle and rubber bung.
3 Incubate the column at 37° for 30 min.
4 Cool to 4° for 30 min before use.
5 Prepare a single-cell suspension of mouse spleen or lymph-node cells (Section 1.15) and deplete of phagocytic cells (Section 1.17). Wash in medium and adjust to 10^7 lymphocytes ml^{-1}.
6 Pipette 1 ml of lymphocytes onto each column.
7 Allow the cells to enter the column bed and re-seal column.
8 Add 1 ml of medium to the column, allow it to enter the column.

Under the conditions described the anti-Ig column will be able to deplete 10 aliquots of lymphocytes. The depleted population may be collected either as individual aliquots or as a pool.

9 After the last aliquot of cells, wash the column through with 15 ml of medium. Collect effluent.
10 Concentrate the effluent cells by centrifugation and count in a haemocytometer.

Technical notes

1 The high non-specific retention by these columns can be minimised by a high flow rate. At a flow rate of $2-3$ ml min^{-1} about $20-30\%$ non-specific loss may be expected.
2 All cell fractionation procedures must be carried out at $4°$.
3 T-lymphocytes prepared by this technique may be contaminated by a variable proportion of null cells (see Fig. 1.3).

9.9.2 Nylon wool columns

Spleen cell suspensions may be fractionated on the basis of their differential adherence to nylon fibers. At $37°$ and in the presence of serum, B lymphocytes will bind avidly to nylon wool columns, giving an effluent population of virtually pure T lymphocytes and 'null' cells.

The technique has the obvious advantages of speed, convenience and low cost.

Materials and equipment
Nylon wool, sterile (Appendix II)
Tissue culture medium (Appendix I) containing 5% fetal bovine serum, FBS
Syringe, 20 ml, plastic, sterile

Method
1 Pack 600 mg of sterile nylon wool (approximately 6 ml) into a 20 ml syringe barrel and wash with tissue culture medium containing 5% FBS.
2 Seal the column and incubate at $37°$ for 1 h.
3 Prepare cells (as in Section 1.15), deplete of phagocytic cells (Section 1.17) and adjust to 5×10^7 lymphocytes ml^{-1}.
4 Flush column with 5 ml of warm tissue culture medium. (This will correct any change in pH during incubation.)
5 Add 2 ml of cell suspension dropwise to the top of the column. After it has all entered, add 1 ml of warm tissue culture medium.
6 Seal the column and incubate at $37°$ for 45 min.
7 Wash the column with 25 ml of warm tissue culture medium and collect the unbound cells in the effluent.
8 Concentrate the cells by centrifugation (150 g for 10 min at $4°$) and determine the number of viable lymphocytes.

The effluent population should be depleted of B lymphocytes, as evidenced by anti-immunoglobulin immunofluorescence (Section 3.5.1), and will consist of T lymphocytes and 'null' cells.

A proportion of the bound cells may be recovered by mechanical elution as follows:

1 Wash the column with 100 ml of warm tissue culture medium and discard the effluent.

2 Seal the column with a needle and rubber bung.

3 Add 2 ml of warm tissue culture medium and squeeze the nylon wool with blunt stainless steel forceps.

4 Unseal the column and wash with 10 ml of warm tissue culture medium. Finally replace the syringe piston and expel all the tissue culture medium.

5 Collect the effluent cells and concentrate by centrifugation (150 g for 10 min at 4°).

6 Count number of viable lymphocytes ml^{-1} (Section 3.4).

The cells recovered by mechanical elution will consist of B lymphocytes (as evidenced by anti-immunoglobulin immunofluorescence, Section 3.5.1) contaminated with a variable number of T lymphocytes and 'null' cells.

9.10 Antigen-specific cell depletion and enrichment

In the previous section, cells were fractionated on the basis of their membrane content of immunoglobulin, i.e. into T and B cells. Because of the nature of the immunoadsorbent, the enriched B cells cannot be recovered in a viable state. In this section, we will describe a technique by which the column matrix may be solubilised and the cells released. The technique as described is used for the fractionation of antigen-reactive lymphocytes; however, an identical technique may be used for the preparation of T and B cells. (Although of course, anti-Ig antibodies must be substituted for antigen.)

9.10.1 Preparation of antigen immunoadsorbent

Materials
Sephadex G-200 (Appendix II)
Cyanogen bromide
0.2 M sodium hydroxide
Phosphate-buffered saline, PBS (Appendix I)
Borate−saline buffer, pH 8.3, ionic strength 0.1 (Appendix I)
Dinitrophenyl−human serum albumin, DNP−HSA (Section 1.6.1)

Method

1 Swell the Sephadex G-200 in water containing sodium azide or in PBS and remove the 'fines' by settling six times in 2 litres of water.

2 Pipette 40 ml of packed Sephadex G-200 into a 150 ml beaker and add 8 ml of water.

All further steps must be carried out in a fume cupboard.

3 Prepare a 50 mg ml^{-1} solution of cyanogen bromide (Section 9.6.1).

4 Adjust the Sephadex to pH 10.5 with 0.2 M sodium hydroxide and add 2 ml of cyanogen bromide solution.

5 Maintain the Sephadex at pH 10.5 for 7 min by dropwise addition of sodium hydroxide.

6 Wash the activated Sephadex with 100 ml of water and then 100 ml of borate–saline buffer. (Use sintered glass funnel. *Do not* use negative pressure.)

7 Allow the Sephadex to settle and remove the supernatant.

8 Add 20 mg of DNP–HSA (in solution at 2.5 mg ml^{-1}) and mix for 4 h at room temperature.

9 Wash away the unbound protein with PBS and store immunoadsorbent at 4° with 0.1 M sodium azide.

9.10.2 Use of immunoadsorbent

PREPARATION IN ADVANCE
Prime five inbred mice with 400 µg dinitrophenyl–fowl γ-globulin (DNP–FγG) on alum with *Bordetella pertussis* (Section 4.6, Protocol) 2–3 months before use.

Materials and equipment
DNP–FγG-primed mice
DNP–human serum albumin, HSA, immunoadsorbent (Section 9.10.2)
Tissue culture medium (Appendix I) containing 5% fetal bovine scrum and EDTA (5 mM)
Dextranase enzyme (Appendix II)
20 ml plastic syringe barrel
Sintered plastic disc for column (Appendix II)

Method

1 Pour 10 ml (packed column) of immunoadsorbent into the syringe barrel fitted with a sintered plastic disc.

2 Equilibrate the immunoadsorbent with 20 ml of medium and incubate at 37° for 30 min.

3 Transfer immunoadsorbent to a 4° cold room for 30 min before use.

4 Prepare a spleen-cell suspension from the immunised mice (Sections 1.15), remove active phagocytic cells (Section 1.17) and wash three times in medium.

5 Count and adjust the cell suspension to 10^7 viable lymphocytes ml^{-1}.

6 Add 10 aliquots of 10^7 lymphocytes to the column as in Section 9.9.1; collect the effluent as a pool (DNP-depleted cells).

7 Add a further 10 aliquots of 10^7 lymphocytes to the column. Do not collect the effluent cells.

8 Finally wash the column with 20 ml of medium and seal the column.

9 Add 500 iu dextranase enzyme to the immunoadsorbent and incubate at 37° for 30 min, with shaking.

The immunoadsorbent should digest completely in this time, however, digestion may be extended for a further 30 min if required.

10 Unseal the column and collect the digest (DNP-'enriched' cells).
11 Wash all the cells in tissue culture medium (without fetal bovine serum or EDTA) and count in a haemocytometer.
12 Calculate the percentage cell recovery for depleted (effluent) and enriched (digest) fractions.

9.10.3 Effector functions in depleted and enriched populations

We will assay the number of DNP plaque-forming cells in each population to estimate the approximate number of DNP reactive precursor lymphocytes. A more precise estimate of the precursor frequency can be determined by limiting dilution analysis (Section 4.13.1).

Materials
X-irradiated mice (Section 1.19.1)
Cells from previous section
Mice primed to keyhole limpet haemocyanin, KLH (Section 4.6, Protocol)
Dinitrophenyl, DNP, on fowl γ-globulin, FγG and KLH (Section 1.6.1)

Method
1 Irradiate the recipient mice with 8.5 Gy from a high energy source and reconstitute them according to the Protocol below.

Protocol

Group no.	Cells primed to:	Fractionation	Number of cells transferred per X-irradiated recipient	Antigen challenge (10 µg soluble antigen)
1	DNP−FγG	None	5×10^6	DNP−FγG
2 (a)	DNP−FγG +	None	5×10^6 +	DNP−KLH
(b)	KLH	None	5×10^6	
3	DNP−FγG	DNP depleted	5×10^6	DNP−FγG
4	DNP−FγG	DNP enriched	*	DNP−FγG
5 (a)	DNP−FγG +	DNP enriched	*	DNP−KLH
(b)	KLH	None	5×10^6	
6	KLH	None	5×10^6	DNP−KLH

* The number of cells per recipient $= \dfrac{\text{total number recovered from digest}}{\text{total number of recipients}}$.

Notes on Protocol
1 The design of the Protocol has been abbreviated from our own experience. Normally groups 1 and 2 would be replaced by a titration curve of transferred cells, for example 2×10^5, 2×10^7 and 2×10^8, to determine the dose−response curve.

2 Group 4 may be omitted. T cells are not bound by these columns and so the B cells alone will not respond.

3 Challenge each group with 10 μg soluble antigen intraperitoneally as shown in Protocol (p. 335).

4 Assay each group of mice 7 days later for DNP plaque-forming cells (PFC) as in Section 4.6.1.

5 Calculate the percentage depletion and enrichment for each group relative to the original population of spleen cells.

It is very important, in any technique of cell separation, to consider and record cell-recovery data, especially when dealing with antigen-specific cell purification. One would not expect, for example, to recover 10% of even a primed lymphocyte population on an antigen-coated column, without being aware of a large non-specific element in the isolation procedure. It is therefore essential, in experimental work, to include another, non-cross-reactive antigen as an internal control of non-specific adsorption.

In addition, the calculation of the factor of enrichment of purified cells from this *in vivo* assay can only be made against a full titration curve of the original population, as the PFC response curve of antigen-stimulated, transferred cells is not linear. Accordingly, the total number of PFC detected in the depleted and enriched populations may exceed the number present in the unfractionated population.

9.10.4 General technique for specific cell fractionation

The various techniques described for affinity fractionation of cells have required the preparation of an immunoadsorbent for each antigen or antibody used. In 1976, Scott described a very elegant technique, with wide application, for the fractionation of cells using antigen or antibody derivatised with fluorescein isothiocyanate. Lymphocytes are treated in suspension with fluoresceinated antigen (or antibody) and antigen-binding cells isolated by anti-fluorescein immunoadsorbent columns. Column-bound cells may then be released by mechanical shear (gentle stirring) in the presence of fluorescein on an heterologous carrier (this prevents re-association of cells after mechanical release).

PREPARATION IN ADVANCE

1 Treat keyhole limpet haemocyanin (KLH) with fluorescein isothiocyanate to obtain 5 moles of fluorescein per KLH molecule (per 100 000 Da) (Section 2.1).

2 Immunise a goat with the fluorescein−KLH conjugate (Section 1.9). Test for anti-fluorescein (Fl) activity (using Fl conjugated to an unrelated carrier; for example, goat γ-globulin) by precipitation in agar (Section 6.7).

3 Isolate anti-Fl antibodies using a Fl-goat γ-globulin immunoadsorbent (Section 9.6.1) and link to Sepharose 6B (Appendix II) using cyanogen bromide (conditions of activation as in Section 9.6.1).

4 Fluoresceinate antigen or antibody to be used for the fractionation of lymphocytes (Section 2.1).

Materials and equipment

As in Section 9.10.1, but in addition:

Sepharose conjugated with anti-fluorescein, anti-Fl, antibodies

Antigen (or antibody) for cell fractionation, conjugated with fluorescein (as in Section 2.1).

Bovine serum albumin, BSA, conjugated with 5 moles mol^{-1} fluorescein (as in Section 2.1)

Tissue culture medium (appendix I) containing 5% v/v fetal bovine serum, FBS

Method

1 Pour 3 ml (packed volume) of anti-Fl derivatised beads into a 10 ml syringe barrel. Equilibrate and incubate column (as in Section 9.10.2).

2 Prepare cell suspension for fractionation (as in Section 9.10.2).

3 Treat cells with Fl-antigen (or antibody) at 100 µg ml^{-1} for 30 min on melting ice.

4 Wash in culture medium containing 5% FBS by centrifugation.

5 Adjust cells to 1×10^8 ml^{-1} and load dropwise onto the top of the anti-Fl column. Experience has shown that a 3 ml anti-Fl column, prepared as above, will retain $1-3\times10^7$ Fl-labelled lymphocytes.

6 Wash the cells into the column with 0.5 ml tissue culture medium and seal column.

7 Incubate for 5 min at 4°. Unseal the column and wash with 20 ml of cold tissue culture medium. Collect the depleted population (cells not binding the Fl-labelled reagent) in the effluent and concentrate by centrifugation (150 *g* for 10 min at 4°).

8 Add 3 ml Fl$_5$-BSA (initial concentration 5 mg ml^{-1} protein) and stir the column gently with a fine stainless steel rod. Collect the eluted cells.

9 Wash the column with 10 ml of Fl$_5$-BSA (initial concentration 500 µg ml^{-1} protein) and then 20 ml of tissue culture medium. Collect the eluted population.

10 Pool eluted populations from steps 9 and 10, and wash three times by centrifugation (150 *g* for 10 min at 4°) in tissue culture medium.

11 Assay the depleted (effluent), enriched (eluted) and original cell suspensions for activity as in Section 9.10.3

9.11 Preparative continuous-flow cytofluorimetery

Continuous-flow cytofluorimetery undoubtedly provides the most powerful and discriminatory means of fractionating cell populations. Each of the analytical parameters described in Section 3.9 may be 'nested' to provide a 'sort profile' for a very particular and very minor cell population. The only limitation to the application of this technique, other than the expense of purchasing the instrument, is the need to work with single cells in suspension.

Cell suspensions are treated with an antigen or antibody labelled with a fluorochrome reagent. In the cytofluorimeter, the labelled cells are injected into a liquid carrier stream in ultradilute suspension and pass through a small orifice which is vibrated to break up the liquid into regularly spaced droplets of uniform size. Cells are irradiated with high intensity monochromatic light from one or more lasers (currently three laser instruments are available, based on krypton, argon and pulsed dye lasers, thus permitting, for example, simultaneous use of a combination of three of the following fluorochromes: fluorescein, phycoerythrin, Texas red and rhodamine). Correlated information on size, granularity, surface topography and fluorescent intensity of each cell is collected by an array of photomultipliers and a photodetector and the digitised information processed by a computer.

In this way, cells may be examined individually and, if specified by the pre-set parameters, may be extracted from the main droplet stream by electrically charging the appropriate set of droplets (usually a constant number of droplets; between 3 and 5, are charged depending on the cell frequency in the droplet stream) which are then deflected as they pass between charged plates (Fig. 9.7). The droplets (and therefore the cells) can end up in one of three places: (a) 'don't care' — no charge placed on droplet which then falls directly into the waste collector; (b) sort left — parameter set A; and (c) sort right — parameter set B.

Although the sorting rate of these instruments (fluorescent activated cell sorter, FACS [Becton–Dickinson], and electronically programmable individual cell sorter, EPICS [Coulter Electronics]) is relatively low, about 10^4 cells sec^{-1}, this is offset by a prodigious increase in the frequency of positively selected cells; for example, cells at an original frequency of 1 in 10^3 or 10^4 may be purified up to a relative purity of 80–90%.

Viable cells are not harmed by the separation process and can be used for *in vitro* culture or *in vivo* transfer experiments. However, in any technique of positive selection, the cells will have been in contact with a ligand (antigen, antibody, lectin, etc.) and so will be altered from their pre-selected state. In practice, this caveat is important to the interpretation of results but is not a barrier to the use of these techniques.

Fig. 9.7 (*Facing page*) **Principles of preparative flow cytometry**. The basic layout of the system is shown in (**a**). When a cell meeting the 'sort right' parameters is detected at position 1, the whole of the buffer stream is given an instantaneous negative (or positive) charge so that droplets formed at this instant carry with them the charge of the stream prior to separation. The charge of the buffer stream then returns to neutral ('don't care' because the droplets run to waste) or its charge may be reversed if a cell meeting the 'sort left' criteria is detected. Deflection of the charged droplets occurs between a pair of charged plates.

As the information is gained at position ① and acted upon at position ②, and the machine can be called upon to control $10^4 - 10^5$ such events per sec, it is easy to see the precision and speed of operation required of the electronic decision making circuits.

(**b**) to (**d**) summarise the deflection process. Droplets carry with them the charge of the stream at their moment of formation. (**b**) The 3 droplets between the deflection plates do not contain cells of interest and so have not been charged. (**c**) Droplets with a negative charge contain one of the required cells and so are displaced laterally from the buffer stream. (**d**) The cell in the droplets between the charged plates are not required so the droplets are allowed to go to waste. The number of droplets sorted as a group, and the number of cells in the group, is crucial to the purity of the end result and the speed with which sorting is achieved. For high-purity sorting, a rapid 'low-purity' sort is often followed by a slow 'high-purity' second sort.

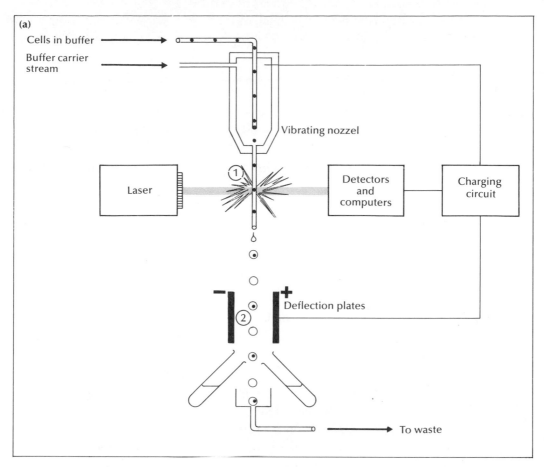

(a)

Cells in buffer

Buffer carrier stream

Vibrating nozzel

Laser

Detectors and computers

Charging circuit

Deflection plates

To waste

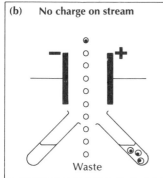
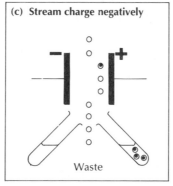
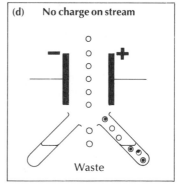

(b) No charge on stream

Waste

(c) Stream charge negatively

Waste

(d) No charge on stream

Waste

9.12

Immunomagnetic bead fractionation

Magnetic beads — polymer beads containing $\gamma\text{-}Fe_2O_3$ — to which antibodies may be coupled are increasingly used to deplete or isolate lymphocyte subpopulations and offer the significant technical advantage that they may be quickly separated by applying a magnetic field. Beads ready-coated with a range of antibodies are available commercially, a particularly useful preparation being beads coated with anti-mouse immunoglobulin. When working with human lymphocytes, for example, cells can be incubated with a mouse monoclonal antibody to a particular phenotypic marker and the antibody coated-cells removed by adding magnetic beads coated with anti-mouse immunoglobulin.

Materials and equipment

Human lymphocytes (isolated by density gradient centrifugation, Section 1.13)
Magnetic beads coated with anti-mouse immunoglobulin (Appendix II)
Samarium magnet (Appendix II)
Mouse monoclonal antibody to lymphocyte subpopulation to be depleted Hank's buffered saline (Appendix I)

Method

1 Wash the cells twice with Hank's buffered saline by centrifugation (150 g for 10 min at 4°).
2 Add monoclonal antibody to the cells to be depleted and incubate in an ice bath for 30 min.
3 Wash the cells twice with Hank's buffered saline.
4 Re-suspend the cells in ice-cold Hank's with 2% fetal calf serum at a concentration of $20-40\times10^6$ ml^{-1}.
5 Add magnetic beads coated with anti-mouse immunoglobulin. The precise number of beads to add will vary with the proportion of cells to be depleted, about 10−20 beads per cell are recommended.
6 Incubate at 4° for 30 min on a roller.
7 Place a samarium magnet on the outside wall of the tube for about 30 sec to collect rosetted cells and free beads.
8 Decant the supernatant containing the cells minus the depleted population.

Technical note

These beads may also be used to adsorb cells but recovery of cells from the beads can be difficult. The addition of excess antibody of the same specificity as that on the beads combined with incubation at 37° with agitation will release a proportion of the cells.

9.13 ## Summary and conclusions

Much of our present knowledge on the functional relations between lymphocytes has been gained by the study of fractionated populations, whether alone or after deliberate recombination. In this chapter, we have described only a small number of the wide variety of affinity techniques that have been used for fractionation of mixtures of cells. Indeed, so many markers are now available for the delineation and potential isolation of lymphocyte subpopulations that they greatly exceed the number of functional attributes available (Figs 12.8−12.11).

Clearly, immunology is once again at a stage analogous to the discovery of T and B lymphocytes; we know there are lots of different types of lymphocytes, but we are not sure what they all do in the cellular complexities that underlie the control and expression of the immune response.

9.14   ## Further reading

Affinity Chromatography — Principles and Methods. Available from Pharmacia LKB Limited (Appendix II).

Dean PDG, Johnson WS and Middle FA (editors) (1985) *Affinity Chromatography — a Practical Approach*. IRL Press, Oxford.

Pretlow TG and Pretlow TP (editors) (1987) *Cell Separation: Methods and Applications*, 5 volumes. Academic Press, New York.

Shapiro HM (1988) *Practical Flow Cytometry*, 2nd edition. Alan R Liss, New York.

10 Immunoassay

Antibodies have been used as diagnostic reagents for most of this century but it is less than 30 years since immunoassay as such was introduced. It is impressive that only 20 years ago clinical investigations such as pregnancy testing relied on the use of live animals and skilled technicians, whereas now a more reliable and sensitive immunoassay can be purchased over the chemist's counter and carried out by anyone in their own kitchen (or wherever!).

In essence, immunoassay simply involves the mixing of antigen with antibody followed by the discrimination of bound from free reactants. To aid this, either the antigen or antibody is labelled, most often with an enzyme or radioisotope. As there is no fundamental difference between assays using antibodies as the analytical reagent and assays involving other reagents, it can be helpful to think in the assayists' terms of the *analytical reagent* and the *analyte* (the substance to be analysed). This can be especially helpful in immunology where frequently it is the antibody which is being assayed and so the antigen becomes, in effect, the analytical reagent.

The basis of all these assays is the formation of a complex between analyte and analytical reagent, followed by estimation of bound versus free components. At virtually every step in the general assay procedure it is possible to choose from a wide variety of different techniques, and therefore enormous methodological flexibility is possible to achieve an optimised system. For example, there are solid versus soluble-phase assays, radioisotope versus enzyme, competitive versus non-competitive assays, etc.

The original immunoassays, introduced in the UK in 1960 by Ekins as an assay for thyroxine and in the USA by Yalow and Berson as an assay for insulin, involved a saturation analysis in which a limiting amount of antibody was reacted with excess labelled antigen. If samples of unlabelled antigen are added to an assay of this type they will inhibit the binding of labelled antigen to the antibody (Fig. 10.1). A set of standards may be used to construct an inhibition curve from which the amount of an unknown analyte may be determined by the degree of inhibition induced. It can be appreciated that, to obtain optimal sensitivity, the concentration of antibody should be as low as possible but, as the concentrations of reactants decrease, other factors such as the speed of reaction and accuracy become limiting. Thus, the sensitivity of competition immunoassays is dependent on a combination of the antibody affinity and the error in determining the bound fraction. Once assay procedures have been optimised, the limiting factor becomes the ability to raise antisera containing high-affinity anti-bodies. Since the affinity is unlikely to exceed 1×10^{12} litre mol^{-1} and as it is impractical to lower the experimental error to less than 1%, this imposes a theoretical limit on sensitivity of 1×10^{14} mol litre^{-1}. Using the Avogadro constant this gives just under 10^7 molecules ml^{-1} as the theoretical lower limit of detection (Ekins, 1981 and 1985, for a fuller discussion of these points see further reading).

Labelled antibody assays introduced by Miles and Hales (1968) depend upon the completely different (immunometric) principle of using an excess of antibody rather

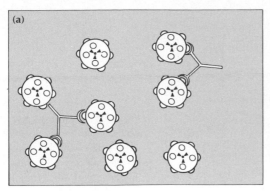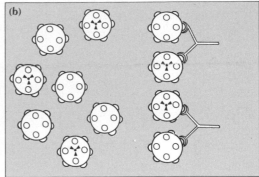

Fig. 10.1 Saturation Immunoassay. An excess of antigen competes for a limiting amount of antibody. Unlabelled antigen inhibits the binding of labelled antigen.

than an excess of antigen. Standard amounts of antigen are reacted with excess labelled antibody then, following separation of bound and free reactants, the bound antibody is estimated. An important feature of this type of assay is that no matter how low the antigen concentration, if sufficient antibody is added, some of the antibody will combine to form a complex within a given time; the rate of complex formation being equal to $K_1[Ag][Ab]$. In principle, therefore, a single molecule of antigen may be detected.

In addition to sensitivity, an equally important consideration is assay specificity. This is a particular problem for immunometric assays where the antibody is in excess and any cross-reactivity in the antiserum could allow side reactions with inappropriate antigens. The propensity of immunometric assays to pick up very weak and possibly spurious cross-reactions has probably been under-estimated in some studies. The need for pure and highly specific antibodies was a considerable hindrance to the widespread application of immunometric assays based on polyclonal antisera. However, the development of highly efficient affinity chromatographic techniques and, more especially, the introduction of techniques for the routine preparation of monoclonal antibodies has reduced this problem to trivial proportions.

A big advantage of immunometric assays is that two analytical reagents can be used to characterise the analyte as long as it has two distinct epitopes. Most frequently, the assay is performed in sandwich form as shown in Fig. 10.2.

This type of analysis may be exploited to great benefit using a combination of an antibody and another analytical reagent to secure specificity, as we did when we estimated circulating IgG-containing immune complexes, using both C1q and rabbit anti-human IgG antibody (Section 7.4).

10.1   # Choice of label

We have already seen that immunometric, antibody excess assays are theoretically capable of detecting one molecule of bound antibody, whereas the detection limits of

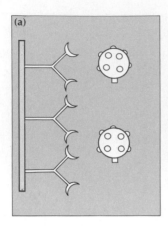 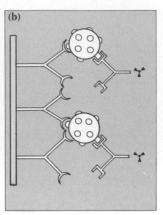

Fig. 10.2 Immunometric assay. An excess of antibody usually on a solid phase, binds to one epitope on the antigen while a second labelled antibody binds to an unrelated epitope and detects the bound antigen.

saturation immunoassay depend upon (experimental error/K, where K is the affinity constant of the antibody used). We must also consider the nature of the label, the characteristics of signal generation and the detection system used to measure it. Although a wide range of substances have been used to label antigen or antibody, only radioisotopes and enzymes have so far found wide application in immunoassay. The type of label chosen is not simply a matter of laboratory convenience; it can also have a marked effect on the maximum sensitivity of the assay system.

Two main factors contribute to the accuracy and sensitivity of signal detection: (a) the level of background; and (b) the number of measurable units of activity generated per unit time for each labelled molecule. Obviously sensitivity will be at its greatest when the background is near zero and each molecule of bound antibody emits an observable signal. For the past 20 years ^{125}I has been the most frequently used label. It has the significant advantages of a low natural background in the environment (and in biological fluids) and its radioactive disintegration is independent of the chemical or physical nature of the assay. Paradoxically, however, this apparently useful isotope imposes a handicap of about six orders of magnitude on assay sensitivity. For example, under normal conditions, the background count in a radioassay is unlikely to be less than 30 c.p.m. Assuming a detection efficiency of 50% of radioactive disintegrations, if each reagent molecule is labelled with a single ^{125}I molecule, we will need about 250000 molecules of antibody to obtain a count rate of 1 c.p.m. Thus, to get a statistically significant result compared to background, many millions of antibody molecules will need to be bound, rather than the theoretical threshold for immunometric assays of a single molecule.

Enzymes offer a distinct advantage over radioisotopes in that each enzyme-labelled antibody can contribute to the signal during the time of the assay, as each enzyme molecule can convert many molecules of substrate to detectable product. However, with current technology, most enzyme assays are limited by the sensitivity of the detection apparatus (photometer, spectrophotometer) and the poor optical and chemical reproducibility of the cuvettes, micro-titre trays, etc. used for the assays. An interesting strategy has been adopted by Harris *et al.* (1979) where an enzyme label (alkaline phosphatase) was used to convert a radioisotopically labelled substrate (^{3}H-adenosine monophosphate), rather than a chromogenic substrate, into a labelled product (^{3}H-adenosine). This procedure permits the sensitivity of radioactive detection to be combined with enzyme amplification thus giving a detection sensitivity of 10^{-21} moles (about 600 molecules); much closer to the theoretical threshold.

In conventional competition immunoassay, as the threshold of detection is high and depends upon antibody affinity, rather than on the ability to detect single molecules of reagent, increases in specific activity only contribute to increased assay speed. Thus conventional radioisotopic methods are still the method of choice in many of these assays.

10.2 Methods for detection of label

The method chosen for detection will, of course, depend on the label. ^{125}I is easily detected in a γ spectrometer scintillation counter and many systems are now available for counting multiple samples at the same time. A big advantage of ^{125}I as a label is that there is no problem with naturally occurring label being present in the sample.

Enzymes are generally used to produce coloured products from colourless substrates. The product can be determined easily in a spectrophotometer or colorimeter. Automated plate readers are now commercially available which make reading large numbers of samples relatively easy.

10.3 Immunoassay procedure

As discussed above, immunoassays may be classified into two main forms: competition assays and excess antibody immunometric assays. Each of these assay systems may utilise radioisotope or enzyme labels. To illustrate the principles of each type of assay we will describe the use of a radiolabel in a competition assay and an enzyme label in an immunometric assay.

10.4 Competition radioimmunoassay

These assays have become very sophisticated with a wealth of literature, but a basic feature common to most of these assays is the need to separate bound from free reactants. Many systems are available to achieve this; for example, molecular sieving, solvent and salt precipitation, second antibodies and solid-phase systems. In the radioimmunoassay for IgG described below, precipitation with polyethylene glycol (PEG) is used to separate bound from free antigen. A problem with this immunoassay is that the antigen (human IgG) and the antibody (rabbit IgG) are of the same molecular weight and precipitability by PEG. This problem is circumvented by the use of human ^{125}I-Fab as the labelled antigen since it is soluble in PEG. Ideally, however, the labelled antigen and the 'cold' antigen to be assayed should be as alike as possible.

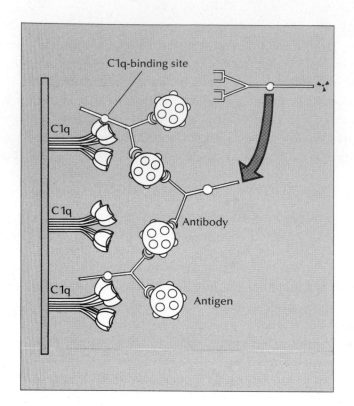

Fig. 10.3 C1q solid-phase immunometric assay for immune complexes. An excess of solid phase C1q binds immune complexes through the Fc region of the IgG. The bound complexes are then detected by labelled antibodies to the rest of the IgG molecule.

10.4.1 Radioimmunoassay of human IgG

PREPARATION OF ^{125}I-Fab

Materials and equipment
Human IgG (either Section 8.5.2 or Appendix II)
Sodium ^{125}I iodide, carrier free (Appendix II)
Bovine serum albumin, BSA, RIA grade
Tris-buffered saline, TBS, pH 8.0 (Appendix I)
Chicken serum (Appendix II)
Whatman GF/B glass-fibre filter

Method
1 Obtain human IgG and prepare the Fab fragment (Sections 8.5.2 and 8.8.1).
2 Label 10 µg protein with 18.5×10^6 Bq ^{125}I (Section 2.5) and store in 5 ml TBS.
3 Immediately before use, dilute with TBS containing 10% chicken serum and filter under gentle pressure through a Whatman GF/B glass-fibre filter.

DETERMINATION OF BINDING CURVE

Materials and equipment
Anti-human IgG (Appendix II)
^{125}I-Fab (prepared as above)
Bovine serum albumin, BSA, RIA grade
Tris-buffered saline, TBS, pH 8.0 (Appendix I)
Polyethylene glycol, PEG 6000 (15% w/v in TBS)
Micro-titre plates (Appendix II)
Cell-harvesting machine (Appendix II)
Whatman GF/B glass-fibre filter strips, for harvester

Method
1   Dilute the anti-IgG serum 1:100 and then prepare a range of two- to three-fold dilutions in TBS containing 0.1% BSA.
2   Add 100 μl of ^{125}I-Fab (dilute to yield 10^5 c.p.m. in TCA precipitable material per well, as in 3 above) to each well of the micro-titre tray. (Use sufficient wells for triplicates of each antibody dilution.)
3   Add 50 μl aliquots of the diluted anti-IgG serum to appropriate wells, mix thoroughly and incubate at room temperature for 16 h.
4   Add 200 μl of 23% w/v PEG solution to each well and incubate at room temperature for 2 h.
5   Collect the contents of each well onto Whatman GF/B glass-fibre filter strips using a cell-harvesting machine.
6   Wash each precipitate with 1.5 ml of PEG, 15% w/v in TBS.
7   Determine number of c.p.m. per sample using a γ spectrometer and plot a curve of c.p.m. against antiserum dilution.

In all future assays with the same reagents use the dilution of antiserum binding 50% of the added radioactivity.

10.4.2   Construction of inhibition curve

Materials and equipment
Human IgG (Appendix II)
Anti-human IgG serum (standardised as above)
^{125}I-Fab (diluted in chicken serum to half dilution used above)
Tris-buffered saline, TBS, pH 8.0 (Appendix I)
Bovine serum albumin, BSA, RIA grade
Polyethylene glycol, PEG 6000, 23% w/v in TBS
Cell-harvesting machine (Appendix II)
Whatman GF/B glass-fibre filter strips, for harvester

Method

1 Prepare a stock solution of IgG, final concentration 0.3 mg ml^{-1} in TBS containing 1% w/v BSA (Aliquot and store at $-20°$ for use.)

2 To perform the assay, prepare standard IgG solutions in the range 2 ng to 2 µg ml^{-1} in TBS containing 0.1% w/v BSA.

3 Add 50 µl aliquots of standard IgG to 50 µl of an appropriate dilution (determined as section above) of anti-IgG serum (in triplicate).

4 Mix samples and incubate for 16 h at room temperature.

5 Add 50 µl of ^{125}I-Fab (diluted in 20% chicken serum to half dilution used above) and incubate for 4 h at room temperature.

6 Precipitate complex by the addition of 200 µl of PEG solution (23% w/v in TBS). Incubate and harvest precipitates as in steps 4−7 section above.

7 Plot the inhibition of binding of ^{125}I-labelled Fab on a linear scale (i.e. c.p.m. in precipitate) against the concentration of unlabelled IgG added on a log scale.

Use this standard curve to determine the concentration of IgG in unknown solutions.

Technical note

If an anti-immunoglobulin antibody is used to enhance complex formation, only a 2% solution of PEG is required in this method. This offers the significant advantage that whole IgG may then be used as a labelled antigen.

10.5 Immunometric assays

Immunometric assays almost invariably require solid-phase systems. They can be performed in many different ways, for example; (a) with antibody on the solid phase to capture antigen, which is then detected by a second labelled antibody directed against another epitope on the antigen; or (b) for the detection of antibody by adsorption of antigen on the solid phase, followed by binding of the antibody to be determined, which, in turn, is detected by the addition of a labelled second antibody directed against the Fc region. We have described a method based on the latter type of assay.

10.6 Enzyme-linked immunosorbent assay (elisa)

Materials and equipment

Antigen; for example, human serum albumin, HSA (Appendix II)

0.05 M carbonate−bicarbonate buffer, pH 9.6 (Appendix I)

Phosphate-buffered saline, PBS (Appendix I) containing 0.05% Tween 20 (PBS−Tween)

Hydrogen peroxide (30%)

0.18 M phosphate−citrate buffer, pH 4.0 (Appendix I)

2,2'-azinobis (3' ethylbenzthiazoline sulphonic acid), ABTS.

Casein (Appendix II)
Bovine serum albumin, BSA
Normal sheep serum
Sodium fluoride (80 mg in 25 ml distilled water)
Horse radish peroxidase—anti-immunoglobulin conjugate; for example, sheep anti-mouse Ig conjugate (Section 2.3.1 or Appendix II)
Test sera; for example, sera from mice immunised with HSA
Enzyme immunoassay micro-titre plates (Appendix II)
ELISA reader (Appendix II)

PREPARATION IN ADVANCE

Preparation of enzyme substrate

Prepare this just before adding to the plates.

1 Add 50 mg ABTS to 100 ml 0.18 M phosphate—citrate buffer, pH 4.0.
2 Add 30 µl of 30% hydrogen peroxide

Hydrogen peroxide is gradually lost from the stock solution with storage. Therefore it is advisable to calculate the exact amount needed to be added each week.

3 Make a 1:1000 dilution of hydrogen peroxide by adding 50 µl H_2O_2 to 50 ml distilled water.
4 Determine the absorbance at 240 nm in a 1 cm cell against a distilled water blank.
5 The % concentration of original H_2O_2 = absorbance $_{240}$ × 77.98.
6 Volume of original H_2O_2 solution needed per 100 ml substrate solution

$$= \frac{1}{\% \text{ concentration}} \text{ ml.}$$

For example, absorbance of 1:1000 dilution of H_2O_2 = 0.37, therefore % concentration = 0.37 × 77.98 = 28.9%, therefore, volume of H_2O_2 needed per 100 ml = 1/28.9 = 0.035 ml.

Method
1 Dissolve the antigen in carbonate—bicarbonate buffer. The optimum concentration should be determined for each antigen but a concentration of 5–10 µg ml^{-1} should give acceptable results for most antigens.
2 Add 200 µl to each well of a micro-ELISA plate and incubate overnight at 4° in a humid chamber.
3 Wash to remove unbound antigen and fill the wells with 250 µl 1% w/v casein to block any remaining protein-binding sites (gelatin, BSA or skimmed milk powder are often used instead of casein).
4 Incubate at room temperature for 1 h.
5 Wash the plates two times with PBS—Tween by filling, then inverting and shaking the plates.

6   Dilute the test sera in PBS–Tween containing 1% BSA. (The optimum dilution must be determined in advance; it will generally be about 1 : 1000.)

7   Add 200 µl diluted test serum and incubate for 2 h at room temperature in a humid chamber.

8   Wash the plates three times with PBS–Tween.

9   Prepare the peroxidase–antibody conjugate by mixing 100 mg casein, 1 ml sheep serum, 100 µl Tween 20 with 50 µl peroxidase–antibody and adjust to a final volume of 100 ml with PBS. Allow to dissolve with gentle stirring. (The exact dilution of conjugate will vary and must be determined by experiment. As a guide, this will generally be between 1 : 1000 to 1 : 10,000 for good antibody preparations.)

10 Add 200 µl diluted conjugate to each well.

11 Incubate at room temperature for 1 h.

12 Wash three times with PBS–Tween.

13 Prepare the substrate solution and add 200 µl substrate to each well. Leave in the dark at room temperature for the colour to develop, usually 10–30 min.

14 Stop the reaction by adding 50 µl sodium fluoride solution to each well.

15 Quantitate the colour reaction in an ELISA reader set at 650 nm.

Technical notes

1   Strictly, each assay should include dilutions of a standard reference serum for the calibration of unknown samples. In practice, however, the test is reasonably reproducible and some workers record their results directly in absorbance units.

2   The same assay could be performed with radiolabelled antibody. In this case flexible polystyrene plates should be used so that each well may be punched out and the bound radioactivity measured in a γ spectrometer after step 12, instead of processing for enzyme activity.

3   An alternative substrate for the peroxidase enzyme is 34 mg O-phenylene diamine and 50 µl hydrogen peroxide (20 volumes) to 100 ml 0.1 M citrate–phosphate buffer, pH 5.0 (Appendix I). The reaction is stopped by the addition of 50 µl 12.5% sulphuric acid and the absorbance measured at 492 nm.

4   If an alkaline phosphatase-labelled enzyme is used, the substrate should be made up as follows: 50 mg 4-nitrophenyl phosphate in 50 ml diethanolamine buffer pH 9.8 (Appendix II). The reaction is stopped by the addition of 50 µl 3 M NaOH and the absorbance is measured at 405 nm.

5   Material from detergent-solubilised cells binds very poorly to ELISA plates because of the surfactant effect; for example, protein dissolved in <0.1% Triton X-100 shows little and variable binding; >0.1% detergent inhibits binding completely. The problem of poor adherence may be overcome (for many antigens) by denaturation with Bouin's fixative: add 50 µl antigen solution to each well (approximately 40 µg ml^{-1} initial protein concentration) and 200 µl Bouin's fluid. Centrifuge at 500 g for 10 min, remove the fixative, wash once with 50% v/v ethanol and twice with phosphate-buffered saline (PBS) (Appendix I). Block plates with PBS containing 3% w/v BSA and 0.01% w/v thiomersal for 1 h. Such plates can be stored at 4° for 1 week. This does not work for all cell-derived antigens and needs to be determined empirically.

10.7 Matrices for solid-phase assays

10.7.1 Plastic surfaces

Although the original work with solid-phase assays involved covalent coupling of antigen or antibody to the solid phase, the majority of assays are now performed with the antigen or antibody passively adsorbed onto a plastic solid phase. Improvements in manufacturing processes have resulted in plastic supports with reproducible binding characteristics, although batch-to-batch variation can be noticed and should be controlled. Various proteins adsorb to differing degrees to the same plastic so trials must be carried out to determine the best support for a particular protein. For radioassays, flexible polystyrene plates which can be easily cut into separate wells for counting should be used, whereas flat-bottomed plates with good optical as well as binding properties are required for enzyme assays (Appendix II).

10.7.2 Particles

Cellulose, Sephadex, Sepharose, Sephacryl and many other particles are available as supports and offer the significant advantage of a large surface area for derivatisation. For assay quantitation, the particles must be recovered from suspension and this has been achieved by centrifugation in the past. Recently, particles containing iron oxide have been introduced and can be rapidly sedimented with a magnet prior to decantation of the supernatant (Section 9.12).

10.7.3 Papers and membranes

Cellulose comes in a convenient form as every-day paper, small discs of which can be coupled with antigen. Nitrocellulose membranes have a strong surface charge and bind proteins tightly, a property taken advantage of in Western blotting (Section 2.11). Samples may be dot blotted onto nitrocellulose; the paper is blocked with non-specific protein such as albumin and then assayed with specific antibodies.

Finally, if using radioisotopes the paper is cut up for counting, or in enzyme assays an insoluble coloured product is deposited on the membrane, which can be quantitated in a densitometer.

10.8 Summary and conclusions

Enormous strides have been made in immunoassay technology. Either antibody or antigen may be determined. Saturation immunoassays involve limiting amounts of antibody to detect, by inhibition, an unknown amount of antigen in excess. Immunometric assays, in contrast, use an excess of antibody. Although the sensitivity of immunometric assays is theoretically greater than for saturation immunoassay this may be hard to achieve in practice. Assays may be performed in solution or on solid phase and a range of detector systems such as enzymes, radiolabels or luminescence may be used to detect the binding.

10.9 ### Further reading

Bolton AE and Hunter WM (1986) Radioimmunoassays and related methods. In *Handbook of Experimental Immunology*, Weir DM (editor), Volume 1, 4th edition. Blackwell Scientific Publications, Oxford.

Chard T (1986) *An Introduction to Radioimmunoassay and Related Techniques: Laboratory Techniques in Biochemistry and Molecular Biology*, 3rd edition. Elsevier, Amsterdam.

Ekins RP (1981) Merits and disadvantages of different labels and methods of immunoassay. In *Immunoassays for the 80's*, Voller A, Bartlett A and Bidwell D (editors). MTP Press, Lancaster, p. 5. Many types of immunoassay and their applications are dealt with in this book.

Ekins RP (1985) Current concepts and future developments. In *Alternative Immunoassays*, Collins WP (editor). John Wiley and Sons, London, p. 219. There are many other useful chapters in this book.

Harris CC, Yolken RH, Krokan H and Chang Hsu I (1979) Ultrasensitive enzymatic radioimmunoassay; Application to detection of cholera toxin and rotavirus. *Proc. Natl. Acad. Sci. U.S.A.* **76**: 5336.

Miles LEM and Hales CM (1968) Labelled antibodies and immunological assay systems *Nature* **219**: 186.

Tijssen P (1985) *Practice and Theory of Enzyme Immunoassays. Laboratory Techniques in Biochemistry and Molecular Biology*. Elsevier, Amsterdam.

11 *In Vivo* Manipulation of the Immune System

Much of our current immunological knowledge has been gained by removing some part of the lymphoid system and observing the result. Initially studies were limited to the intact animal deprived of some major lymphoid organ; for example, the thymus or bursa. More recently techniques have been developed for the reconstitution of immunologically deprived mice; the mouse is immunosuppressed by X-irradiation and then used as a life-support system for the cells under test.

Suppression of the immune response by X-irradiation

The dose of X-rays required to kill most types of non-dividing cells is much greater than that required to kill actively dividing cells. One of its major effects is to induce chromosomal breaks and so the cells are unable to complete mitosis. Lymphocytes, however, are unusual among mammalian cells in being susceptible to X-ray-induced death in G_0. They have a D_{37} of only 1.0 Gy.

The dose-dependent immunosuppressive effect of X-irradiation can be demonstrated in a primary immune response against sheep erythrocytes. This experiment is also designed to determine the lethal and immunosuppressive X-ray doses of recipient animals for other experiments (see Technical notes).

Materials and equipment
Mice (preferably inbred, see Section 1.19.1)
Sheep erythrocytes, SRBC (Appendix II)
Irradiation source
Materials for haemolytic plaque assay (Section 4.5.1)

Method
Irradiate and prime the mice according to the Protocol.

Protocol

	Group (3−5 animals per group)							
	1	2	3	4	5	6	7	8
Irradiation dose (Gy)	0	0	2	4	6	8	8.5	9
Immunising antigen-SRBC intravenously	0.2×10^7 ————————————————→							

1 Challenge the animals with antigen immediately before or after X-irradiation.
2 Assay the anti-SRBC haemolytic plaque response 5 days after antigen challenge (Section 4.5.2).

3 Calculate the total number of plaques per spleen for each animal and the geometric mean for each group.

4 Plot a graph of the X-ray dose against the log mean plaque response.

Technical notes

1 See Section 1.19.1 for changes in blood leucocytes following whole-body irradiation.

2 For most laboratory strains of mice there should be very few deaths during the period of assay due to X-irradiation over the range indicated. For long-term survival, however, it is necessary to reconstitute the mice with bone marrow as X-irradiation not only suppresses lymphoproliferation, but also proliferation of the haemopoietic system. Bone marrow reconstitution is dealt with in Section 11.3.

11.1.1 Radioresistance

Experiments suggest that T and B cells show a differential radioresistance in the whole animal. Thus, if an animal is primed with sheep erythrocytes and X-irradiated 4 days later, functional T cells remain, whereas B-cell activity is suppressed.

Materials and equipment
Inbred mice (Section 1.19.1)
Sheep erythrocytes, SRBC (Appendix II)
Materials for haemolytic plaque assay (Section 4.5.2)

Method

1 Prime recipient mice with 2×10^7 sheep erythrocytes intravenously. X-irradiate (8–8.5 Gy) 4 days after priming.

2 Prepare spleen and thymocyte suspensions from normal donor mice.

3 Treat aliquots of the spleen suspension with anti-Thy-1 and complement or an irrelevant monoclonal and complement (Section 7.5).

4 Reconstitute the X-irradiated mice according to the Protocol.

Protocol

Group	Recipients per group	Previous treatment	Cells transferred	SRBC challenge
1	3–5	2×10^7 SRBC+8 Gy*	None	2×10^7
2	3–5	2×10^7 SRBC+8 Gy*	Thymocytes	2×10^7
3	3–5	2×10^7 SRBC+8 Gy*	Spleen treated with anti-Thy-1 + complement	2×10^7
4	3–5	2×10^7 SRBC+8 Gy*	Spleen treated with irrelevant monoclonal + complement	2×10^7

* 8.0 Gy 4 days after SRBC challenge.

5 Assay all mice for anti-SRBC haemolytic plaques 8 days after cell transfer (Section 4.5.2).

6 Calculate the total plaque-forming cells per spleen for each individual and the geometric mean for each group.

Knowing the cell phenotype specificity of the anti-Thy-1 serum, you should be able to identify the radiosensitive and radioresistant lymphocyte populations.

This is an extremely useful method by which to prepare helper cells (cf. Section 5.6).

Technical notes

1 We have assayed at only one time point; both T and B cells have phases of relative radioresistance after antigen stimulation.

2 Differential radioresistance is not shown by T and B cells *in vitro*.

11.2 Surgical and chemical manipulation of the lymphoid system

Removal of a central lymphoid organ during embryonic or early post-natal life results in a severe depression or complete absence of the dependent peripheral lymphoid population. Historically, the chicken was a very important model for this type of investigation as its sites of T and B differentiation are anatomically distinct; the thymus and bursa of Fabricius, respectively.

The central lymphoid organs are active during embryonic life and so at birth there is a well-established peripheral lymphoid population. Accordingly, any technique concerned with the ablation of the central lymphoid organs must be carried out as early as possible in ontogeny. If ablation is delayed until the pre- or post-natal period, it must be accompanied by generalised immunosuppression, usually X- or γ-irradiation. The remaining central lymphoid organ is then allowed to re-populate the peripheral lymphoid tissue, with or without bone marrow therapy to overcome the X-irradiation.

11.2.1 Surgical bursectomy

This technique can only be used on birds, an anatomically distinct site of B-cell differentiation does not exist in mammals.

Method

1 Anaesthetise the chick with ether and squeeze abdomen between finger and thumb to void faeces.

2 Remove feathers between tail and cloaca, and swab area with 70% alcohol.

3 With the chick on its abdomen, hold its tail with forceps and make a small incision with fine-pointed scissors in the centre line, midway between tail and cloaca.

4 Insert the closed scissors firmly into the incision, keeping the points up.

5 Open the scissors *in situ* (horizontally). This will enlarge the original incision and free the bursa from its dorsal attachment.

6 Pull the bursa through the incision using blunt forceps and dissect away the surrounding tissue with fine forceps until the bursa is attached to the rectum alone. (Take care to identify and avoid the ureters which run close to the bursa).

7 Cut the bursa free, close to the rectum. Cautery is not necessary.

8 Close the incision with three single sutures.

9 X-irradiate the chicks 1 day after surgery. An X-ray dose of 7—8 Gy through 1 mm Al and 1 mm Cu is usually sublethal for chicks and is successful in suppressing peripheral lymphocytes.

Technical notes

1 There should be no post-operative death. Mortality results only from X-irradiation. It may be necessary to vary the X-ray dose used depending on strain, health and housing conditions of birds.

2 If the bursa breaks during reflection it is inadvisable to complete the operation as organ remnants are able to reform a dwarf, but fully functional, bursa.

3 Bursectomised birds are usually used for experimentation at 8 weeks of age, when the T-cell system has regenerated.

4 Although bursectomised birds are usually immunosuppressed for a primary response the magnitude of the secondary response is often near normal, presumably due to the expansion of a residual population of peripheral B cells.

Hypo- or agammaglobulinaemic birds may be selected on the following basis:

(a) Serum immunoglobulin levels as determined by Mancini single radial diffusion in agar (Section 6.6) using rabbit anti-chicken immunoglobulin.

(b) Anti-sheep erythrocyte haemagglutination titre (Section 6.14). Often bursectomised birds have near normal levels of serum immunoglobulins, but are unable to produce an antibody response to antigenic challenge.

(c) Percentage of immunoglobulin-bearing lymphocytes in blood, as detected by immunofluorescence (Section 3.5.1).

The above tests may be used to screen live birds for further experiments. At eventual sacrifice; however, a macroscopic examination should be made for bursal rudiments.

A similar technique has been developed for the surgical bursectomy of 17—18 day old embryos *in ovo*, but it requires considerable skill.

11.2.2   ## Surgical thymectomy

Surgical removal of the thymus is the only technique available for thymectomy in both birds and mammals.

Neonatal thymectomy of the mouse

The operation must be performed within the first 24 h of neonatal life for maximum effect on peripheral T-lymphocyte populations.

Materials and equipment
Neonatal mice, and mothers
Surgical instruments

Method
1 Cool the mouse in a refrigerator until it stops moving. (An anaesthetic is not used as the difference between the anaesthetic and lethal dose is marginal in neonatal mice.)
2 Support the animal in a harness as shown in Fig. 11.1.
3 Open the skin by a longitudinal incision in the midline overlying the sternum.

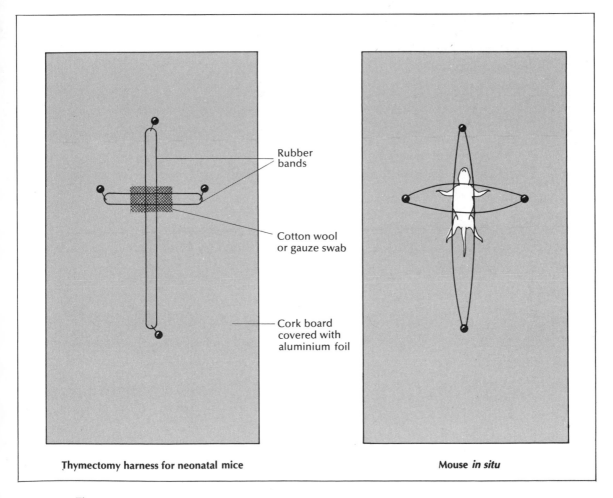

Rubber bands

Cotton wool or gauze swab

Cork board covered with aluminium foil

Thymectomy harness for neonatal mice

Mouse *in situ*

Fig. 11.1 Harness for the thymectomy of neonatal mice.

4 Make a triangular cut in the rib cage at the anterior end of the sternum. Remove the underlying fibrous tissue to expose the thymus.

5 Suck out both thymus lobes using a fine-glass tube attached to a vacuum line. (Do not suck too hard or enter too deeply to avoid the heart following the thymus into the suction tube).

6 Close the wound with 2 or 3 fine-silk sutures.

7 Warm the mouse gently under a lamp.

With practice, post-operative mortality is low. Cannibalism may be reduced by fostering the operated mice onto docile mothers.

Neonatal thymectomy of chickens

The anatomical distribution of the avian thymus is quite unlike that of the mammal. It consists of a series of six to eight paired lobes running beside the carotid arteries in the neck. In addition, there is often a thymic infiltrate of the thyroid gland.

Materials and equipment
Chicks, on day of hatch
Surgical instruments
Irradiation source

Method

1 Anaesthetise the chick using 0.1 ml of a 12 mg ml^{-1} solution of sodium pentobarbital given intraperitoneally.

2 Remove the feathers from either the dorsal or ventral surface of the neck and swab the area with 70% alcohol.

3 Open the neck via either a dorsal or ventral incision. (If a ventral incision is made, it is necessary to reflect the crop and oesophagus).

4 Expose the carotid arteries and identify the thymus lobes to their anterior and posterior extent.

5 Using a glass tube connected to a vacuum line, break the fascia covering the thymus lobes and suck out each lobe.

It is advisable to remove all subcutaneous fat to ensure that no thymic tissue remains.

6 Close the wound with a series of single sutures.

7 Allow the chicks to recover in an incubator.

8 X-irradiate the next day, as in Section 11.1.

Technical note
Because of their high body temperature, chicks are sensitive to hypothermia while under anaesthesia. It is advisable, therefore, to perform the operation under a lamp.

The effectiveness of thymectomy may be assessed in the following ways, in addition to a macroscopic examination once the chicks are killed:

(a)   Ability of immunised birds to give a positive wattle test to PPD (Section 4.2, page 129).

(b)   High percentage of immunoglobulin-bearing lymphocytes in the blood assessed by indirect immunofluorescence (Section 3.5.1).

(c)   Poor or absent skin graft rejection. In the chicken it is convenient to graft onto the scaly part of the leg to avoid the problem of feathers.

11.2.3   Adult bursectomy and thymectomy

Adult bursectomy and thymectomy is without immediate general effect in both mammals and birds. After 1−2 years some of the B or T lymphocyte-mediated functions decline. The effectiveness of adult thymectomy in the mouse has been increased by treating the operated animal with two injections of anti-lymphocyte serum (Section 3.8.1) or by combining lethal X-irradiation with bone marrow reconstitution (Section 11.3).

THYMECTOMY — MOUSE

Materials and equipment
Mice
Surgical instruments
Ethanol, 70% v/v in water

Method

1   Anaesthetise the mouse with a safe inhalation anaesthetic.

2   Stretch the animal out on an operating board (as in Fig. 11.1, but adjust harness to fit an adult animal). Attached a pinned wire loop to the upper incisors to hold the head back.

3   Swab the ventral surface of the upper thorax and neck with ethanol.

4   Make a midline longitudinal incision (about 2 cm long) through the skin just above the anterior end of the sternum.

5   Open the skin, separate and deflect the salivary glands (handle gently to avoid bleeding).

6   Make an anterior−posterior cut through the right clavicle just adjacent to the sternum.

7   Repeat for the left clavicle, deflect and cut off the triangular piece of anterior sternum.

8   Remove the fascia overlying the thymus.

9   Place a thumb under the mouse's diaphragm and press so that the contents of the thorax force the thymus into a more convenient position for manipulation.

10   Remove the left and right lobe of the thymus using a wide-mouthed pipette attached to a vacuum line.

11   Release the mouse's arms and pinch the skin together with the finger and

thumb, thus exerting a slight lateral pressure on each side of the thorax. This will prevent air entering the thoracic cavity.

12 Close the incision with a Michel clip.

Technical notes

1 Once the triangular piece of anterior sternum has been removed it is necessary to work rapidly. If too much air enters the thoracic cavity lung collapse will occur.

2 Post-operative mortality should be less than 10%.

11.3 Reconstituted mice

Historically the 'B-mouse' (thymus deprived, X-irradiated and bone marrow reconstituted) was of great importance but has now been replaced by inbred nu/nu mice and severe combined immunodeficient (SCID) mice (Section 1.18.1) which are effectively devoid of mature T cells or total lymphocytes respectively.

Materials and equipment
6-week old CBA male mice (Appendix II)
CBA donors for bone marrow cells
Irradiation source

Method

1 Thymectomise the recipient mice (as above).

2 Between 3–6 weeks after thymectomy irradiate the mice; use highest possible X-ray dose. This can be up to 11 Gy under 'clean' conditions.

3 Prepare a suspension of bone marrow cells from the femurs of the donor mice. Remove each femur, cut off the ends and blow out the marrow with tissue culture medium from a syringe and needle. Disperse the cells with a pasteur pipette.

4 Count the cells and treat with anti-Thy-1 and complement to remove any mature T lymphocytes (Section 7.5).

5 Warm the mouse under a bulb for 20–30 min to enlarge its tail vein.

6 Inject 5×10^6 syngeneic bone marrow cells into the tail vein of each thymectomised, irradiated mouse.

7 The mice may be used 8–10 weeks later.

Assay the effectiveness of B-cell reconstitution and T depletion using anti-immunoglobulin membrane immunofluorescence (Section 3.5.1) and complement-mediated anti-Thy-1 killing (Sections 3.8.3 and 7.5.1).

11.4 Thoracic duct cannulation of mice

There is a continuous circulation of small lymphocytes from the blood into other peripheral organs and thence into the tissues in general. From here the cells finally return to the blood via the lymphatic vessels; the most important of which is the thoracic duct. Cells in the thoracic duct are part of the so-called re-circulating pool of lymphocytes and represent non-dividing, G_0 cells that are either virgin or memory cells. There is doubt at present as to whether the virgin cells are permitted to enter the re-circulating pool for any prolonged period of time or whether it is purely the abode of memory cells. It is known, however, that cells selectively leave the re-circulating pool if the animal is challenged with antigen and congregate at the site of greatest antigen concentration.

Much of the information on cell 'trafficking' patterns has been gained by thoracic-duct cannulation as a means of obtaining re-circulating lymphocytes, principally in the mouse, rat and sheep. Strictly speaking the cysterna chyla, rather than the thoracic duct, is cannulated in mice. This is a relatively wide, flaccid vessel lying behind the kidney between the inferior vena cava and the lumbar muscles.

PREPARATION IN ADVANCE
1   Give each mouse 0.1 ml of cream by injection into the oesophagus 20 min before the operation. The lipid soon appears as a translucent milkiness in the lymph and enables the cysterna chyla to be more easily visualised.
2   Prepare anaesthetic as follows: dissolve 10 g tribromomethanol in 10 ml of amyl alcohol and store in a light-tight bottle at 4°. Dilute this solution 1:50 in PBS and use 0.01 ml^{-1} total body weight, given intraperitoneally, to induce anaesthesia.

Materials and equipment
Mice, 6–8-week old
Boak cannulas (Appendix II)
Cotton buds or Q tips (Appendix II)
Surgical instruments and Michel clips
Tissue adhesive (Appendix II)
Tissue culture medium and balanced salt solution, BSS (Appendix I)

Method
1   Shave the left flank of the anaesthetised mouse.
2   Place the mouse on a cork board (under an adjustable light) with the shaved side uppermost and with the head to the left.
3   Swab the flank with alcohol, lift the skin with forceps and excise a strip of skin from the thigh region to the costal margin of the rib cage. It is important to make the excision both extensive and in the mid-lateral region.
4   Open the peritoneal cavity with a 2–3 cm incision in the abdominal musculature parallel to the inferior border of the spleen.
5   Place four retractors (made from the wire holding Michel clips, and attached to the heads of dissecting pins) in the incision and pin out so that the abdominal cavity is exposed through a square hole measuring about 2 × 2 cm.
6   Free the kidney from the fatty tissue holding it onto the lumbar muscle by blunt dissection using two cotton buds. Draw the kidney ventrally to expose the cysterna

chyla. It lies in a furrow between the inferior vena cava and the lumbar muscles.

7   Prepare the cannula by cutting the tip with a scalpel blade at a point just after the short arm becomes parallel with the long arm. Optimum lymph flow is obtained if the tip is cut to produce an 'arrow shape'.

8   From the right, place an 18 gauge needle through the posteriorly retracted abdominal muscles and insert, from the left, the uncut (long) arm of the cannula. Withdraw the needle so that the cannula can be drawn into position with the cut (short) arm overlying the duct and the long arm over and parallel with the mouse's tail.

9   Fill the cannula with BSS from a syringe and 25 gauge needle; be sure to avoid air bubbles. Remove the syringe and keep the cannula horizontal with the hooked end under the upper-left retractor.

10 Make a small hole in the cysterna chyla using a pair of sharp-tipped jeweller's forceps; with the forceps closed, place the tips just through the wall of the vessel and open the tips slightly, at the same time pulling the mesentery ventrally with a cotton bud. The hole produced should be about 1 mm in diameter and will be clearly seen if air can be drawn into the hole by firm ventral traction with the cotton bud.

11 Hold the curved end of the cannula with the jeweller's forceps and place the tip into the hole made in the vessel.

12 Hold the cannula in position with a cotton bud and test whether lymph can enter the cannula freely by lowering the long arm below the horizontal. The siphoning effect of the saline in the cannula should draw the lymph into the cannula. Return the cannula to a horizontal position and apply 1 drop of tissue adhesive over the general region where the cannula enters the duct. Exercise great care in applying the adhesive which will 'set' in about 20−30 sec; do not let it enter the lymph vessel.

13 Remove the retractors and close the wound with 3−4 Michel clips through the skin. For an overnight collection of lymph, it is not necessary to close the abdominal musculature separately.

14 Place adhesive tape around the mouse's abdomen, but not around the cannula, so that the mouse can be suspended from above and allowed to run on the outside of a vertical wheel (see Technical note).

15 Infuse the mouse via the tail vein with a balanced salt solution at $0.5−1.0$ ml h^{-1} to promote lymph flow.

16 Collect the thoracic duct lymph into 2 ml of tissue culture medium containing 10% fetal calf serum and 2 drops of preservative-free heparin. Use 15 ml plastic tubes standing on ice in a thermos flask.

17 Check cannulas constantly within the first 3 h of the operation to see that the lymph is flowing — remove fibrin clots with a horse hair or a fine nylon thread. A simple test that the lymph is flowing is to raise the cannula — this should cause the lymph to run backwards freely.

During a 16 h collection it should be possible to obtain between 2.0 and 10.0×10^7 lymphocytes per mouse, depending on its age, health, etc.

Technical note

If the mice are allowed to run on the outside of a treadmill during drainage this promotes lymph flow and increases cell yield. It is also essential that mice are kept warm and given water and food *ad libitum*.

11.5 Grafting techniques

Graft rejection *in vivo* was used classically to investigate cell-mediated immunity, in particular to demonstrate that T, like B lymphocytes, showed specificity and memory (Section 4.17.1) and to investigate transplantation genetics controlled by the major histocompatibility complex (H-2 mouse, HLA in man and B locus in rats) and experimental tolerance (Section 5.7).

11.5.1 Skin grafts

Grafts of flank skin can be exchanged between mice; although this involves some surgical skill to get a good 'take'; the results look more impressive than the technique we describe below. Our technique requires only skill with a razor.

Materials and equipment

Mice: inbred recipients and at least one allogeneic donor
Safety razor blades
4–5 cm glass tubes, internal diameter slightly larger than the mouse's tail
Michel clips

Method

1 Anaesthetise the recipient mouse with ether.
2 Hold the mouse's tail over your forefinger with the mouse pointing away from you.
3 Place the razor blade horizontally on the tail, about 2 cm from the base of the tail, and press slightly to indent the skin. Draw the blade towards you with a slicing action. Do not cut too deeply or the tail will bleed; this will not make a good 'bed' for a recipient graft.
4 Cut off a piece of skin about 0.5 cm long, and leave the skin on the blade.
5 Move about 1 cm down the tail and cut off a second piece of skin.
6 Replace one of the pieces of skin on the wound to form an autograft (and discard the other), be sure to turn the graft through 180° so that the hairs are facing the wrong way. The success of this graft will depend purely upon your surgical technique, it should have no immunological consequences.
7 Use a gauze swab to press the graft firmly in place to exclude all the air. If there is bleeding around the graft, pressure must be applied until haemostasis is achieved.

8 Anesthetise the donor mouse and prepare pieces of tail skin for grafting as above.

9 Place one piece of donor skin on each recipient graft bed and press in place as in 5 above. Each recipient mouse should have an auto- and an allograft on its tail.

10 Protect the grafts with glass tail tubes. These should be about 4–5 cm long and wide enough to slide easily over the mouse's tail. (The cut edges of the glass must be flame polished to avoid injury to the mouse.)

11 Place a Michel clip through the tail to hold the tube in place. (The tube must not be attached too near the base of the tail or it will become fouled with faeces and urine).

12 Remove the tail tubes 24–36 h after grafting.

11.5.2 Thymus grafts

Immune deficient *nu/nu* and severe combined immunodeficient (SCID) mice lack an effective immune response and so are highly susceptible to lethal infection with environmental pathogens. This presents a particular problem for breeding programmes as expensive clean and ultraclean areas, which are technically difficult to operate, are required. Once congenic strains of these mice became available, the problem of immune deficiency was neatly overcome by thymus grafting breeding pairs.

Materials and equipment
Mice, 3–4 weeks old
Neonatal thymus donors of a congenic strain (Section 1.19.1)
Tissue culture medium (Appendix I)
Cotton buds or Q tips (Appendix II)
Surgical instruments and Michel clips
Vacuum line

PREPARATION IN ADVANCE

1 Kill one of the neonatal thymus donors.
2 Support the animal in a harness as shown in Fig. 11.1.
3 Open the skin by a longitudinal incision in the midline overlying the sternum.
4 Make a triangular cut in the rib cage at the anterior end of the sternum. Remove the underlying fibrous tissue to expose the thymus.
5 Use a fine pipette attached to a minimal vacuum to hold thymus lobes while freeing them by blunt dissection. (Do not let the vacuum suck too hard otherwise you will rupture the lobes.)
6 Remove and store the lobes in tissue culture medium on ice until they are required for grafting.

Method
1 Anaesthetise and shave the left flank of the recipient mouse.
2 Place the mouse on a cork board (under an adjustable light) with its shaved side uppermost and head to the left.

3 Swab the flank with alcohol, lift the skin with forceps and open the skin from the thigh region to the costal margin of the rib cage, in the mid-lateral region.
4 Open the peritoneal cavity with a 1–2 cm incision in the abdominal musculature parallel to the inferior border of the spleen.
5 Free the kidney from the fatty tissue holding it onto the lumbar muscle by blunt dissection using two cotton buds.
6 With a fine pair of forceps, pick up the kidney fascia and make an incision with a pair of scissors.
7 Place three neonatal thymus lobes into the hole and gently massage them away from the hole, so that they are held firmly between the kidney and its fascia.
8 Sew up the abdominal musculature with silk sutures and finally close the wound with 3–4 Michel clips through the skin.

The T lymphocytes seem to find their way out of the kidney just as easily as from under the sternum, and populate the peripheral lymphoid tissue.

11.5.3 Bone marrow grafts

In clinical medicine, allogeneic or autologous bone marrow grafting has become a routine and highly successful therapy for myelosuppression during treatment of certain childhood leukaemias. In experimental immunology it is often used to allow mice to overcome the effects of whole-body irradiation or to set the 'ontological clock' of the immune system back to zero (Section 11.1).

Materials and equipment
CBA mice, 6 weeks old (Appendix II)
Syngeneic donors for bone marrow cells
Irradiation source

Method
1 Kill the donor mice and remove their right and left femurs (Fig 1.2) onto a gauze pad soaked in tissue culture medium.
2 Cut off the ends of each femur and blow out the marrow with tissue-culture medium from a syringe and needle into a petri dish.
3 Disperse the cells with a Pasteur pipette.
4 Count the cells and adjust 10^7 ml^{-1} in tissue culture medium.
5 Warm the recipient mice under a bulb for 20–30 min to enlarge their tail veins.
6 Inject 5×10^6 syngeneic bone marrow cells into the tail vein of each mouse.
7 The marrow and immune system of the mice should be re-populated 8–10 weeks later.

11.6 Summary and conclusions

The majority of the techniques described in this section are noteworthy because of their historical associations with the growth of experimental immunology and our understanding of the immune system. Indeed, the observations made on thymectomised and bursectomised animals are at the very basis of the discovery of T (thymus-dependent) and B (bursa-dependent) lymphocytes.

We have included these techniques in the current edition of the book not because of their past importance, but because the *in vivo* situation is still the 'highest court of appeal.' Work on an *in vitro* assay with no *in vivo* relevance or counterpart might be intellectually stimulating, but, like the completion of crossword puzzles, it is an essentially sterile pursuit.

11.7 Further reading

Universities Federation for Animal Welfare (1987) *The UFAW Handbook on the Care and Management of Laboratory Animals*, 6th edition. Churchill Livingstone, Edinburgh.

12 B and T Hybridomas and Cell Lines

With hindsight, it is impressive that immunological research was able to operate with precision and discrimination using a tool so ill-defined as an antiserum, where the active ingredient, antibody, is a minor component in a complex mixture of serum proteins. In addition, unless one used antigens that stimulated a very limited number of lymphocyte clones, the antibodies were a heterogeneous mixture of molecules with a wide range of binding affinities. It is not surprising, therefore, that an antiserum lacks the degree of definition required for many of the current molecular techniques, where an increase in assay sensitivity is often counteracted by a decrease in serological specificity.

The non-specific or cross-reactive binding reactions shown by antibody or other components in an antiserum can be a serious problem when antisera are used to identify or quantitate antigens either in research, for example the study of differentiation or tumour antigens, or in the clinical laboratory for immunodiagnosis. Although it is possible to ensure that an antiserum is 'monospecific' by careful controls or cross-absorption, such standardisation is usually limited to one test system and indeed, often only to one laboratory.

The need for homogeneous antibodies as reproducible reagents was fulfilled by the rescue and propagation of hybrid-cell tumours representing clones of single plasma cells. Köhler and Milstein fused plasmacytoma cells with normal plasma cells to produce hybrid cells (later called hybridomas) that secreted both myeloma and antibody immunoglobulin and grew as a transplantable tumour. By antigen-specific screening of culture supernatants and cloning of secreting cells, these investigators were able to produce potentially immortal cell lines synthesising homogeneous antibody of exquisite specificity.

To counteract the impression that we are discounting a role for polyclonal antisera in the future advance of immunology, it is worth noting that in many instances a cycle of purification of a rare antigen from a complex mixture may start with a monoclonal antibody, graduate to 'gene product fishing' in an expression library (Section 2.13.2) but then obtain a polyclonal antiserum as soon as possible. Polyclonal sera are excellent for routine affinity purification of the native antigen or to relate an expressed partial gene sequence to the mature gene product (Section 2.13.3). The fact that a polyclonal antiserum can 'see a particular antigen from so many different perspectives' is of great technical advantage.

12.1 Outline of technique for B-hybridoma production

Spleen cells, prepared from immunised mice or rats, are induced to fuse with murine plasmacytoma cells using polyethylene glycol. Many cells show cytoplasmic fusion; a lower proportion complete the nuclear fusion required to produce tetraploid hybrids

367

(or a greater ploidy, depending upon the number of fusing cells). Although this procedure results in a heterogeneous mixture of fused and unfused cells, there is a preferential association of ontogenetically similar cells: plasmacytoma cells tend to 'rescue' large, recently activated B lymphocytes.

After dispensing into culture wells, the cell mixture is cultured in a selective medium that positively selects for fusion hybrids. The culture supernatants are tested for antibody activity after 1–3 weeks and positive cultures cloned by conventional cell cloning techniques.

12.1.1 Basis of fusion and selection

To understand the choice of cells and manipulation of the system it is necessary to consider the contribution of each component of the hybrid cell:

(a) The plasmablast parent is terminally differentiated, dies in culture but provides the genetic information for the required antibody.

(b) The plasmacytoma parent confers potential immortality on the hybrid cell, but will itself grow in culture.

(a)

(b)

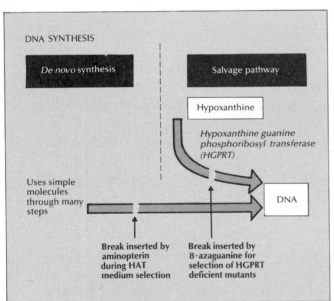

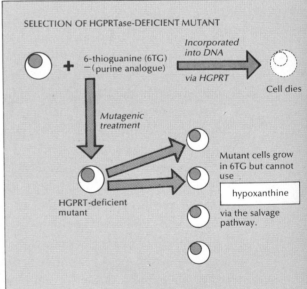

Fig. 12.1 DNA synthesis and the selection of HAT-sensitive mutants. (a) Most cells can make DNA either by *de novo* synthesis or via the so-called 'salvage' pathway, using an endogenous or exogenous source of pre-formed bases. (b) Cells grown in the presence of the lethal purine analogue 8-aza- or 6-thioguanine die, until HGPRT deficient mutants arise. Although these mutants no longer die, they cannot make DNA by the salvage pathway. (c) The tumour 'parent' used in the hybridoma technique (x63) is HGPRT deficient and so is unable to grow in HAT medium; HAT contains the folic acid analogue aminopterin which blocks *de novo* synthesis; as these cells cannot use hypoxanthine — they die. Hybrid cells grow out from HAT medium because DNA from the normal partner provides the information to synthesise HGPRT and the tumour cell DNA provides the 'message' for unrestricted proliferation.

(c)

CELL SELECTION IN HAT MEDIUM

x63 : HGPRTase deficient   but immortal

Normal lymphocyte : has HGPRT   but has normal growth control

Fusion mixture

Polyethylene glycol

Unfused tumour	Unfused lymphocyte	Tumour/tumour fusion	Lymphocyte/lymphocyte fusion	Tumour/lymphocyte fusion
Dies in HAT	No message for immortality	Message for immortality but not HGPRT	Lots of HGPRTase but no immortality	HGPRT and immortality
	Dies anyway	Dies in HAT	Dies in HAT	Tumour – lymphocyte hybrids proliferate in HAT medium. Functional selection now required to find cells producing the required antibody

Fig. 12.1 (continued)

Thus, once plasma cells from an appropriately immunised animal have been fused with tumour cells *in vitro* it is necessary to eliminate unfused tumour cells (or tumour—tumour hybrids) and then select those hybrid cells secreting antibody of the required specificity.

12.1.2 Elimination of plasmacytoma cells

This problem was overcome by the use of a plasmacytoma cell line deficient in the enzyme responsible for incorporation of hypoxanthine into DNA.

By way of explanation, cells can synthesise DNA in two ways, either by *de novo* synthesis or via the so-called 'salvage' pathway using exogenous or endogenous sources of pre-formed bases, as summarised in Fig. 12.1a. If plasmacytoma cells are grown in the presence of a purine analogue, for example 8-azaguanine or 6-thioguanine, the HGPRT enzyme catalyses the incorporation of the purine analogue into DNA where it interferes with normal protein synthesis and so the cells die.

The gene coding for the HGPRT enzyme is on the X chromosome and so only a single copy per cell is expressed. Eventually cells will arise that are deficient in the HGPRT gene and therefore do not incorporate the purine analogue. These HGPRT-deficient cells are unable to utilise hypoxanthine and so synthesise ribonucleotides only by *de novo* synthesis (Fig. 12.1b).

In 1967 Littlefield introduced a selective medium containing aminopterin (or amethopterin, methotrexate), hypoxanthine and thymidine (HAT medium). Aminopterin is an analogue of folic acid and binds very tenaciously to folic-acid reductase, thus blocking the coenzymes required for *de novo* synthesis of DNA. To grow in this medium a cell must make DNA via the 'salvage' pathway.

Thus, if the plasmacytoma cells, deficient in HGPRT, are fused with normal lymphoid cells and then placed in HAT medium, only the hybrids between plasmacytoma and normal cells will grow; the plasmacytoma cell provides immortality and the plasma cell provides the HGPRT enzyme (Fig. 12.1c).

12.1.3 Origin of plasmacytoma lines for fusion

The vast majority of fusion experiments have been performed using sublines of P3/X63-Ag8, which is itself an 8-azaguanine-resistant subline of the plasmacytoma MOPC 21 (induced in a BALB/c mouse by the injection of mineral oil). This cell line is special in that it tends to fuse spontaneously (with itself) and can grow at very low cell densities, thus facilitating the recovery of fusion hybrids. However, this line has the disadvantage that it synthesises and secretes the MOPC 21 myeloma protein (a fully sequenced IgG1, κ) and so hybrid cells will secrete myeloma and antibody molecules, as well as inactive hybrid molecules.

Spontaneous variants of P3/X63-Ag8 have been selected that neither synthesise nor secrete immunoglobulin molecules, but still retain the ability to rescue normal antibody—producing cells. These are listed below, all are resistant to 8-azaguanine:

(a) *NS1-Ag4—1*. Synthesises, but does not secrete, κ light chain. Hybrids can still secrete a mixed molecule of antibody heavy chains with myeloma light chains.
(b) *P3/X63-Ag8—6.5.3*. Does not synthesise or secrete immunoglobulin chains.
(c) *SP2/0—Ag14*. Non-synthesising and non-secreting variant of a hybrid cell formed by the fusion of a lymphoid cell (secreting anti-sheep erythrocyte antibody) with P3/X63-Ag8.

For obvious reasons we recommend one of the non-synthesising, non-secreting variants for any fusion work. Although there are commercial suppliers (Appendix II), it is often possible to beg the 'parent' cell lines from one of the many laboratories doing routine fusions. Commercial suppliers have the advantage that their cells are routinely cloned and passaged through 6-thioguanine to maintain their HAT sensitivity.

12.2
Maintenance of plasmacytoma cells for fusion

The efficiency of fusion and recovery of hybrids is greatest when the plasmacytoma 'parent' cells are uniformly viable and growing exponentially. The times and cell densities given below should only be used as a guide; it is necessary to determine the growth characteristics of each plasmacytoma line upon receipt.

Materials and equipment
Plasmacytoma line (Appendix III) (if necessary, recover from frozen state)
Tissue culture medium with serum supplement (Appendix I)
Plastic culture flasks (Appendix II), 10 ml culture volume
Incubator, humidified and gassed with 5% CO_2 in air

Method
1 Add 10^5 plasmacytoma cells to 10 ml of tissue culture medium and place in a humid incubator gassed with 5% CO_2 in air.
2 Each day, re-suspend the cells and determine the number ml^{-1} using a haemocytometer.
3 Plot a growth curve of cell number versus time (as for Fig. III.1, Appendix III).
4 As soon as the growth rate starts to decline, dilute the cells by transferring 0.2—1.0 ml aliquots of the re-suspended culture to flasks containing 10 ml of fresh medium.
5 When the cells have again reached their exponential growth phase, select viable cultures for storage under liquid nitrogen.

Technical notes
1 These cell lines will reach a maximum density of approximately 10^6 cells ml^{-1}. Exponential growth should be maintained by diluting the culture 1:10 with fresh medium every 3—5 days. Under these conditions the cells will have a doubling time of 16—20 h.
2 The plasmacytoma cells grow either in suspension or lightly adherent. Release the adherent cells by gently tapping the culture flask or by gentle pipetting.
3 Check by phase-contrast microscopy that the cells are 'healthy'. They should be

phasebright and of regular shape with clear outlines. Even in cloned lines size variation is common. Cell viability (Section 3.4.2) should be between 90 and 95%.

4 As with all cell lines in long-term culture care must be taken to avoid cross-contamination between cultures.

5 The rate of reversion to HAT resistance varies with cell lines and is a relatively rare event. Eliminate revertants by culturing the cells in medium containing 8-azaguanine or 6-thioguanine (2×10^{-5} M) every 3–6 months. Alternatively, import a 'seed' culture from a commercial supplier; grow up into a large batch in the minimum number of subpassages and freeze for cryopreservation.

6 As with all long-term maintenance of cell lines *in vitro* it is advisable to check periodically for *Mycoplasma* infection. Commercial kits are available (Appendix II) for the demonstration of *Mycoplasma* DNA using a fluorescent dye. A rapid, but non-specific, indication of potential *Mycoplasma* contamination may be obtained by culturing supernatant, obtained by centrifugation (150 g for 15 min) of a 5 ml sample of the suspected culture, with 3.7×10^3 Bq ^{3}H thymidine (Appendix II) overnight at 37°. Incorporation of label into TCA precipitable material (Section 2.5.2) indicates contamination.

12.3 Target cells for fusion

Most of the plasmacytoma cells used as fusion 'parents' have a BALB/c haplotype, but will fuse efficiently and productively with mouse or rat cells without regard to histocompatibility barriers. It is important to note, however, that if it is intended to propagate the hybridoma cells *in vivo*, it is technically simpler to use immunised BALB/c mice as spleen-cell donors. In addition, although the murine plasmacytoma lines can fuse to almost any species, for example human, frog or carrot, stable hybrid lines are only rarely obtained in other than rodent–rodent fusions (see Technical notes below).

Immunisation protocols should be determined empirically and are likely to vary not only with the type of antigen used but also with the 'folklore' of the laboratory. Plasmacytoma cells seem to fuse preferentially with recently activated B lymphoblasts, rather than plasma cells, so one might expect that the immunisation scheme giving the highest serum antibody titres might not necessarily give the highest rate of positive hybrids. Few problems have been encountered with immunisation against cell or particulate antigens, almost any immunisation scheme will give a 10–20% recovery of positive hybrids (percentage calculated as a function of total wells showing cell growth hybrid). For soluble antigens, for example human IgG or γ-globulin, we have found that the following immunisation protocol works well: 100 µg i.p. human IgG in Freund's complete adjuvant (Section 1.7.1) 7 days before fusion, followed by i.v. boost with 100 µg soluble IgG 4 days before fusion.

Most investigators tend to fuse 2–4 days after a final intravenous injection of antigen on the rationale that this should localise recently activated B lymphocytes in the spleen. The ultimate splenic localisation protocol is the so-called 'intrasplenic immunisation': the spleen of an anaesthetised mouse is exposed through an incision parallel to the costal margin of the ribs and soluble antigen is injected directly into the organ via a fine 23 gauge needle. The wound is closed with two discontinuous sutures or Michel clips, and the spleen used for fusion 3–5 days later. This procedure is similar to the classical intra lymph-node injections practiced to spare precious antigen and boost the immune response.

In practice, however, the potential advantages of intrasplenic injection are outweighed not only by the cumbersome injection route but also the disadvantage that it tends to favour IgM producing hybrids.

12.4 Fusion protocol

PREPARATIONS IN ADVANCE

Materials and equipment
Plasmacytoma cells in culture
Tissue culture medium (Appendix I)
Serum (Appendix I)
Tissue culture flasks (Appendix II)
Polyethylene glycol, PEG 1500
Phosphate-buffered saline, PBS (Appendix I)

Animals and cells

1   Immunise mice against required antigen.
2   Prepare plasmacytoma cell cultures for fusion by centrifugation (150 g for 10 min at room temperature) followed by re-culture in an equal volume of tissue culture medium plus serum supplement. (Set up a sufficient culture volume to yield 10^7 cells for each spleen to be fused.) For efficient fusion, the plasmacytoma cells should be uniformly viable and in the exponential phase of growth. To ensure that this is so we routinely replace the culture medium, at the same cell density, the day before the cells are used for fusion.

Preparation of polyethylene glycol solution
1   Add 50 g PEG to warm PBS (in a 37° water bath) and adjust to 100 ml.
2   Dispense 5 ml aliquots into 10 ml glass bottles and autoclave at 120° for 15 min.
3   Store at 4° for use.

TECHNIQUES

Materials and equipment
Mice (immunised as above)
Plasmacytoma cells in culture (as above)
Tissue culture medium and serum (Appendix I)
L-glutamine (200 mM initial concentration)
Polyethylene glycol, PEG 1500, 50% w/v in phosphate–saline buffer (as above)

Ethanol, 70% v/v in distilled water
Water bath at 37°
Culture plate, 96 micro-wells (Appendix II)
Conical test tubes, 50 ml, sterile
Conical test tubes, 15 ml, sterile
Petri dishes, 5 cm, sterile
Pasteur pipettes, sterile
Scissors, two pairs, sterile
Forceps, fine, sterile
Forceps, blunt, two pairs, sterile
Time clock

12.4.1 Preparation of spleen cells

1 Prepare tissue culture medium as follows:
   a 100 ml medium, add 10 ml serum and 1.0 ml L-glutamine.
   b 200 ml medium, add 2.0 ml L-glutamine.
2 Kill mouse by cervical dislocation and swab its left side with ethanol.
3 Open skin to expose peritoneum, discard scissors and forceps.
4 Use fresh forceps and scissors to open the peritoneum and remove the spleen, transfer to a Petri dish containing serum-free tissue culture medium.
5 Prepare a suspension of spleen cells free of clumps (Section 1.15).
6 Wash spleen cells three times by centrifugation (250 g for 10 min at 4°) and re-suspend in 5 ml of serum-free tissue culture medium.
7 Determine the number of viable lymphoid cells ml^{-1} (Section 3.4.2).

12.4.2 Preparation of plasmacytoma cells

1 Re-suspend the cells and pool the suspensions into a 50 ml conical tube.
2 Wash the cells three times by centrifugation (250 g for 15 min at room temperature) in serum-free tissue culture medium.
3 Re-suspend the final pellet in serum-free tissue culture medium, count the number of viable cells (Section 3.4.2) and adjust to 1×10^6 cells ml^{-1}.

12.4.3 Fusion

1 Mix 10^8 spleen cells with 10^7 plasmacytoma cells in a 50 ml conical tube and centrifuge at 500 g for 7 min at room temperature.
2 Decant the supernatant carefully, finally inverting the tube to drain completely.
3 Mix cell pellet by gently tapping the tube and allow to equilibrate to 37° in a water bath. Similarly allow PEG solution and tissue culture medium with 10% serum to equilibrate to 37°.
4 Add 0.8 ml of PEG to re-suspended cells, mix gently and incubate at 37° for 1 min.

5   Add 1.0 ml of serum-free medium over 1 min with gentle shaking.

6   Add 20 ml of serum-free medium over 5 min. Dilution must be done very slowly as the cells are very sensitive to mechanical damage when in the PEG solution.

7   Centrifuge at 200 g for 10 min at room temperature.

8   Remove supernatant and re-suspend the cell pellet in 10 ml of tissue culture medium containing 10% serum.

9   Dispense 50 µl aliquots of cell suspension into each well of a 96-well culture plate.

10 Dilute the remaining cell suspension with 2 volumes of medium containing 10% serum and dispense 50 µl aliquots into each well of a second 96-well culture plate.

11 Dilute the remaining cell suspension with 2 volumes of medium containing 10% serum and dispense 50 µl aliquots into each well of a third 96-well culture plate.

12 Place all the plates in a humid 37° incubator gassed with 5% CO_2 in air.

The plates are now incubated for 24 h before the addition of the HAT selective medium.

Technical notes

1   Although murine plasmacytoma cells have been fused with avian, amphibian and human lymphocytes in a similar manner, they rarely produce stable, antibody-secreting hybrids because of a rapid loss of chromosomes. Indeed, in mouse–human hybrids, the elimination of human, but not mouse, chromosomes occurs so frequently that this technique has been extensively used for mapping the human genome.

2   The method of plating out the fusion mixture may be varied depending on the frequency of hybrid formation, the frequency of hybrids secreting the desired type of antibody and the method of detecting antibodies. If the frequency of hybrids is low, as with soluble proteins for example, then 2 ml cultures can be dispensed into 24-well culture plates. We have found that dilution plating as described above limits the number of independent clones that grow out and so reduces the chance of a positive clone (secreting the desired antibody) being lost by 'overgrowth' of non-secreting hybrids.

12.4.4   Preparation of stock solution of HAT medium

Materials

Hypoxanthine (6-hydroxypurine) (molecular weight 136.1) 10×10^{-2} M

Thymidine (molecular weight 242.2) 1.6×10^{-3} M

Aminopterin (4-amino-folic acid; 4-aminopteroyl glutamic acid) (molecular weight 440.4) 4.0×10^{-5} M

Note: aminopterin is highly toxic and a potent carcinogen.

Method

A   100-fold concentrated stock solution of hypoxanthine and thymidine.

1   Dissolve 136.1 mg hypoxanthine and 38.8 mg thymidine in 100 ml twice-distilled water at 50°.
2   Sterilise by membrane filtration and store in 2—5 ml aliquots at −20°.

The hypoxanthine might precipitate out of solution during storage. Re-dissolve by heating in a boiling water bath.

B   100-fold concentrated solution of aminopterin.

1   Add 1.76 mg aminopterin to 90 ml of twice-distilled water.
2   Add 1 M sodium hydroxide dropwise until the aminopterin dissolves and then titrate to pH 7.5 with 1 M HCl.
3   Adjust final volume to 100 ml with twice-distilled water.
4   Sterilise by membrane filtration, dispense into 2—5 ml aliquots and store at −20°.

Technical notes
1   Aminopterin must be protected from light.
2   This stock can be frozen and thawed several times for use, provided sterility is maintained.
3   Aminopterin may be purchased as a sterile 10^{-4} M solution from Flow Laboratories (Appendix II).

12.4.5   Use of HAT medium

Materials and equipment
Stock solution of hypoxanthine and thymidine, HT, as above.
Stock solution of aminopterin (A), as above
Tissue culture medium containing L-glutamine (Section 12.4.1) and 10% serum (Appendix I)
Plates containing fused cells (Section 12.4.3)

Method
1   Add 2 ml of HT and 2 ml of A stock solutions to 100 ml of tissue culture medium containing 10% serum.
2   Add 50 µl of HAT medium to each well containing fused cells.
3   Return plates to 37° incubator.

Technical notes
1   The HAT medium used above is double strength so that the final concentration in the cultures is as follows:
    hypoxanthine 1.0×10^{-4} M
    thymidine 1.6×10^{-5} M
    aminopterin 4.0×10^{-7} M.
    This medium will appear to kill all the cells in the plate but do not despair, hybrids usually grow without any problem.

2 You will need to feed each well with 25 μl of single strength medium only once per week. Prepare single strength medium by adding 1 ml of each of the HT and A stock solutions to 100 ml of tissue culture medium containing 10% serum.

3 Vigorously growing hybrids are usually visible in the high cell density plates, i.e. those prepared from the undiluted suspension of fused cells, at 1−2 weeks after fusion (indicated by a change in the pH indicator dye). Examine all the plates under an inverted microscope and select the plate containing the cell dilution that shows growth every second to third well. Discard the plates that received the more concentrated cell suspensions, they will probably have several clones per well.

4 After the 'selection phase' is complete, it is necessary to grow the hybrids on to normal tissue culture medium. However, do not transfer the hybrids directly from HAT to normal tissue culture medium as sufficient aminopterin may be carried over to prevent a resumption of *de novo* synthesis of DNA. Instead, grow the cells in HT and tissue culture medium for 3−5 days before transferring to tissue culture medium alone. Depending on the source of plasmacytoma cells and the frequency of fusion, hybrids may not show optimal growth when cultured alone. This problem may be overcome by plating onto feeder layers of macrophages.

12.4.6 Preparation of macrophage feeder layers

Materials and equipment
Mice
Tissue culture medium containing 10% serum (Appendix I)
Micro-culture plates, flat bottomed, 96 wells (Appendix II)
Incubator, humidified and gassed with 5% CO_2 in air

Method
1 Prepare a suspension of peritoneal exudate cells from untreated mice (Section 1.18.1)
2 Wash the cells once in tissue culture medium by centrifugation (150 *g* for 10 min at room temperature).
3 If the cells are not histocompatible with the fusion hybrids, irradiate the peritoneal exudate cells with 20 Gy.
4 Count (Section 3.4.2) and adjust the cells to 2×10^5 ml^{-1}.
5 Dispense 100 μl aliquots into each well of a micro-culture plate.
6 Incubate in a humid 37° incubator gassed with 5% CO_2 in air.

The feeder layers may be used for plating out of fusion mixtures after 24 h or up to 7 days.

Technical note
Each mouse should yield about 5×10^6 peritoneal exudate cells of which about 50% will be lymphocytes.

12.4.7 Screening of fusion wells for antibody activity

The initial screen for antibody activity should be carried out as soon as growth of hybrid cells is seen under the microscope or when the pH indicator dye has become yellow.

Although we have diluted the cells to limit the number of independent hybrid cells per well, it is important to realise that several hybrids may grow, perhaps at different rates, each producing their own clone of cells. This might affect the screening assay in two ways:

(a) A positive clone (secreting the desired antibody) may be detected soon after fusion, but then might be lost by overgrowth of a negative or other positive clones.

(b) No activity may be detected during the first assay due to the cells of a positive clone being in a minority. It is therefore essential to test negative supernatants from actively growing cultures on two or three occasions.

Once antibody activity has been detected in any particular well, it is essential to clone and re-test the cells as soon as possible.

The type of assay to be used to detect antibody is determined by the nature of the antigen and the type of antibody desired. During the initial screening, for the selection of positive hybrids for cloning, speed, convenience and reproducibility are essential. Positive wells must be detected rapidly and then cloned out immediately to avoid overgrowth. Technically simple and convenient assays are required so that a large number of supernatants can be screened to identify the wells containing the antibody with the required properties.

It is absolutely essential that the screening assay be established and standardised before any hybridisation is undertaken.

Binding assays have the advantage that they will, by definition, detect all antibody activity against a particular antigen and can be modified for the use of isotype specific anti-immunoglobulin antibodies. Thus, unless one wishes to select for a particular effector function, for example agglutination or complement fixation, solid-phase radio- or enzyme-linked immunoassays are preferable (discussed in detail in Chapter 10). We will describe a radioimmunoassay developed in our laboratories for the detection of antibodies to surface components of *Trypanosoma cruzi* (the causative agent of South American sleeping sickness); however, the same assay may be used to detect any cell-associated antigen. Modifications of this assay for soluble antigens are given in the Technical notes section.

The early determination of antibody isotype is important; particularly if you wish to select for or against specific isotypes, and also to ensure that you use an appropriate antibody-purification protocol.

12.5 Solid-phase radioimmunoassay for cell-surface antigens

12.5.1 Preparation of cell-coated assay plates

Materials and equipment
Cells carrying antigen of interest
Glutaraldehyde
Phosphate-buffered saline, PBS (Appendix I)
PBS containing bovine haemoglobin, 5% w/v and sodium azide, 0.2% w/v
Micro-titre plate with U-shaped wells, flexible polyvinyl chloride (Appendix II)

Method
1 Harvest the cells and wash three times in PBS by centrifugation (150 g for 10 min at 4°).
2 Count (Section 3.4.2) and adjust the cell numbers to 2×10^7 ml^{-1}.
3 Dispense 50 µl aliquots of fresh 0.25% glutaraldehyde in PBS into each well of the micro-titre plate.
4 Add 50 µl of cell suspension to each of 95 wells of the plate and centrifuge at 100 g for 5−10 min at 4°. The 96th well is used as a control for non-specific binding in the final assay.
5 Remove the glutaraldehyde solution by tapping the inverted plate over a sink.
6 Flood the plate with PBS and roll a glass rod over the surface to remove air bubbles. Washing may also be performed by immersing the plate in a beaker of PBS.
7 Flood the plate with PBS containing bovine haemoglobin (5% w/v) and sodium azide (0.2% w/v). Again, roll a glass rod over the surface to remove air bubbles.
8 Incubate the plate for 1 h at room temperature. This will saturate the protein-binding sites on the plastic.
9 The plates may be used immediately or stored up to 10 weeks without removing the haemoglobin buffer.

Technical notes
1 Soluble proteins will adsorb directly to these polyvinyl plates. Add 50 µl of protein solution (at 50−200 fmol ml^{-1}) in PBS to each well and incubate for at least 1 h at room temperature. Remove the supernatant (keep for re-use) and wash the plate three times with PBS containing bovine haemoglobin (5% w/v) and sodium azide (0.2% w/v). The protein solution must be free of detergent as this will inhibit binding.
2 Antibody may also be linked to the plate and used to adsorb viable cells which are then fixed with glutaraldehyde.
3 The relatively low concentration of glutaraldehyde used to fix the cells does not seem to alter surface antigens.

12.5.2 Radioiodinated anti-mouse immunoglobulin antibody

Prepare antibody to mouse immunoglobulin by affinity chromatography (Section 9.6) and label with ^{125}I using 'Iodogen' (Section 2.5.3).

Alternatively label anti-mouse immunoglobulin antibody while it is still attached to the affinity column (Section 9.6) using the Chloramine T technique (Section 2.5.1). Elute the ^{125}I-labelled antibodies with 0.2 M glycine−HCl buffer, pH 2.5 (Appendix I) containing carrier protein.

12.5.3 Binding assay

Materials and equipment
Cultures of fused cells (Section 12.4.5)
Assay plates coated with cells
Phosphate-buffered saline, PBS (Appendix I)
PBS containing bovine haemoglobin (5% w/v) and sodium azide (0.2% w/v).
^{125}I-labelled anti-mouse immunoglobulin antibody (Sections 1.7.2, 9.6 and 2.5.2).
Plate sealers (Appendix II)
Vacuum trap for radioactive washings
Nichrome wire, electrically heated, for cutting up plates
γ spectrometer

Method
1   Remove the haemoglobin buffer by tapping the inverted test plate.
2   Remove 50 μl of supernatant from each hybrid well to be tested and transfer to the assay plate according to the following Protocol:

Well number	Test antigen	Antibody	^{125}I-anti-mouse immunoglobulin
1	+	Hybrid supernatant	+
↓		↓	
93	+	Hybrid supernatant	+
94	+	Positive control*	+
95	+	Negative control*	+
96	−	Positive control*	+

* See Technical notes, item 3.

3   Incubate for 1 h at room temperature.
4   Wash the plate three times by immersing it in PBS and emptying it into a sink.
5   Add 25 μl of haemoglobin buffer containing 5×10^4 c.p.m. ^{125}I labelled anti-mouse immunoglobulin antibody to each well and incubate for 1 h at room temperature.
6   Remove the unbound radioactive antibody using a Pasteur pipette attached to a suction trap.

7   Wash five times by adding 3 drops of PBS to each well and then suck the solution into a vacuum trap.

8   Leave the plates to dry in a fume cupboard.

9   Cut up the tray with an electrically heated Nichrome wire to release the wells. For convenience, a plate sealer can be stuck to the bottom of the tray during cutting.

10 Load the wells directly into γ counter tubes with forceps and determine their radioactive content.

Technical notes

1   The baseline counts in wells 95 and 96 should be less than 200 c.p.m.

2   Provided the baseline counts are reproducible, a count of more than 500 c.p.m. usually indicates antibody activity in the test supernatant.

3   Because hybridoma supernatants have low total protein concentrations they give much 'cleaner' results in these assays compared with conventional antisera. Accordingly, the best controls are positive and negative supernatants from already established hybrids. Although it is often possible to beg hybrid supernatants with unrelated antibody activity to serve as controls in initial experiments, it is usually necessary to use diluted conventional antisera as positive controls.

4   When working with parasites we have found that monoclonal antibody defined antigens are sometimes not expressed uniformly by all members of a population. Under these conditions it is necessary to use a binding assay that gives information on the population distribution of binding; for example, indirect immunofluorescence using either a UV microscope (Section 3.5.1) or a fluorescence-activated cell sorter (Section 3.9).

5   As soon as positive cultures have been identified the cells should be cloned and, if possible, some of each uncloned positive well should be expanded and stored in liquid nitrogen as an insurance against a failure during cloning.

6   This is intended as a screening assay. Quantitation may be achieved as explained in Section 10.4.

12.6   Cloning of hybrids

Antibody-secreting hybrid cells from positive culture wells must be cloned to ensure that the antibody is homogeneous and monospecific. In practical terms, cloning is necessary to ensure that non-producers, arising either in the original fusion wells or as spontaneous variants, do not outgrow the antibody-secreting hybrids. If continuous growth of a hybrid line is required, it will be necessary to repeat the cloning and positive selection procedure at regular intervals. Alternatively, prepare a large batch of cryopreserved cloned cells, and discard and replace growing lines at regular intervals.

Cloning, the initiation of a cell line from a single progenitor, may be achieved: (a) in soft agar; (b) by limiting dilution; or (c) if the hardware is available, by using the continuous-flow cytofluorimeter (Section 9.11).

12.6.1   Cloning in soft agar

PREPARATION OF SOFT AGAR STOCK SOLUTION

Materials
Agarose (Appendix II)
Water, twice distilled

Method

1   Prepare a 2% w/v solution of agarose in twice-distilled water and dispense into glass bottles.
2   Autoclave at 120° for 15 min and store at 4° for use.

TECHNIQUE

Materials and equipment
Hybrid cells
Agarose solution, 2% w/v, as above
Tissue culture medium, double strength, with 20% serum (Appendix I)
24-well culture plates (Appendix II)
Water bath at 44°
Microwave oven

Method

1   Melt the agarose in the microwave oven and allow it to equilibrate in a 44° water bath. Similarly, equilibrate the tissue culture medium to 44°.
2   Mix equal volumes of agarose and tissue culture medium, and return the mixture to the water bath. The agarose will solidify if this is not done rapidly.
3   Dispense 1 ml of the agarose tissue culture medium into each well of the tissue culture plate and allow it to solidify. Allow two cloning wells for each positive hybrid culture.
4   Count the hybrid cells (Section 3.4.2) and prepare suspensions at 2×10^3 cell ml^{-1} and 1×10^3 cells ml^{-1}.
5   For each cell suspension: mix 0.5 ml of cells with 1.0 ml of the agarose–tissue culture medium mixture.
6   Add 0.6 ml of the cell–agarose mixture to each of two subbed wells.
7   Repeat for all cells to be cloned.
8   Allow the agarose to solidify and incubate the plate in a humid incubator gassed with 5% CO_2 in air.

Cell colonies will grow within 1–2 weeks and will be visible as white spots in the agarose, each discrete spot represents an individual clone.

9   Pick off 10 discrete colonies per well using sterile Pasteur pipettes and transfer to separate 200 µl micro-cultures (Section 12.7).

Technical notes

1　The underlay agarose is used to ensure that the cell colonies grow away from the well bottom. This aids manipulation of clones during isolation.

2　Only discrete cell colonies must be isolated.

3　The cloning efficiency of this technique is usually between 20 and 70% (percentage of original cells that grow as colonies). If optimal growth is not achieved a feeder layer of macrophages may be used, under the agarose (Section 12.4.6).

4　Not all of the colonies isolated will grow to produce lines of antibody-secreting cells. It is necessary, therefore, to screen and select for antibody activity (Section 12.4.7). If the screening assay can be designed around the agar-cloning plate, for example a modification of the Jerne plaque assay (Section 4.5), it is possible to select antibody-secreting clones directly.

5　The precision of cloning can be greatly enhanced by the direct selection of single hybrid cells from colonies growing in an antibody positive, primary fusion well. Cells can be picked by means of a micro-manipulator (Appendix II) and grown up either in agarose, as here, or in macrophage-supplemented micro-cultures (Section 12.6.2).

12.6.2　Cloning by limiting dilution

This technique is a direct counterpart of the limiting dilution technique used to estimate the frequency of antigen-reactive lymphocytes (Section 4.13) and is based on the same principle of random dispersion of rare elements, in this case hybrid cells, according to the Poisson distribution.

PREPARATION IN ADVANCE

Prepare macrophage feeder layers in 96-well, flat-bottom micro-culture plates (Section 12.4.6); allow one plate for each positive hybrid well to be cloned.

Materials and equipment

Hybrid cells for cloning

Micro-culture plates with macrophage feeder layers

Incubator, 37°, humidified and gassed with 5% CO_2 in air

Method

For each positive hybrid well:

1　Harvest and count the cells.

2　Prepare cell suspensions at 10 and 5 cells ml^{-1}.

3　Add 100 µl aliquots of the 10 cells ml^{-1} suspension to each of 48 wells. Repeat into remaining wells for the suspension at 5 cells ml^{-1}.

4　Incubate the plates in a humid 37° incubator gassed with 5% CO_2 in air. Colonies should be visible after 1−2 weeks.

5 Test supernatants for antibody activity (Section 12.4.7) and select positive wells for culture.

Technical notes

1 The initial distribution of cells per well follows Poisson statistics (Section 4.13), thus although about 40% of the wells will receive only one cell (and therefore initiate a true clone), a significant proportion will receive two or more cells. Cloning must be repeated to ensure the homogeneity of any interesting hybrid line.

2 It is advisable to re-clone both the plasmacytoma and hybridoma lines at regular intervals. This will eliminate any variant cells, especially spontaneous non-secreting variants, before they overgrow the culture.

12.7 ## Initiation and maintenance of B-hybridoma cell lines

Freshly isolated hybrid cell cultures often grow slowly and are less tolerant of low cell densities than their plasmacytoma parent. The volume of the cell culture must be expanded slowly, at a rate that can only be determined empirically because hybrid lines show different growth rates. In general, colonies or cloning wells should be transferred to a maximum of 0.2–0.5 ml of medium (again with a feeder layer if necessary) and diluted with an equal volume of fresh medium as the pH indicator dye just begins to turn an orange–yellow.

If hybridoma lines are allowed to grow up to stationary phase in static flasks or spinner culture vessels they can produce up to 1 μg ml^{-1} of antibody protein. Although the antibody is pure, the spent medium contains many other serum proteins.

Large amounts of hybridoma-derived antibody may be prepared by injecting these tumorigenic lines into histocompatible (or immunoincompetent) mice.

Materials
Mice (histocompatible with hybridoma or nude, athymic, Section, 1.19.1)
Hybridoma line from *in vitro* culture
Pristane (2,6,10,14-tetramethylpentadecane) (Appendix II)

Method
1 Inject 0.5 ml Pristane into the peritoneal cavity of each mouse.
2 After 7 days, inject 10^7 hybridoma cells i.p. into each mouse.

Most hybridoma lines will produce solid tumours or ascites within 2–3 weeks.

3 Use a syringe and 19 gauge needle to drain off the ascitic fluid. Clarify the ascitic fluid by centrifugation (500 g for 15 min at 4°).
4 If desired, screen the ascitic fluid from individual mice by electrophoresis (Section

6.9.1), store those samples showing a prominent peak of paraprotein in the γ-globulin region.

5 Repeat steps 3 and 4 for the lifetime of the mouse.

Technical notes

1 Ascitic fluid often contains up to 1 mg ml^{-1} of specific antibody protein. There are, of course, other proteins, including immunoglobulins of unknown specificity.

2 The serum of these tumour-bearing mice also contains large quantities of hybridoma-derived antibody.

3 It is inadvisable to maintain a hybridoma by serial passage in mice because of the risk of accumulating non-secreting cells. Instead, inject large batches of mice with recently cloned cells from *in vitro* culture.

4 Immunoincompetent nude or severe combined immunodeficient (SCID) mice will also be required if the hybrid line was derived from a mouse−rat fusion. Some investigators prefer to immunise rats, rather than mice, for fusion, as it is possible to obtaiı significant volumes of antisera in test bleeds prior to fusion.

12.8 Antibody purification

Although culture or ascitic fluid containing a high titre of monoclonal antibody is sufficiently pure for many applications, it still contains many irrelevant proteins, some of which, in the latter case, will be immunoglobulin molecules of unknown specificity. If the appropriate antigen is available, the most direct way to isolate antibody is to use affinity chromatography. Alternatively total immunoglobulin, or individual isotypes, may be isolated by the techniques described either in Sections 8.2−8.5, or below.

12.8.1 Antigen immunoadsorbents

Protein antigens (not necessarily in a pure form) may be linked to a support matrix, such as cyanogen bromide-activated Sepharose (Section 9.6.1) and packed into a column. Ascitic fluid or culture supernatant is then simply allowed to filter through the column, which is then washed to remove unbound proteins and the antibody eluted under the most gentle conditions compatible with antibody release. (See Section 9.6.4 for choice and advantages of elution buffers.)

12.8.2 Cell-surface immunoadsorbents

The purification of antibody against cell-surface components is technically more difficult than for soluble antigens. If the appropriate cells can be immobilised on a support matrix and cross-linked by glutaraldehyde, it is possible to use cell-column chromatography for the isolation of specific antibody.

Preparation of cellular immunoadsorbent

Materials and equipment
Cells carrying appropriate antigen
Concanavalin A, Con A (Appendix II)
Glutaraldehyde
Phosphate-buffered saline, PBS (Appendix I)
Sephadex G-50 (Appendix II), coarse, swollen and equilibrated with PBS (Section 1.5.1)

Method
1 Add 50 mg of Con A in PBS to Sephadex and stir at room temperature.
2 After 30 min allow the Sephadex to settle and remove the excess Con A by decantation.
3 Add packed cells and mix slowly for 15 min at room temperature. The exact proportions of cells and matrix will vary according to the availability of the cells and the concentration of antigen at the cell surface. Typically, use 4 ml of packed cells to 50 ml of swollen Sephadex.
4 Add 100 ml of glutaraldehyde solution (3% in PBS) and stir gently for 1 h at room temperature.
5 Wash Sephadex−cell mixture with PBS by three cycles of mixing and decantation.
6 Pour mixture into a column and wash overnight with PBS for use.

Isolation of antibody

1 Add ascitic fluid or culture supernatant to the top of the affinity column and allow it to filter through slowly (5−10 ml h^{-1}).
2 Wash with PBS until the absorbance of the effluent is less than 0.01 at 280 nm.
3 Elute antibody with 0.05 M glycine−HCl, 0.5 M NaCl, pH 3.0, and adjust pH and concentration of eluate (as in Section 9.6.2).
4 Re-equilibrate the column with PBS containing sodium azide (0.2% w/v).
5 Test eluted antibody for activity (Section 12.4.7) and store at −20°.

Technical notes
1 The cell columns may be stored at 4° in PBS containing sodium azide (0.2% w/v) and re-used over several weeks. Before use, pre-elute the column with acid buffer and re-equilibrate with PBS.
2 Antibodies prepared by acid elution from an immunoadsorbent invariably contain soluble complexes formed by denaturation under acid conditions. If required, these may be removed by gel chromatography (Section 8.2).

12.9 ## Isolation of monoclonal immunoglobulin

If purified antibody cannot be isolated directly by antigen binding, it is possible to prepare an immunoglobulin fraction of the ascitic fluid using either affinity or ion-exchange chromatography. The purification of monoclonal immunoglobulin from a tissue culture supernatant poses fewer problems.

12.9.1 Problems and solutions

Purification of monoclonal antibodies follows the same general procedures outlined for polyclonal antibodies. As each monoclonal antibody is unique, an individual determination will be required to establish the particular conditions for the isolation of each antibody. Obviously different considerations will apply to hybridoma antibodies to be isolated from tissue culture medium compared with those from ascitic fluid. Antibodies in tissue culture supernatants must first be concentrated, either in a membrane concentrator or by ammonium sulphate precipitation (Section 8.1) before they can be isolated, whereas ascitic fluids can be treated in a similar manner to serum immunoglobulins.

Hybridoma antibodies grown in serum-free medium contain little immunoglobulin other than that of hybridoma origin, but they do contain a lot of albumin. Consequently the problems of antibody purification are essentially the same for serum-supplemented or serum-free media. Concentration and partial purification can be obtained by precipitation at a 50 % saturation with ammonium sulphate, using solid ammonium sulphate to avoid excessive increase in volume (Section 1.3.1). Ascitic fluids frequently contain appreciable quantities of lipid which should be removed at the beginning of the isolation procedure by treatment with Aerosil (Section 8.5.4).

Excess albumin may be conveniently removed by affinity chromatography on Cibacron blue dye affinity gel before attempting ion-exchange chromatography. A combination of Cibacron blue with diethylaminoethyl (DEAE) is available from Biorad (Appendix II) which allows albumin removal and ion-exchange in one step. DEAE and quarternary aminoethyl (QAE) ion-exchangers are suitable for purification of IgG monoclonal antibodies (Section 8.5). As monoclonal antibodies have a unique isoelectric point and charge density it is best to use gradient elution from the ion-exchanger.

Monoclonal IgA is rather more difficult to prepare but can be isolated by ammonium sulphate precipitation, followed by ion-exchange chromatography. Using gradient elution, the IgA should elute after IgG but before the albumin fraction.

IgM antibodies are most readily prepared by gel filtration using a high-resolution gel such as Ultrogel AcA 22 or Sephacryl S-300 (Section 8.2.6).

12.9.2 Anti-immunoglobulin affinity columns

The IgG (Section 8.5) or antibody (Section 9.6) fraction of goat or rabbit anti-mouse immunoglobulin may be linked to Sepharose (Section 9.6.1) and the affinity column so formed used to isolate hybridoma immunoglobulin.

Materials and equipment
As for Section 9.6.2, but in addition:
Anti-mouse immunoglobulin, goat or rabbit (Section 1.7.2)

Mouse immunoglobulin (Section 1.3.2)
Hybridoma-derived antibody

Method

1 Isolate the antibody (Section 9.6.2) or IgG (Section 8.5.2) fraction from the anti-mouse immunoglobulin serum.
2 Link anti-immunoglobulin to Sepharose (Section 9.6.1) and pack into a column.
3 Add 100 mg normal mouse immunoglobulin prepared by ammonium sulphate precipitation (Section 1.3.2) and allow it to filter slowly through the column.
4 Elute with glycine–HCl buffer (Section 9.6.2) and re-equilibrate the column with PBS until the absorbency of the effluent is less than 0.01 at 280 nm.

These columns are pre-cycled with normal mouse IgG and eluted with acid buffer to saturate the high-affinity anti-immunoglobulin antibodies that would otherwise bind the precious monoclonal antibody virtually irreversibly. In any case, these columns should always be pre-eluted with acid buffer and re-equilibrated before use to remove any loosely bound material.

5 Add solution containing hybridoma-derived antibody, wash and elute as above.

To minimise denaturation, elution should be accomplished with the most gentle conditions compatible with the release of antibody (Section 9.6.4).

Mouse immunoglobulin may also be isolated by ion-exchange chromatography (Section 8.5.2) or by affinity chromatography on staphylococcal protein A–Sepharose (subclass IgG2a, IgG2b and IgG3, Section 9.3). (Rat immunoglobulins, with the exception of the minor subclass IgG2c, do not bind to protein A, but may be prepared by streptococcal protein G, Appendix II.)

12.10 Enzymic fragmentation of monoclonal antibodies

Removal of the Fc region of monoclonal antibodies, to leave a divalent fragment which is no longer able to bind to Fc receptors or to activate the complement pathway, is often desirable but, in practice, is often difficult, or impossible, to achieve. Amongst the IgG subclasses there is a differential sensitivity to proteolysis; with pepsin, for example, IgG2b is most sensitive followed by IgG3 > IgG2a > IgG1, while for papain, IgG1 is most sensitive followed by IgG2a > IgG3 > IgG2b. Superimposed over this there are individual sensitivities unique to each monoclonal antibody. Thus, as it is impossible to use one set of conditions that will apply optimally to all antibodies, it is essential to perform a range of trial digests on each antibody preparation. For most purposes a single set of IgG and enzyme concentrations can be used at constant pH, in which case time provides the experimental variable. Unfortunately, for some monoclonal antibodies this will not provide sufficient scope for optimisation and it will be necessary to repeat the digestions under conditions where enzyme concentration and pH are varied, in addition to time. Fortunately, as each batch of the same monoclonal antibody will be structurally identical, once the digestion conditions are determined they will not need to be varied.

In the experiment described below, a batch of purified antibody is mixed with the enzyme, under digestion conditions and samples taken for fragment analysis by SDS-PAGE to determine the optimal time of incubation, i.e. that which gives maximum yield of the desired fragment with minimum subfragmentation to smaller peptides. Generally, as only small amounts of monoclonal IgG will be available, slightly lower concentrations are used than for rabbit or human IgG.

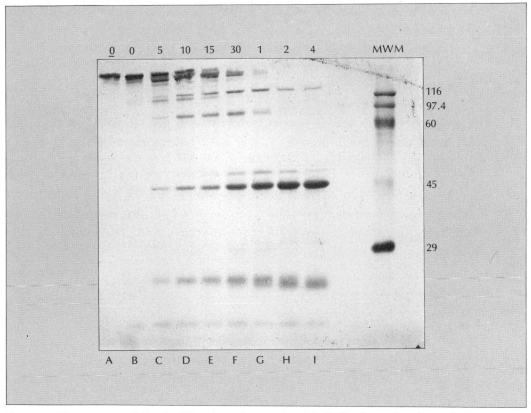

Fig. 12.2 Time course of papain digestion of monoclonal IgG. To determine the optimum conditions for the papain digestion of a monoclonal antibody a time course experiment was performed. Samples were taken, at intervals, and run on a SDS-PAGE system in non-reducing conditions.

0   Sample prior to digestion.
0   Reaction stopped immediately on addition of papain.
5   Reaction stopped 5 minutes after addition of papain.
10   Reaction stopped 10 minutes after addition of papain.
15   Reaction stopped 15 minutes hour addition of papain.
30   Reaction stopped 30 minutes after addition of papain.
1   Reaction stopped 1 hour after addition of papain.
2   Reaction stopped 2 hours after addition of papain.
4   Reaction stopped 4 hours after addition of papain.

Easily detectable digestion products are visible at first sampling at 5 minutes. The reaction proceeds through a number of intermediates, such as one Fab linked to Fc, before arriving at the 50 000 kD products. With prolonged incubation small molecular weight degradation products begin to appear. Choosing an optimum time is a balance between efficient usage of starting material and not too much degradation.

12.10.1 Pepsin digestion

Materials and equipment
0.1 M citrate buffer, pH 3.5 (Appendix I)
IgG, monoclonal antibody
Pepsin (1 mg ml^{-1}) (Appendix II)
SDS-PAGE (Section 2.10)

Method
1 Dissolve or dialyse the IgG in the citrate buffer and adjust concentration to 1 mg protein ml^{-1}.
2 Place 300 μl in a small tube and add 6 μl of a 1 mg ml^{-1} solution of pepsin in the same buffer and incubate at 37°.
3 Immediately (time 0) and then at 5, 10, 15, and 30 min, 1, 2, 4, 8, 16, and 24 h, remove a 20 μl aliquot.
4 The pH of each aliquot should be adjusted to just above 7.0 to stop the reaction.
5 At the end of the time course, analyse the fractions by SDS-PAGE under reducing and non-reducing conditions.

From an examination of these gels, for example Fig. 12.2, it should be possible to select a suitable set of conditions to apply to a bulk preparation of the monoclonal antibody. The fragments may then be separated by a combination of gel filtration and protein A chromatography (Sections 8.2 and 9.2).

12.10.2 Papain digestion

Papain needs activation by cysteine; this can be accomplished by either incorporating cysteine in the reaction mixture or by pre-activating the papain prior to addition to the digestion mixture. Using pre-activated papain with mouse IgG sometimes gives a F(ab)$_2$ fragment similar to the pepsin F(ab')$_2$. If cysteine is present during the enzyme reaction the fragmentation proceeds to give Fab and Fc.

PRE-ACTIVATED PAPAIN

Materials and equipment
Papain (Appendix II)
Phosphate-buffered saline, PBS (Appendix I)
IgG monoclonal antibody (1 mg ml^{-1} in PBS)
PBS containing 0.002 M EDTA
Cysteine, 0.5 M in PBS
0.002 M ethylene diamine tetra-acetic acid, EDTA, disodium salt
0.1 M iodoacetamide

Method
1 Place 100 μg papain in a small tube containing 50 μl 0.002 M EDTA and 10 μl 0.5 M cysteine in PBS.

2   Incubate at 37° for 30 min.

3   Prepare a small Sephadex de-salting column (Section 1.5). A disposable 10 ml pipette with glass or nylon wool at the bottom would be suitable. The column should be filled with Sephadex G-25 and equilibrated with PBS containing 0.002 M EDTA.

4   Apply the activated papain to the column and elute with PBS—EDTA. Collect 0.25 ml fractions and determine their protein content (Section 1.4) to locate the papain peak. Use the peak tube for the digestion, this should contain about half the total absorbance units of enzyme.

5   Add the papain to 1 mg IgG in 0.5 ml PBS containing 0.002 M EDTA.

6   Incubate at 37°.

7   Immediately remove 20 μg IgG and mix with 0.1 M iodoacetamide to a final concentration of 0.025 M to stop the reaction.

8   Remove further 20 μg samples at 5, 10, 15 and 30 min, 1, 2, 4, 8 h and each time stop the reaction with iodoacetamide.

9   Analyse the fractions by SDS-PAGE in both non-reducing and reducing conditions. As the samples contain iodoacetamide, add 2-mercaptoethanol to a concentration of 0.02 M before proceeding to the normal sample preparation conditions for the reducing gel (Section 2.10).

Having established the optimal conditions for digestion, proceed with the bulk preparation and isolate the resultant fragments by gel filtration and protein A affinity chromatography (Sections 8.2 and 9.1).

12.11   Characterisation of monoclonal antibodies

Frequently, the isolation of a novel monoclonal antibody has been the first step in the identification of a minor, but functionally important, component in a complex mixture of antigens. Fortunately, it is possible to determine many of the chemical properties and biological attributes of the molecule thus defined in advance of purification or gene cloning, even though the molecule might reside in a cell's surface membrane. The value of this information is obvious; for example, there would be little point taking a DNA cloning route to characterisation if the antibody defined a carbohydrate epitope on a glycoprotein.

12.11.1   Chemical nature of monoclonal antibody-defined epitopes

One of the most appealing features of monoclonal antibody technology is its ability to provide highly discriminatory ligands which are able to define and detect epitopes present in trace amounts in a complex mixture of antigens. Further, even though the antigen might be present as a minor determinant on a minority cell population, it can still be regarded as a valid target for hybridoma production.

With current techniques, characterisation of the antibody in terms of isotype, biological activity (complement fixation, agglutination, precipitation, etc.) or the subpopulations of cells which it defines poses no real problems. Similarly, determination of apparent molecular weight and isoelectric point of the antigen (by immuno-precipitation [Section 2.9] or immunoblotting [Section 2.11]) requires little advance purification as these determinations can be made using the discriminatory power of the antibody. Antigen isolation by immune affinity chromatography (Section 9.7) undoubtedly provides the definitive route to antigen isolation and its characterisation by standard chemical means (structural, composition and sequence analysis) but, even if the type of antibody lends itself to this approach, many laboratories do not possess the necessary time, expertise or inclination to attempt a full characterisation. Flow cytometry using monoclonal antibodies provides a reproducible means of measuring the relative amount of antigen (through antibody binding) in its native state and environment, often in heterogeneous cell mixtures (the cell population of interest need only be delineated at the time of analysis, see Section 9.11). Thus, using techniques which modify antigen expression (enzymes, metabolic inhibitors, chemical treatment, etc.) it is possible to quantitate their effect and so gain some limited information on the chemical nature of the antigen carrying the monoclonal antibody-defined epitope, as summarised in Fig. 12.3.

12.11.2 Modification of cell-surface antigens

These procedures use a continuous-flow cytofluorimeter to quantitate antibody binding to cell surfaces after various manipulations that are designed to yield information about the nature and distribution of the target molecule and therefore rely on efficient detection of the maximum number of cell-surface epitopes at all times. It is essential, therefore, that the antibody be titrated for saturation binding (shown by plateau staining as in Fig. 2.2) with minimum non-specific binding (Section 2.1.7), both before and after each treatment. In addition, few of the treatments are totally devoid of side reactions; for example, enzymes often contain other contaminating enzymes in significant amounts. Thus, for maximum reliability, it is usually essential to link a degradation experiment with re-synthesis in the presence of specific inhibitors. Re-synthesis experiments are not limited to permanent cell lines grown *in vitro*; even normal cells are capable of extensive short-term re-synthesis of membrane components *in vitro*.

The connectivity pathways in Fig. 12.3 should give useful and related information; however, not all the assays are necessary for each monoclonal antibody. The information to be gained from this general approach could be increased by extending the range of useful reagents; for example, by inclusion of specific glycosidases, inhibition of antibody binding by mono- or oligosaccharides, lipases, etc.

The letter of each subheading below refers to the relevant assay shown on Fig. 12.3.

A BINDING SITE DISTRIBUTION
Determine the distribution of antibody-binding sites on the cell population of interest, both in terms of the proportion of total cells carrying the epitope and the relative distribution of binding sites per cell in the positive population. This is most

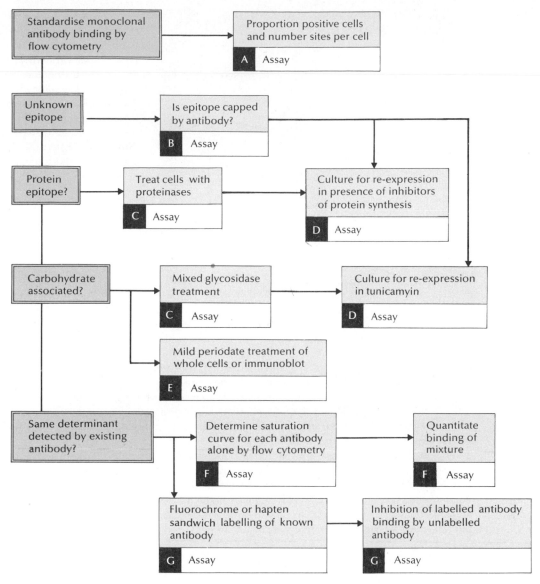

Fig. 12.3 Determination of chemical nature of unknown monoclonal antibody-defined epitope using flow cytometry. Assay letter refers to the technique in Section 12.11.2 for the measurement of antibody binding following the indicated treatment. The applicability of this general approach could be extended, where appropriate, by the inclusion of lipases and glycosidases or inhibition of antibody binding by mono- or oligosaccharides.

conveniently done using a continuous-flow cytofluorimeter (Section 3.9). An illustrative example is shown in Fig. 12.4.

B ANTIBODY-INDUCED CAPPING

This is a useful technique: (a) because the observation that the antibody can induce capping or that the antigen can be capped (or not!), can be informative (see for example Fig. 3.14); and (b) it is a gentle and highly selective way to initiate

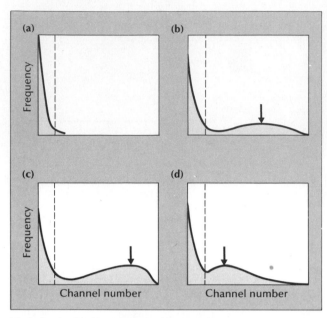

Fig. 12.4 Distribution of fluorescence intensity in lymphocytes stained with monoclonal antibodies. Four illustrative histograms of flow cytometry data (detailed in Section 3.9) are shown — the horizontal logarithmic scale is divided into intervals of increasing fluorescence intensity, the vertical scale shows the frequency of cells at each level of relative fluorescence.

(a) When cells are reacted with an irrelevant monoclonal antibody, about 95% of the total population sampled (usually 10 000 cells) should fall within the first few channel numbers (to the left of the vertical line) and so define the proportion of lymphocytes that bind the irrelevant monoclonal antibody and fluorescent conjugate (if an indirect staining technique is used) non-specifically.

(b) Lymphocytes in this sample have been stained with a monoclonal antibody which binds to their surface membrane. To analyse the distribution, it is arbitrarily divided into two by placing the cursor (vertical line) in the same position as in histogram A; channels to the left of the line contain the 'non-specifically' stained population whereas channels to the right contain 'specifically' stained cells, in this case about 50% of the total population sampled (value obtained by integrating the area under the curve). The modal or peak relative fluorescence, indicated by the arrow, is that showing the greatest frequency in any one channel.

(c) and (d) These histograms show different populations of lymphocytes stained with the same monoclonal antibody as in B. Although approximately the same proportion of lymphocytes are positively stained, the population in C is brightly stained (modal fluorescence shifted to the right) whereas the population in D is weakly stained (modal fluorescence shifted to the left). Supposing the antibody defined a lymphocyte receptor, then 50% of both populations in C and D have this receptor but cells more frequently have receptors in C than in D.

re-synthesis of the molecule of interest (compared, for example, to proteinase treatment). Incubate the cell population with antibody at 37° for varying time periods as described in Section 3.7. If modulation is incomplete or absent with the monoclonal antibody alone, add an anti-immunoglobulin antibody as well as the monoclonal in a parallel assay. Even so, modulation of surface-antigen expression does not occur with all monoclonal antibodies.

C PROTEINASE- OR GLYCOSIDASE SENSITIVE EPITOPES

Materials
As in Section 3.5, but in addition:
Cells carrying the antigen of interest
Proteinases or glycosidases, as Fig. 12.5

Enzyme	Working concentration	Specificity
Proteinases		
Pronase	0.5 mg ml^{-1} ⎫	Multiple sites of hydrolysis along the polypeptide chain
Papain*	0.3 mg ml^{-1} ⎭	
Glycosidases[†]		
Neuraminidase	0.5 iu ml^{-1}	N terminal sialic acid
Endoglycosidase H	5.0 iu ml^{-1}	Linkage between oligosaccharide and protein

Fig. 12.5 Enzymes for modification of cell-surface antigens on viable cells.
* Add also 5 mg ml^{-1} cysteine–HCl to activate the enzyme.
† Use preparations of mixed glycosidases with caution, lack of modification of staining might be due to an insufficient concentration of a crucial glycosidase. In any case, Endoglycosidase H has now largely replaced crude mixtures of glycosidases for this treatment, because the latter is frequently contaminated with proteinases.

Tissue culture medium (Appendix I)
Fetal bovine serum, FBS (Appendix II)
Phosphate-buffered saline, PBS (Appendix I), containing 10 mM sodium azide

Method
1 Count cells and determine their viability by dye exclusion (Section 3.4.2), adjust to 5×10^6 ml^{-1} in serum-free tissue culture medium. If necessary remove dead cells as in Section 1.16.
2 For each time point of the assay, mix 1 ml cell suspension with 1 ml enzyme (see Fig. 12.5) or 1 ml serum-free medium alone.
3 Incubate for 60 min in 37° water bath with occasional mixing.
4 Add 8 ml ice-cold tissue culture medium containing 10% FBS to stop the reaction.
5 Wash twice by centrifugation (150 *g* for 10 min at 4°) and label by indirect immunofluorescence for flow cytometry (Sections 3.5 and 3.9).

Technical note
Always purchase the enzyme in its purest available form; this limits the number of contaminating enzymes and therefore the number of confusing side reactions.

D INHIBITION OF RE-SYNTHESIS

Materials
As C above, but in addition:
Inhibitors as Fig. 12.6
Bovine serum albumin, BSA (Appendix II)

Inhibitor	Stock solution	Working concentration	Specificity
Paramycin dihydrochloride	1.0 mg ml^{-1} in water	1.5 µg ml^{-1}	Disrupts RNA Forms amino acyl puromycin resulting in premature chain termination
Cyclohexaimide	1.0 mg ml^{-1} in water	20 µg ml^{-1}	Blocks peptide synthesis by interfering with the ribosome
Tunicamycin	1.0 mg ml^{-1} in DMSO*	1.0 µg ml^{-1}	Prevents addition of sugars to hydroxyl and amino groups of polypeptides
Monensin	1 mM in water	100 nM	Blocks processing of polypeptides by the Golgi apparatus, thus preventing secretion

Fig. 12.6 **Inhibitors of protein synthesis, glycosylation and secretion.**
* This inhibitor is dissolved in dimethyl sulphoxide (DMSO), add an equal volume of DMSO alone to a parallel cell culture to control for potential non-specific inhibition of re-synthesis.

Method

1 After enzyme or antibody treatment, wash cell suspensions three times by centrifugation (150 g for 10 min at room temperature) in tissue culture medium containing 10% FBS.
2 Determine cell viability by dye exclusion (Section 3.4.2) and adjust to 10^6 cells ml^{-1}.
3 Prepare separate aliquots of enzyme treated cells alone, enzyme-treated cells plus appropriate inhibitor (Fig. 12.6) and, where necessary, enzyme-treated cells plus solvent used to dissolve the enzyme inhibitor.
4 Culture overnight at 37° in a humidified atmosphere containing 5% CO_2 in air.
5 Harvest the cells and wash twice by centrifugation using PBS containing 1% w/v BSA and 10 mM sodium azide
6 Label by indirect immunofluorescence for flow cytometry (Sections 3.5 and 3.9).

E PERIODATE TREATMENT

Materials
As C above, but in addition:
Sodium metaperiodate

Method

1 Dissolve sodium metaperiodate in PBS to 0.1 M, use fresh and keep in the dark.
2 Determine cell viability (Section 3.4.2) and adjust to 10^6 cells ml^{-1}.
3 For each time point, allow 2×1 ml aliquots of cells.

4   Add 10 µl stock periodate solution to 1 aliquot, the other will serve as untreated control.

5   Incubate at 4° between 30 min and overnight.

6   Recover and wash cells by centrifugation (150 g for 10 min at room temperature) in PBS containing 10 mM sodium azide and 1% w/v BSA.

7   Label by indirect immunofluorescence for flow cytometry (Sections 3.5 and 9.11).

Technical note

Under the mild conditions described here, cell-surface sialic acid residues are specifically oxidised and cell viability should be virtually unaffected. However, the reaction is relatively inefficient. If you are still in doubt, having obtained a negative result, we recommend that you use low pH periodate pre-treatment of an immunoblot (Section 2.11), thus permiting the efficient oxidation of *cis*-vicindal diol groups.

F DOUBLE ANTIBODY BINDING

For a proper assessment of additive or competitive binding, both antibodies should be used under saturating (plateau) conditions, and so must have been titrated as described in Section 2.1.6. Aliquots of cells carrying the antigen of interest should be reacted with either antibody alone or with the two as a 1:1 mixture (label by indirect immunofluorescence for flow cytometry, Sections 3.5 and 3.9). Non-competitive binding of the two antibodies should result in a positive displacement of modal fluorescence intensity (peak staining shifted right), whereas competitive binding should result in the antibody mixture having a peak intensity equal to the peak of the brighter of the two antibodies alone. These findings are illustrated in Fig. 12.7.

Although this approach can yield useful data, it is beset by pitfalls for the unwary. For example, it is desirable to label with each antibody at a consistent dilution, whether it is used alone or in an antibody mixture, and yet maintain an equivalent protein concentration in each case. This may be achieved for all practical purposes by diluting the monoclonal antibodies into an irrelevant protein solution; for example, 0.1% fetal bovine serum. Similarly, it is not valid to compare different isotypes in this way. It can be readily appreciated that IgM and IgG antibodies with precisely the same variable regions would not react with the same binding avidity or permit the same specificity and sensitivity of detection.

G COMPETITION WITH LABELLED STANDARD

Once a labelled reference monoclonal has been prepared, either by direct conjugation to a fluorochrome (Section 2.1) or by hapten conjugation (Section 1.6) for hapten sandwich labelling (Section 2.2), then it is possible to carry out a more precise assessment of competitive or non-competitive binding (Fig 12.7) using different concentrations of the monoclonal as required for proper immunoassay (Section 10.4).

In some instances, for example where one is trying to compile a reference set of new monoclonal antibodies, there is a desire to avoid re-selection of commonly occurring monoclonal antibodies. With forethought and ingenuity in assay design, it is often possible to incorporate recurring antibodies into the primary screen and so favour the detection of less immunodominant clones. For example, a binding assay

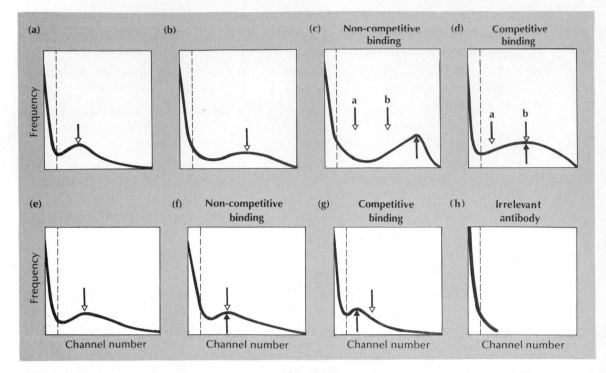

Fig. 12.7 Competitive and non-competitive binding of monoclonal antibodies detected by indirect immunofluorescence. Histograms are labelled and analysed as in Fig. 12.4.

In (a) to (d), two samples of the same cell population have been stained with two uncharacterised IgG monoclonal antibodies. Distribution (a) shows a relatively low peak fluorescence (open arrow) whereas distribution (b) shows an intermediate peak fluorescence (open arrow). If (a) and (b) do not compete for the same binding site, then staining with a mixture of (a) and (b) will result in more antibodies bound per cell and a shift in the modal fluorescence towards a higher channel number (filled arrow in (c)). If (a) and (b) compete for the same binding site, but in this case (b) detects it more efficiently, the modal fluorescence of the antibody mixture (filled arrow in (d)) will coincide with the peak channel number defined by (b) alone.

Competition studies with a single directly labelled monoclonal antibody, histograms (e) to (g), are more sensitive, as they may be conducted at say 50% maximum binding, and are easier to interpret. The modal fluorescence seen for directly labelled antibody E used alone (open arrow) is not affected by an unlabelled monoclonal antibody binding to unrelated epitopes (filled arrow in histogram (f)). However, there is a clear shift to lower channel numbers when an unlabelled antibody binds to the same sites (filled arrow in histogram (g)).

In each case, however, that competitive binding might result from steric hinderance due to two spatially close, rather than identical, epitopes. This equivocal finding could be resolved by evidence from antibody-induced capping (Section 3.7.2).

designed to detect IgG monoclonals by the use of a labelled anti-IgG Fc reagent could be 'spiked' by the addition of the $F(ab')_2$ fragment of an already banked monoclonal (Section 12.10.1).

Technical notes

1   The use of a control for non-specific binding (fluorescein-conjugated irrelevant monoclonal antibody of the same isotype) is crucial throughout all the manipulations described above. Chemical or enzyme treatment of a cell population might increase or decrease non-specific binding in an unpredictable manner.

2 Results from these assays must be interpreted with the same caution as any data using these highly sensitive antibody probes. For example, lack of binding to a test-cell population might mean that the epitope is absent or merely inaccessible. Similarly, enzyme treatment of a cell surface could increase or decrease antibody binding by changing the accessibility of the binding site rather than through a direct effect on the epitope.

12.12 ## Practical applications of monoclonal antibodies

The production, selection and maintenance of hybridoma clones synthesising antibody of a required specificity is so time consuming that, before starting, one must be convinced that hybridoma technology is the best way to achieve the desired result. Under some circumstances, for example for the production of antibodies for the class-specific precipitation of immunoglobulins or screening of recombinant DNA expression libraries, the limited perspective of monospecific antibody is a distinct disadvantage. In general, these antibodies bind to only one determinant per molecule when used with non-polymeric antigens, thus precluding the formation of a matrix for precipitation.

There are however, numerous examples where the availability of monoclonal antibody has greatly improved existing technology or has been fundamental for the generation of new techniques. This is to be expected when one considers their advantages compared with conventional antisera:

(a) Because they are monospecific, hybridoma-derived antibodies can be used for the estimation of degree of structural homology between antigens. For example, with influenza virus, antibodies against chemically defined antigens have been used to investigate strains of virus for the presence of identical or closely related antigens.

(b) In solid-phase binding assays, these antibodies can be used at very low concentrations. This is of particular advantage because these assays are essentially affinity independent and can detect the very low-affinity non-specific protein—protein interactions often found with conventional sera. However, as the degree of non-specific binding shown by an unrelated monoclonal antibody is much less than would be found with a normal control serum or unrelated antiserum the results can be interpreted with greater confidence.

(c) The production of hybridoma-derived antibody is highly reproducible. If one prepares a hybrid cell using a non-synthesising plasmacytoma cell line, then the hybridoma line will produce only one type of antibody. Thus, whenever a new batch of antibody is produced from the same cloned cell line, it will have the same specificity.

In general the use of monospecific antibody is still limited to research and diagnostic applications. Of particular interest is the use of monospecific antibodies for the definition of cell-surface markers for the investigation of specialised or abnormal cell function (Section 14.2). This should continue to yield new information on the development and control of the immune system, and has given powerful diagnostic, and in some cases prognostic, tools for the study of tumours.

Monospecific antibodies have several potential applications in clinical medicine both diagnostic and, once a suitable human plasmacytoma parent line has been discovered, therapeutic. (This latter application was previously discounted because of the possible co-purification of viral oncogenes from hybridoma supernatants. However, an analogous situation now exists with the production of interferon from human cell lines. The safeguards developed for the production and use of interferon are applicable to hybridoma-derived antibodies.)

Monospecific antibodies produced by mouse fusion hybrids have many immediate applications in the clinical laboratory as diagnostic or immunoassay reagents.

(a)   Tissue typing (Section 14.8). Current typing techniques rely on antisera derived from multi-parous women or from patients who have received multiple blood transfusions. They are of low titre and often contain several specificities. A programme has been established in the USA for the production of typing reagents using hybridoma techniques, although it seems likely that this approach will be overtaken by the use of gene probes.

(b)   Blood group typing (Section 6.14.7). A range of standard reagents are now available through national blood banks.

(c)   Immunoassay of hormones, etc. Fusions can be performed with spleen cells from mice immunised with relatively impure antigen. The need for antigen purification is circumvented by the selection of appropriate cell lines from cloned populations. This, and the monospecificity of the antibody thus obtained, has greatly enhanced the range and sensitivity of immunoassay techniques (Chapter 10). For example, an improved 'pregnancy test' has been introduced using hybridoma-derived antibody for the immunoenzymatic detection of human chorionic gonadotrophin (HCG). These tests are now sensitive, rapid, accurate and unequivocal in their interpretation. In one variant, the enzyme substrate develops a minus sign in the event of a negative test; the anti-HCG antibody is so disposed that it then adds an additional bar, to create a plus sign, in the event of a positive test. Monoclonal antibody technology has transformed this test from a highly specialised laboratory technique to a 'home-based' immunoassay.

(d)   Immunodiagnosis of infectious disease. Immunoassays using monoclonal antibodies are sufficiently sensitive to allow the diagnosis of infectious disease by the detection of microbial antigen rather than antibody. This is of much greater clinical value as it is a direct measure of the current state of the patient. Antibody detection has the disadvantage that it is practically impossible to distinguish between a past or present infection using a single blood sample. The ability to select monospecific antibodies also avoids the diagnostic imprecision due to cross-reactivity between serologically related organisms.

In general, attempts to produce human monoclonal antibodies have met with only limited success. In addition to the major limitation that peripheral blood is the only readily available source of lymphocytes (which must be activated *in vitro* as deliberate immunisation *in vivo* would be unethical), there are really no human tumour parents equivalent to the MOPC-21 sublines used in the murine system. Attempts have been made to circumvent these deficiencies; for example, EBV lines used both alone and fused with B-cell tumours (Section 14.9), but no generally applicable technique has emerged.

Fortunately, recombinant DNA techniques have been brought to bear on the problem of antigenicity of murine antibodies destined for clinical use. It has been possible to fuse the DNA sequence encoding murine variable regions with human constant regions thus producing a minimally antigenic molecule. Although the problem of an anti-idiotypic response (Section 6.15) still remains, there appears to be a sufficiently great time window to achieve therapeutic potential. This approach has also been applied to the production of novel hybrid molecules in which the combining site of antibody is used to target a secondary effector function; for example, an enzyme active site.

Antigen				
Human	Mouse	Rat	Distribution	Function
CD2	Ly-37	Ox49/50?	T and B cells	T-cell activation
CD3			T cells	All T cells
CD4	L3T4	W3/25	T helper/inducer cells	Binds class II-restricted T cells
CD5	Ly-1	W3/13	T cells, B-cell subset	
CD6			T cells	
CD7			T cells	Fcμ receptor
CD8a	Ly-2	Ox-8	Cytotoxic T cells	CTL adhesion
CD8b	Ly-3		Cytotoxic T cells	CTL adhesion
CD9			Monocytes, pre-B cells platelets	
CD10			Pre-B cells, cAll	
CD11a	Ly-15 (LFA-1)		T and B cells, stem and NK cells	CTL adhesion
CD11b	Ly-40		Macrophages, Ly-1 B cells, granulocytes	C3bi receptor
CD18			Leucocytes	LFA-B
CD20	Ly-44		B cells	
CD23	Ly-42		B cells	Receptor for IgE Fc
CD25	Ly-43	Ox-39	T and B cells	Receptor for IL-2
CD32	Ly-17	B myeloid and Langerhans' cells	Fc IgG2b/1 receptor	Fc IgG2b/1 receptor
CD45	Ly-5	Ox-1, Ox-29, Ox-30	Pan-leucocyte, erythroblasts, FDCs, thymocytes	L-CA, T-200; role in B-cell maturation
CD45R	Ly-5 (B220)	Ox-22, Ox-31 Ox-32	Pre-B cells, B, subset of CTL	Restricted T-200

Fig. 12.8 Functional equivalence of human, mouse and rat cell-surface antigens defined by monoclonal antibodies.

Antigen	Distribution	Functions
CD1a	Thymocytes (Langerhans, cells)	
CD1b	Thymocytes	
CD1c	Thymocytes	
CD2	T cells	T-cell activation
CD3	T cells	T-receptor complex
CD4	Helper/inducer T cells	Binds MHC class II-restricted T cells
CD5	T cells, B-cell subset	
CD6	T cells	
CD7	T cells	
CD8	T-cell subset	Cytotoxic T-cell adhesion
CD9	Macrophages, pre-B cells platelets	
CD10	Pre-B cells, cAll	
CD11a	Leucocytes	Cytotoxic T-cell adhesion
CD11b	Macrophages, granulocytes some B cells	Receptor for C3bi
CD11c	Macrophages, (granulocytes)	
CD12	Macrophages, granulocytes, platelets	
CD13	Granulocytes, macrophages	
CD14	Macrophages, (granulocytes), follicular dendritic cells	
CD15	Granulocytes, macrophages	
CD16	Granulocytes	
CD17	Granulocytes, macrophages, platelets	
CD18	Leucocytes	
CD19	B cells	LFA-B
CD20	B cells, follicular dendritic cells	
CD21	B cells, follicular dendritic cells	Receptor for C3d
CD22	B cells	
CD23	B-cell subset, follicular dendritic cells	Receptor for IgE Fc
CD24	B cells, granulocytes	
CD25	Activated T cells, activated B cells	IL-2 receptor
CD26	Activated T cells	
CD27	T cells, plasma cells	
CD28	T-cell subset	
CD29	T-cell subset	
CD30	Activated lymphocytes	
CD31	Macrophages, granulocytes, platelets	

Fig. 12.9 Human haematopoietic cell-surface antigens.

Antigen	Distribution	Functions
CD32	Macrophages, granulocytes, platelets, B cells	
CD33	Myelogenous leukaemia	
CD34	Myeloid and lymphoid leukaemia	
CD35	Granulocytes, macrophages, follicular dendritic cells	
CD36	Macrophages, platelets	
CD37	B cells	
CD38	Restricted multiple lineage cells	
CD39	B cells, macrophages	
CD40	B cells, interdigitating reticulum cells, carcinomas	
CD41	Platelets	
CD43	T cells, granulocytes, erythrocytes, brain	
CD44	Pre-B cells, brain	
CD45	Leucocytes	T-200, LCA B cell maturation
CD45R	B cells, T-cell subset, granulocytes, macrophages	Restricted T-200

Fig. 12.9 (continued)

12.13 Cell phenotyping and immunohistochemistry with monoclonal antibodies

Monoclonal antibodies against cell-surface antigens have made important contributions to our understanding and manipulation of the immune response. On current evidence, it seems likely that each mammalian species will have an analogous set of these antigens; whose distributions correspond with functionally distinct subpopulations of cells involved in the immune response. The chaos that reigned when the nomenclature for these antigens was derived from the designation of the relevant monoclonal antibody has now been largely resolved by the definition of 'cluster determinants' for human antigens. Groups of antibodies are now referred to antigen molecules by so-called cluster analysis. We have listed the analogous antigens for human, mouse and rat in Fig. 12.8. Figures 12.9–12.11 give further information for each of these species separately.

The use of monoclonal antibodies against cell-surface markers in leukaemia phenotyping is described in Section 14.2. Indeed, a rapid and accurate diagnosis of some tumours can only be achieved by the use of monoclonal antibodies; for example the use of antibodies against cytoskeletal components for the typing of brain tumours. This approach is particularly useful as some of the monoclonal antibodies react with epitopes that are preserved even after paraffin embedding; one may therefore derive

Antigen	Synonym	Distribution	Functions
Ly-1	Lyt-1	T cells, B-cell subset	
Ly-2	Lyt-2	Cytotoxic T cells	Cytotoxic T-cell adhesion
Ly-3	Lyt-3	Cytotoxic T cells	Cytotoxic T-cell adhesion
Ly-4	L3T4	Helper T cells	Binds class II-restricted T cells
Ly-5	T-200	Pan-leucocyte erythroblasts, stem cells, FDCs, thymocytes	B-cell maturation
Ly-6		T and B cells, granulocytes	T-cell activation
Ly-7		T and B cells, subset of thymocytes, some BM cells	
Ly-8		Thymocytes	
Ly-9	Lgp-100 T-100	T and B cells, thymocytes, BFU-E, some CFU-E and CFU-GM, -M	
Ly-10		T and B cells, thymocytes	
Ly-11		T-cell subset, NK cells	
Ly-12		T and B cells	
Ly-13		T and B cells, erythrocytes	
Ly-14		T and B cells	
Ly-15	LFA-1	T and B cells, myeloid cells, NK cells, stem cells	Cytotoxic T-cell adhesion
Ly-16	Ly-18	Cytotoxic T cells	
Ly-17	Lym-20	B cells, myeloid cells, Langerhans' cells	Fc IgG2b/I receptor
Ly-18	Lym-18	T and B cells, some bone marrow, thymocytes	
Ly-19	Lym-19	T and B cells, some bone marrow	
Ly-20		T-cell subset	
Ly-21		T and B cells	
Ly-22	Lym-22	Suppressor T cells	
Ly-23		T and B cells	
Ly-24	Pgp-1	Non-T leucocytes, bone marrow, memory T cells, pro-thymocytes	
Ly-25		B cells, thymocytes, T-cell subset, bone marrow	
Ly-26		B cells, some bone marrow	
Ly-27		Subset of T and B cells, thymocyte subset	
Ly-28		T cells, thymocytes, B cell subset	

Fig. 12.10 Mouse haematopoietic cell-surface antigens.

Antigen	Synonym	Distribution	Functions
Ly-29		B cells, T-cell subset, thymocyte subset, some bone marrow	
Ly-30		B cells, T-cell subset, bone marrow	
Ly-31		T- and B-cell subset, thymocyte subset, some bone marrow	
Ly-32		B cells, T-cell subset, some bone marrow	
Ly-33		T and B cells, thymocytes, some bone marrow	
Ly-34		Thymocytes, T cells, some bone marrow	
Ly-35		Thymocytes, T-cell subset	
Ly-36		Thymocytes, T and B cells	
Ly-37		Thymocytes, T and B cells	T-cell activation E-rosette receptor
Ly-38		Thymocytes	
Ly-39		Activated B cells	
Ly-40	Mac-l	Macrophages, granulocytes, Ly-l B cells	C3bi receptor
Ly-41	PC-l	T and B cells	
Ly-42		B cells	IgE Fc receptor
Ly-43		T and B cells	IL-2 receptor
Ly-44		B cells	
Lyb-2		B cells	B-cell activation IL-4 like response
Lyb-3		B cells	
Lyb-4		B cells	
Lyb-5		B-cell subset	
Lyb-6		B cells	
Lyb-7		B cells	
Lyb-8		B cells	
Thy-1		T cells, epithelial cells, fibroblasts, neurons, stem cells	T-cell activation
Thy-2		Thymocytes	
F4/80		Monocytes, macrophages	
ThB		B cells, thymocytes	
HSA		B cells, myeloid and erythroid cells, thymocyte subset, some bone marrow	
BP-1, 6C3		Pre-B, early B cells	
Mac-2		Thioglycollate elicited peritoneal macrophages	
Mac-3		Peritoneal macrophages	

Fig. 12.10 (continued)

Antigen	Distribution	Functions
Ox-1	Leucocyte common	
Ox-2	Thymocytes, brain, B cells, dendritic cells	
Ox-3	Ia polymorphic antigen	
Ox-4	Ia common non-polymorphic	
Ox-5	Ia common non-polymorphic	
Ox-6	Ia common non-polymorphic	
Ox-7	Thy-1.1	
Ox-8	T-cell subset, CTL, NK cell, thymocytes	
Ox-9	T-cell subset, thymocytes, NK cells	
Ox-10	T-cell subset, thymocytes	
Ox-17	Ia (Ox-4 negative)	
Ox-18	RT1A (non-polymorphic)	
Ox-19	T cells, thymocytes	
Ox-22	B cells, some T cells, NK cells	LCA
Ox-26	Transferrin receptor	
Ox-31	Same as Ox-22, competes with Ox-22	
Ox-32	Same as Ox-22, but does not compete	
Ox-33	B cells	LCA
Ox-35	Same as W3/25, competes with Ox-36	
Ox-36	Same as W3/25, competes with Ox-35	
Ox-37	Same as W3/25, competes with W3/25 and Ox-38	
Ox-38	Same as W3/25 competes with W3/25 and Ox-37	
Ox-39	Activated T cells, thymic dendritic cells	IL-2 receptor
Ox-40	Activated cells	
Ox-41	Most macrophages, polymorphs, some dendritic cells, brain	
Ox-42	As Ox-41	
Ox-43	Resident and splenic macrophages, red cells, endothelium	
Ox-44	Some thymocytes, mature T and B cells	
Ox-45	Thymocytes, T and B cells, endothelium	
Ox-46	Same as Ox-45, competes	
Ox-47	Thymocytes, T and B cells macrophages, dendritic cells	
Ox-48	Activated T and B cells	
Ox-49	Thymocytes, T cells and some B cells	

Fig. 12.11 Rat haematopoietic cell-surface antigens. The designation Ox is derived from the Oxford series of monoclonal antibodies used to define the majority of these antigens.

Antigen	Distribution	Functions
Ox-50	Same molecule as Ox-49	
Ox-51	Same as Ox-22	
Ox-52	Pan T cell	
W3/13	Thymocytes, T cells, plasma cells, polymorphs	
W3/15	Thymocytes, bone marrow (erythroid)	
W3/25	Thymocytes, T-cell subset, macrophages	Binds class II-restricted T

Fig. 12.11 (continued)

information both from the discriminatory power of antibodies and the descriptive power of classical histology.

12.13.1 Monoclonal antibody staining of paraffin-embedded sections

Materials and equipment
Mouse IgG monoclonal antibody
Rabbit anti-mouse IgG conjugated with horse radish peroxidase (RAM−HRP)
Swine anti-rabbit IgG−HRP (SAR−HRP)
Diaminobenzidine, DAB
Hydrogen peroxide, H_2O_2
Methanol
0.025 M Tris−HCl buffer, pH 7.6 (Appendix I)
Phosphate-buffered saline, PBS (Appendix I)
Normal human serum
Harris' haematoxylin (Appendix II)
DePeX mounting medium
Latex gloves
Coplin staining jar
Glass slide staining jars
Magnetic stirrers

PREPARATION IN ADVANCE

Stock solutions
Prepare a series of de-waxing and re-hydrating solutions:
Xylene and ethanol − 100%, 90%, 70%, 50% v/v in water.
RAM−HRP and SAR−HRP (latter, if needed, as explained below) diluted 1 : 40 in PBS containing 5% normal human serum.

H_2O_2, 0.3% in methanol made up immediately prior to use.

DAB–H_2O_2 — dissolve 24 mg DAB in 40 ml of 25 mM Tris–HCl, pH 7.6, and add 14 µl of H_2O_2, filter and use immediately.

Method

1 De-wax the sections by immersing the slides in the xylene for 2 min.
2 Re-hydrate the sections by immersing the slides for 1 min sequentially in absolute alcohol, 90% alcohol, 70% alcohol and 50% alcohol.
3 Finally, immerse in PBS for 2 min with gentle agitation, then wipe off excess PBS from around the edge of the section.
4 Overlay the section with mouse monoclonal antibody (see Technical note 2), and incubate in a humidified box at room temperature for 1 h.
5 Wash the slides three times in PBS, gently agitating the slides to ensure thorough washing.
6 Immerse the sections in 0.3% H_2O_2 in methanol for 1 h at room temperature to inactivate endogenous peroxidase.
7 Wash thoroughly in PBS and wipe dry around the edge of the section.
8 Overlay with RAM–HRP diluted 1:40 in PBS containing 5% normal human serum and incubate in a humidified box at room temperature for 30 min.
9 Wash and wipe dry around the section.
10 If amplification is required, for example if the antigen of interest is present in trace amounts only, overlay with SAR–HRP diluted 1:60 in PBS containing 5% normal human serum. Incubate in a humidified box at room temperature for 30 min.
11 Wash and wipe dry around the section.
12 Add DAB solution to the sections, and incubate at room temperature for 30 min.
13 Wash the sections under running tap water to stop the reaction.
14 Counterstain with Harris' haematoxylin for 30 min and then wash under running tap water for 2 min.
15 Dehydrate the sections through the graded alcohol solutions; 1 min in each through the ascending series, and finally dip into xylene.
16 Mount under a coverslip using DePeX and examine by transmitted light microscopy.

Results

Areas where the antibody has bound should be stained brown while the cell nuclei should be stained blue.

Technical notes

1 *Diaminobenzidene is a carcinogen and should be handled with care.* Always wear latex gloves, and do not inhale the powder.
2 Monoclonal antibodies should be titrated to achieve both specific staining and economy of use. (The principles explained in Section 2.1.6 also apply here.)

Propagation of antigen-responsive normal T lymphocytes lines

Under the conditions described below, normal T lymphocytes may be expanded into lines capable of extensive *in vitro* proliferation and yet still retain their effector capacity and antigen selectivity. The immunogens used range from allogeneic cells, processed antigen expressed by MHC-compatible antigen-presenting cells or viral antigens expressed on infected autologous host cells. The literature abounds with different methods for isolating antigen-specific T-cell clones *in vitro*. We will describe methods which we have used for the isolation of murine and human antigen-reactive T-cell lines and clones.

12.14.1 Murine T-lymphocyte lines

Dose—response curve for antigen

Materials and equipment

Inbred mice for immunisation (it is important to use inbred mice of known haplotype as Ia-identical animals have to be used as a source of feeder cells)

Antigen

Freund's complete adjuvant

Tissue culture medium

Fetal bovine serum

2-mercaptoethanol

Antibiotics — streptomycin and penicillin

96-well culture plates (Appendix II)

^{3}H-thymidine (Appendix II)

Automated cell harvester (Appendix II)

β-spectrometer

Method

1 Immunise mice by a subcutaneous injection at the base of the tail with antigen emulsified in Freund's complete adjuvant (200 μl total volume, see Section 1.7.1 for details).

2 Anaesthetise the mice 3—4 days after the last injection and bleed for serum (Sections 1.10 and 1.12.1).

3 Kill the mice by cervical dislocation and remove the paraortic and inguinal lymph nodes (draining the base of the tail) using aseptic technique.

4 Prepare a sterile single-cell suspension as described in Section 1.15.

5 Wash the cell suspension twice by centrifugation and re-suspend the cells in complete medium (containing 10% FBS, 2×10^{-5} M 2-mercaptoethanol, 100 U ml^{-1} penicillin and 100 μg ml^{-1} streptomycin) and re-suspend at 2×10^6 cells ml^{-1}.

A control population should be prepared in an identical manner using cells from mice immunised with Freund's complete adjuvant alone.

6 Dispense 100 μl aliquots of cells into the wells of a 96-well micro-titre tray (U-shaped wells) and add a range of antigen concentrations in triplicate, each in 100 μl of medium.
7 Incubate for 4−6 days, depending on the peak of the mitogenic response (Section 4.9), and during the last 18 h of incubation add 37×10^3 Bq per well of ^{3}H-thymidine.
8 Harvest with an automated cell harvester and measure radioactive incorporation using a β scintillation counter.
9 Calculate the proliferation index according to the equation:

$$\text{Stimulation index} = \frac{\text{c.p.m. cells with antigen} - \text{c.p.m. cells without antigen}}{\text{c.p.m. cells without antigen}}.$$

Repeat the calculations for cells from animals immunised with Freund's adjuvant alone to check that the antigen being used reacts specifically with the cells primed with antigen *in vivo*.

10 Plot a dose−response curve for the antigen to determine the optimum concentration for *in vitro* stimulation.

Technical note
The immunisation protocol must be varied to take account of the antigen being used. A single injection of a highly immunogenic antigen is often sufficient. However, for some antigens a booster injection 7 days after the first (or an even more extensive boosting) may be advantageous. In any case harvest the lymph nodes 3−4 days after the last injection.

Murine T-lymphocyte line production

1 Immunise 4−6 mice as described above and prepare a single-cell suspension of lymph-node cells (Section 1.15).
2 Re-suspend the cells in tissue culture medium containing 10% FBS and aliquot at $2-5 \times 10^6$ cells well^{-1} in 24-well culture plates.
3 Add antigen at the optimum concentration (determined above) to achieve a total culture volume of 1.5 ml and incubate for 4−6 days at 37° in a humidified incubator gassed with 5% CO_2 in air.
4 Harvest the cells by centrifugation (150 *g* for 10 min at room temperature) and isolate the blast cells by density gradient centrifugation (Section 1.13.2).
5 Wash the cells twice by centrifugation, re-suspend in tissue culture medium containing 5% FBS and count in a haemocytometer.
6 Prepare a single-cell suspension from the spleens of syngeneic mice (Section 1.15) for use as feeder cells.

7   Irradiate the normal spleen cells with 25 Gy irradiation, wash and re-suspend in tissue culture medium containing 5% FBS.
8   Plate $1-2\times10^6$ irradiated feeder cells with 1×10^5 T-cell blasts per well in a total volume of 2 ml.
9   Incubate for 7–14 days.
10 Repeat steps 3–6 and plate $1-2\times10^6$ irradiated feeder cells with $1-2\times10^5$ T cells plus antigen at the optimum concentration.
11 Incubate for 4 days.
12 Repeat steps 3–7.

T-cell lines can be maintained long-term by this regime of regular stimulation and 'rest'. When larger numbers of cells are required for assays, the cells can be expanded in tissue culture flasks (start with 25 cm² growth area flasks). To maintain maximum cell density at the beginning of an expansion phase, incubate the flasks upright or at a slight angle to vertical. It is possible to maintain antigen-reactive T-cell lines in culture for up to about 14 days without antigen stimulation by adding exogenous IL-2 to the medium. Activated (antigen-stimulated) T-cell lines which express IL-2 receptors will respond by vigorous growth and proliferation. However, growth declines rapidly within a few days because of a decrease in the expression of the IL-2 receptor. Re-stimulation with the appropriately presented antigen or a mitogen is then required to induce re-expression of high levels of the IL-2 receptor.

Laboratories vary in their techniques for production of T-cell lines and many factors can influence the outcome; persistence is obligatory and 'green fingers' are helpful.

T-lymphocyte cloning

Materials and equipment
Antigen-reactive T-cell line
Syngeneic irradiated feeder cells
Antigen
Tissue culture medium (Appendix I) containing 5% fetal bovine serum (Appendix II)
96-well micro-culture plates (flat wells) (Appendix II)
Interleukin 2, IL-2 (see Technical note)

Method
1   Prepare T-cell blasts as described in previous section.
2   Dispense 5×10^5 irradiated feeder cells in tissue culture medium containing IL-2 and the optimum concentration of antigen into the wells of the micro-titre trays.
3   Prepare suspensions of the T-cell blasts at: (a) 100 cells ml^{-1}; (b) 33 cells ml^{-1}; (c) 10 cells ml^{-1}; and (d) 3.3 cells ml^{-1}.
4   Dispense aliquots of 100 μl of each suspension, preparing one plate each for (a) and (b), and three plates each for (c) and (d). The higher concentrations are used to check that the cells will grow.

5 Examine the plates under an inverted microscope with phase-contrast optics after 7 days.

6 Wells in which T lymphocytes have grown can easily be identified as the phase-bright T cells grow as a clump amongst the dying, phase-dark feeder cells.

7 Positive wells should be transferred into 24-well culture plates containing fresh, irradiated syngeneic feeder cells (2×10^6 per well), the optimum concentration of antigen and IL-2.

8 To ensure that monoclonality is obtained the selected 'cloned lines' should be re-cloned by plating at 1 cell ml^{-1}.

Once cloned populations have been selected and expanded, aliquots should be cryopreserved against accidental loss or clonal exhaustion. By this stage the T-lymphocytes will have adapted (probably been intensively selected) to the *in vitro* conditions and so can be maintained relatively easily by repeated cycles of antigen stimulation and 'rest'. Some T-cell clones can be maintained in IL-2 supplemented medium alone for several days but will need stimulation with antigen plus feeder cells to sustain proliferation and their differentiated function.

Technical note

It is preferable to use recombinant IL-2 for technical convenience: titrate the units of activity to determine the optimum concentration in your system. This is likely to be around 2000 U ml^{-1}. Alternatively, IL-2-containing supernatants can be prepared from T-lymphocyte lines (MLA-144 [gibbon line] for use with human cells or EL4 for use with murine cells) or from normal lymphocytes (for example, rat spleen) stimulated in bulk with concanavalin A (mitogenic stimulation as for phytohaemagglutinin, PHA, in Section 4.12.4). IL-2 is constitutively produced by the cell lines; however, its production may be maximised by growing the cells to their plateau density, washing them into serum-free medium and incubating overnight at 37° in a humidified atmosphere containing 5% CO_2 in air.

Interleukin-2 from any of these sources will maintain murine T-lymphocytes, but human T-lymphocytes need primate IL-2.

12.14.2 Human T-lymphocyte lines

The procedures for deriving human T-lymphocyte lines are essentially similar to those described for the mouse (Section 12.14.1). However, there are some important differences and limitations; for example, human lines are usually derived using either ethical (vaccination) or fortuitous (usually an infection) immunisation, and invariably need repeated donations from the same individual both to provide T lymphocytes (a minor requirement) and feeder cells (a massive requirement). Although it is possible to select a panel of HLA-D matched individuals to supply feeder cells or to transfect the required major histocompatibility complex (MHC) molecules into antigen-presenting cells, this requires sophisticated laboratory back up. Attempts have been made to establish lines of Epstein–Barr virus-transformed autologous B cells (Section 14.9) from the T-lymphocyte donor and use these as antigen-presenting cells, but without uniform success.

Materials and equipment
Peripheral blood drawn from an antigen-sensitised individual (see Technical note)
Antigen
Tissue culture medium (Appendix I)
Pooled normal human serum, NHS
^{3}H-thymidine (Appendix II)
96-well micro-culture plates, U-shaped wells (Appendix II)
24-well culture plates (Appendix II)
Tissue culture flasks, 25 cm^2 (Appendix II)
Automated cell harvester (Appendix II)
β spectrometer

Method
As with the murine T cells, it is important to establish a dose—response curve for the antigen to be used.

1 Fractionate peripheral blood mononuclear cells (PBMC) from heparinised blood by density gradient centrifugation (Section 1.14.1).
2 Wash the cells twice by centrifugation and re-suspend in tissue culture medium containing 10% pooled normal human serum.
3 Dispense 100 μl aliquots of cells (2×10^6 ml^{-1}) into the wells of U-shaped well micro-titre plates. Add 100 μl aliquots of antigen in doubling dilutions in 100 μl medium.
4 Incubate at 37° in a humidified atmosphere of 5% CO_2 in air for 5 days.
5 Add 37×10^3 Bq of ^{3}H-thymidine to each well and incubate for a further 6 h.
6 Harvest the wells using an automated cell harvester and measure isotope incorporation using a β counter.
7 The results are expressed as an index of stimulation, as defined for murine lymphocytes above.
8 Plot a dose—response curve to determine the optimum antigen concentration required to give maximum T-lymphocyte proliferation.

Technical note
Although many of the antigenic constituents of human vaccines or common infectious organisms have been used to produce T-lymphocyte lines, those of the influenza virus have been particularly useful because parallel developments in molecular biology have made a wide range of defined 'flu peptides readily available.

Human T-lymphocyte line production

Materials and equipment
Heparinised human peripheral blood
Tissue culture medium (Appendix I)

Pooled normal human serum, NHS

Source of IL-2, either supernatant from the cell line MLA-144, or recombinant human material

Antigen

96-well micro-culture plates, flat wells (Appendix II)

Tissue culture flasks, 25 cm^2 growth area (Appendix II)

24-well culture plates (Appendix II)

Method

1 Prepare human peripheral blood lymphocytes from heparinised blood by density gradient centrifugation (Section 1.14.1) and re-suspend in tissue culture medium containing 10% pooled NHS.

2 Adjust the cell concentration to $1-2\times10^6$ ml^{-1} and dispense in 10 ml aliquots into 25 cm^2 tissue culture flasks or in 2 ml aliquots in 24 well-cluster plates. Add the required antigen at its optimum concentration.

3 To maintain high cell density incubate the flasks upright at 37° in a humidified atmosphere of 5% CO_2 in air for 6-7 days.

4 Harvest the cells and separate the blasts by density gradient centrifugation (Section 1.14.1) and wash the cells in tissue culture medium by centrifugation.

The T-cell lines can be maintained in IL-2 containing medium with repeated rounds of stimulation with antigen and feeder cells. They are much easier to grow than their murine equivalents; to the extent that they can be cloned at or soon after primary plating.

Human T-lymphocyte cloning

Materials and equipment

As previous section, but including phytohaemagglutinin, PHA (Appendix II)

Method

1 To prepare autologous irradiated feeder cells, separate leucocytes from heparinsed blood (Section 1.14.1), wash and irradiate with 40 Gy from a high energy source.

2 Adjust the cell concentration to 1×10^6 ml^{-1} in medium containing 10% pooled NHS, IL-2, antigen at the optimum concentration and a submitogenic concentration of PHA; for example, 1 μg ml^{-1}.

3 Re-suspend fractionated T-cell blasts after *in vitro* stimulation as described in the previous section. Prepare suspensions at 100, 33, 10, 3.3 and 1 cell ml^{-1} in tissue culture medium containing 10% human serum. Prepare sufficient for 48 micro-cultures of each of the three higher concentrations and 96 cultures for each of the two lower concentrations.

4 Plate out 100 μl aliquots of the T-lymphocyte suspensions and incubate at 37° in a humidified atmosphere of 5% CO_2 in air for 7 days.

5 Examine the plates under a phase-contrast inverted microscope for growth. The clones tend to grow in clumps and so are very easy to identify.

6 Positive wells can be expanded into 24-well cluster plates containing 1×10^6 irradiated autologous feeder cells per well in medium supplemented with serum, IL-2, antigen and PHA.

7 After a further 7 days incubation the T-cell blasts can be further expanded on an irradiated feeder layer grown in 25 cm^2 culture flasks with antigen stimulation.

To ensure monoclonality, repeat steps 1–6. T-cell clones can be maintained for short periods in IL-2 containing medium but will need stimulation with antigen and feeder cells every 6–14 days.

12.15 T-lymphocyte hybridomas

Following the success of monoclonal B-lymphocyte hybrid cells, similar principles were applied to T-lymphocytes in order to study their effector functions. T-cell hybridomas have been used for studies on the T-cell receptor and as a source of T-cell-derived cytokines and other regulatory effector molecules, particularly suppressor factors. They have also proved useful in evaluating cell-recognition reactions. The methods used to prepare T-cell hybridomas are essentially the same as for B-cell hybrids; an activated population of T cells primed to respond to a particular antigen, or activated with mitogen (phytohaemagglutinin, PHA, or concanavalin A, Con A) are fused with a tumour-cell line of T-cell origin, usually the murine AKR thymoma BW-5147. Fusion products are assessed for phenotype and karyotype (to determine that they are true T lymphocyte–tumour cell hybrids); and finally cloned and functionally selected depending upon the activity(ies) desired.

Materials and equipment
Activated murine lymphocytes (Technical note 1)
8-azaguanine-resistant variant of the murine AKR thymoma BW-5147 (but see also Technical note 3).
Tissue culture medium (Appendix I), alone or with 10% fetal bovine serum, FBS
Polyethylene glycol solution, PEG 1500 (prepared as Section 12.4)
Concentrated HAT medium (Section 12.4.4)
96-well micro-titre plates (Appendix II)
24- and 48-well tissue culture plates (Appendix II)
Irradiated (25 Gy) spleen cells and thymocytes, syngeneic with the lymph-node donor

Method

1 Mix 2×10^7 washed BW-5147 cells in serum-free medium with 1×10^8 washed stimulated murine lymphocytes in a 50 ml conical tube and centrifuge (150 *g* for 15 min at room temperature).

2 Carefully remove the supernatant by aspiration and tap the tube to re-suspend the cells.

3 Place the tube in a water bath at 37° and add 1 ml of a 1:1 mix of PEG 1500 in serum-free medium; add dropwise over 45 sec.

4 Allow the tube to stand for 45 sec and then over 5 min add 50 ml of serum-free medium pre-warmed to 37°, with gentle mixing.

5 Leave the cell suspension at 37° for 5 min and then centrifuge to pellet the cells (150 g for 15 min at room temperature).

6 Remove and discard the supernatant before re-suspending the cells in serum-free medium. Centrifuge and re-suspend in tissue culture medium containing 10% FBS.

7 Dispense in 100 μl aliquots into 96-well micro-titre plates.

8 Incubate at 37° for 24 h, and then add 50 μl of threefold concentrated HAT medium to each well.

9 Every 5 days, remove half of the supernatant and replace with fresh single strength HAT medium; for at least 3 weeks.

The first hybrids will begin to appear after about 10 days and new ones will continue to appear for the next 3 weeks. Growing hybrids should be karyotyped, phenotyped and screened for antigen reactivity as soon as possible. T-cell hybrids tend to be unstable in the expression of their selected function and so positive lines should be cloned by limiting dilution once their hybrid status has been confirmed. Cloning may be facilitated by the addition of 1×10^5 per well irradiated syngeneic spleen cells, these feeder cells also act as antigen-presenting cells if required by an antigen-specific response. The cells should be freshly prepared and irradiated immediately before they are required.

Samples of each clone of interest should be cryopreserved after screening, as an insurance against accidental loss and also population drift resulting in loss of function.

Technical notes
1 Activate T-lymphocytes by:
(a) Priming *in vivo* by injection of antigen in adjuvant subcutaneously at the base of the tail, re-stimulate *in vitro* and expand in IL-2 containing medium to achieve the required cell numbers, or
(b) Stimulating with mitogen (PHA or Con A); stimulation *in vitro* followed by expansion in IL-2 containing medium.
Hybridomas derived from these cell populations would not be expected to show antigen specificity.

2 The BW-5417 line should be cultured every 2–3 months in 2×10^5 M 6-thioguanine to maintain sensitivity to aminopterin in HAT.

3 Other murine tumour-cell lines such as FS6-14.13 (Kappler JW *et al.* [1981] can also be used for fusion to murine T-cells to produce T-cell hybridomas. Human T-lymphocyte hybridomas can be produced using appropriate human T-tumour cell lines; for example, MOLT-4.

4 The activated lymphocyte population may be enriched for T cells by nylon wool column fractionation (Section 9.9.2) under sterile conditions prior to fusion.

5 To facilitate phenotypic analysis (Section 12.15.3), it is convenient to use a T-lymphocyte donor that expresses the Thy-1.2 gene product (Section 3.8.3), in contrast to the Thy-1.1 expressed by the AKR-derived BW-5147 line.

12.15.1 Screening for functional T-hybrids

The techniques used to analyse the T-hybridomas will depend upon the effector function rescued and whether the cells are antigen-specific. In general, any of the techniques described in Section 4.8 may be adapted for use with T-hybrid lines. T-cell hybrids tend to be unstable, often exhibiting very high ploidy numbers immediately after fusion (Fig. 12.12) but rapidly losing chromosomes thereafter. Clones of interest should be cryopreserved and growing clones checked and re-cloned to maintain their antigen-specific effector function.

12.15.2 Karyotype analysis

Materials and equipment
Actively growing T-hybrids
Colchicine (usually supplied as Colcemid) 0.1% w/v solution (Appendix II)

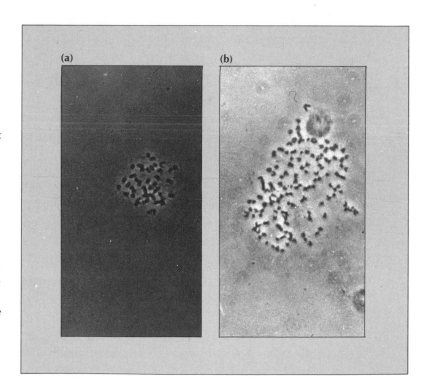

Fig. 12.12 Chromosomal spreads from BW-5147 and T-hybrid cell lines. Although the T-hybrid cell in (b) does not have the total sum of the chromosome of its parents (tumour parent shown in (a)), there has been a convincing increase in the number of chromosomes following cell fusion. The hybrid line continued to loose chromosomes during the next 8 weeks of culture, at which point it became stable. Chromosome loss is random in mouse–mouse hybrids and can result in the loss of the chromosome encoding the hybrid effector function.

Trypsin, 1.0% w/v solution (Appendix II)
Potassium chloride, 0.5% solution
Buffered Giemsa stain, freshly made prior to use (see Section 3.3)

Method

1   Transfer about 10^7 actively growing and dividing T-hybridoma cells into a tissue culture grade conical centrifuge tube. Add 0.1 ml of 0.1% colchicine and incubate at 37° for 2 h. This arrests the cells in mitosis.
2   Centrifuge to pellet the cells and remove the supernatant.
3   Re-suspend the cells vigorously, using a vortex mixer, add 10 ml of 0.5% potassium chloride and incubate for 10 min to allow the lymphocytes to swell and burst.
4   Centrifuge to pellet the contents of the tube, remove the supernatant and slowly re-suspend the pellet in 1 : 3 solution of glacial acetic acid and methanol to fix the nuclei.
5   Repeat the centrifugation and fixing twice and finally re-suspend the pellet in about 10 drops of fixative.
6   Wash a clean microscope slide with a few drops of fixative and wipe dry with a clean tissue to completely de-grease.
7   Breathe onto the slide to warm and moisten it. Using a Pasteur pipette deposit a single drop of the cell suspension onto the slide from a height of 15−30 cm. Tilt the slide to drain the fixative away and allow the slide to dry.

This procedure ruptures the nuclei and allows the chromosomes to spread. It requires a certain amount of practice to achieve good separation of the chromosomes.

8   Dip the slide in the trypsin for 20 sec and wash with tap water.
9   Stain with buffered Giemsa (Section 3.3).
10 Wash with tap water.
11 Observe under a transmitted light microscope; at ×40 magnification to select a suitable nuclear spread and then to ×100 magnification for counting.

12.15.3   Phenotypic analysis

Although karyotypic analysis (Section 12.15.2) provides the definitive demonstration of hybrid status, in the initial stages it is convenient to select on the basis of a hybrid cell-surface phenotype. Most strains of mice express the Thy-1.2 gene product, whereas AKR mice, from which the tumour-cell line BW-5147 was derived, express Thy-1.1. Thus hybrids are HAT resistant, express the Thy-1.2 antigen and sometimes co-express Thy-1.1. Lines selected after HAT treatment which express only Thy-1.1 should be discarded as they are probably HAT-resistant revertants of the tumour-cell line.

Materials and equipment

Anti-Thy-1.1 and anti-Thy-1.2 monoclonal antibodies (for direct or indirect immuno-fluorescent staining, Section 2.1.5)

Phosphate-buffered saline, PBS (Appendix II) containing 2% fetal bovine serum, FBS
U.V. microscope or continuous-flow cytofluorimeter

Method
1 Wash 6×10^6 of the hybrids by centrifugation and divide into 3 aliquots.
2 Process for direct or indirect immunofluorescence using anti-Thy-1.1, anti-Thy-1.2 and irrelevant (control) antibodies (Section 3.5.1).
3 Examine by fluorescence microscopy or by flow cytometry (Section 3.9).

12.16 Characterisation of antigen reactivity

Although monoclonal antibodies and normal or hybrid T-lymphocyte lines can be produced against well-characterised and purified antigens, these techniques also have enormous potential for the analysis of complex mixtures of antigens.

This potential may be appreciated, for example, by reference to the study of an exotic pathogen. A detailed knowledge of its epitopes (which are recognised by B and which by T lymphocytes?) or its immune susceptibilities (can it be killed by antibody-related mechanisms, does it require T lymphocyte-mediated mechanisms or a combination of both?) could be invaluable in the design of a candidate vaccine.

The production of B hybridomas from the spleen of an infected or immunised mouse provides a direct route for the identification and evaluation of antibody-based mechanisms. Protection gained by the passive administration of antibody to an experimental animal, prior to infectious challenge, not only identifies antibody as being important in protection but also provides a valuable tool for the isolation and characterisation of the specific epitope involved (via immunoprecipitation [Section 2.9], immunoblotting [Section 2.11], affinity chromatography [Section 9.7], recombinant DNA technology [Section 2.13], etc.).

It is possible to use syngeneic cell-transfer experiments (Section 4.6) to investigate whether helper, cytotoxic, suppressor or lymphokine-producing cloned T lymphocytes (or their secreted products) are involved in the immune response to infection with the pathogen. It is then possible to use a combination of one- or two-dimensional SDS-PAGE fractionation (Section 2.10) and an *in vitro* T-lymphocyte assay (Section 4.8) to identify the polypeptide involved. Current evidence suggests that the majority of T-lymphocytes recognise sequence, rather than conformation, determinants (cf. Section 2.12) which should therefore survive the denaturing conditions of SDS-PAGE without problem, as described below.

Materials and equipment
As Sections 2.10, 2.11 and 4.8, but in addition:
Lymphocytes, lines or *ex vivo*, for analysis
Antigen mixture
Phosphate-buffered saline, PBS (Appendix I)
Dimethyl sulphoxide, DMSO (Appendix II)
0.05 M Carbonate−bicarbonate buffer, pH 9.5 (Appendix I)

Tissue culture medium (Appendix I)
Fetal bovine serum, FBS (Appendix II)
Tween 20 (Appendix II)
Aurodye (Appendix II)
Eppendorf tubes, 1.5 ml, sterile, conical, plastic
Orbital mixing platform (Appendix II)
Vortex mixer
Microcentrifuge (Microcentaur) (Appendix II)

Method

1 Fractionate the antigen mixture by one- or two-dimensional PAGE (Section 2.10) and transfer electrophoretically onto nitrocellulose (Section 2.11).
2 Wash the nitrocellulose membrane in a large volume of PBS containing 0.3% v/v Tween 20 on an orbital mixing platform. Wash once for 60 min at 37° and twice for 30 min at room temperature.
3 Incubate overnight in Aurodye, according to the manufacturer's instructions, to identify the polypeptide bands.
4 Cut and divide the membrane as required by the analysis (see experimental design at end of section), and dissolve strips individually in DMSO. A volume of 250 µl of DMSO is required to dissolve 20 mm^2 of nitrocellulose membrane.
5 Leave the dissolved membranes in DMSO at room temperature for at least 60 min to ensure chemical sterilisation is complete. This avoids having to run the initial fractionation and blotting under aseptic conditions.
6 Add an equal volume of carbonate−bicarbonate buffer to the DMSO solution; add the buffer dropwise while vortexing the mixture vigorously.
7 Transfer the particle suspensions to sterile Eppendorf centrifuge tubes and wash twice in tissue culture medium containing 10% FBS by centrifugation (10 000 g for 10 min at 4°).
8 Re-suspend the final pellet in a convenient volume of tissue culture medium and either use immediately or store at −20°.

Technical notes

1 Although other organic solvents may be used to dissolve the nitrocellulose (for example, acetone, pyridine, etc.), DMSO has the advantage of low toxicity during the cell-based stages of the analysis. However, once opened, it is good practice to use the DMSO for only 3−4 weeks or alternatively to re-distill it frequently.
2 The staining methods described for immunoblots in Section 2.11.1 are not compatible with lymphocyte assays. If Aurodye proves too expensive for routine use, use a preparative SDS-PAGE slot gel, blot over and cut off a sample strip of nitrocellulose for staining as in Section 2.11.1. Use this to locate 'regions of interest' on the remaining unstained part of the membrane, which may then be used for preparation of antigen.
3 The particle suspensions may be stored at −20° for several weeks without diminution of antigen activity. Disperse by gentle ultrasonication after thawing, if required.

EXPERIMENTAL DESIGN

Material prepared in this way is easily phagocytosed by antigen-presenting cells *in vitro* and often gives a better mitogenic response than an equivalent amount of soluble protein. A single polypeptide band on a slot blotted gel can produce enough material for the stimulation of 30–60 lymphocyte micro-cultures.

This method of analysis offers the significant advantage that it can be used to study protein and carbohydrate-based epitopes with equal facility: identify the former by proteinase treatment of the strips prior to DMSO solubilisation (Fig. 12.5) and the latter by glycosidase digestion (Fig. 12.5) or periodate oxidation (Section 12.11.2). Initial analysis may be carried out on mini-gels divided into a relatively few fractions. Once the approximate molecular weight region has been established, discrimination may be increased by the use of a longer and/or gradient gels, by alteration of the percentage of polyacrylamide, and ultimately, by a combination of isoelectric focusing and SDS-PAGE into a two-dimensional analysis (Section 2.10).

Although this technique may be adapted as a 'front end' analytical step for any of the T-lymphocyte assays in Section 4.8, it is particularly suited to the mitogenic response assay (Section 4.9) carried out on whole populations, cloned lines or hybridomas or even for the determination of frequency data on *ex-vivo* lymphocyte populations (Section 4.13).

12.17 Summary and conclusions

Although the production of functional lymphocyte clones, lines and hybrids is very time consuming, it is technically no more demanding than normal *in vitro* cell culture. The most difficult and rate-limiting step in the isolation of functional hybridoma lines is the need to screen large numbers of cultures. For this reason, it is essential to establish and standardise the screening assays before attempting to produce hybrids.

On a practical level, the maintenance of normal or hybridoma lines requires:

(a)   A well-ordered technique to enable the operator to maintain several lines without cross-contamination, otherwise all lines will eventually be overtaken by the one with the fastest growth rate.

(b)   Facilities for the cryopreservation of cells. This is essential as a source of replacement cells, if cultures are lost by microbial contamination or overgrowth by non-secreting variants, and also to avoid having to maintain the many different cell lines that are rapidly produced (Appendix III).

12.18   Further reading

Fathman CG and Fitch FW (editors) (1982) *Isolation, Characterisation and Utilisation of T Cell Clones.* Academic Press, New York.

Feldman M, Lamb JR and Woody JN (editors) (1985) *Human T Cell Lines.* Humana Press.

Goding JW (1986) *Monoclonal Antibodies: Principle and Practice*, 2nd edition. Academic Press, New York.

Kappler JW, Skidmore B, White J and Marrack P (1981) *J. Exp. Med.* **153**: 1198.

Köhler G and Milstein G (1975) Continuous cultures of fused cells secreting antibody of predefined specificity. *Nature* **256**: 495–497.

Littlefield JW (1984) Selection of hybrids from matings of fibroblasts *in vitro* and their presumed recombinants. *Science* **145**: 709–710.

13 Lymphokines and Cytokines

There now exists a vast array of published information about the immunoregulatory molecules known as lymphokines. Although a lymphokine is simply a cytokine produced by lymphocytes, the term can be restrictive and misleading. For example, the so-called lymphokine interleukin 6 is produced by many cell types in addition to leucocytes: fibroblasts, epithelial cells, keratinocytes, monocytes, microglial cells, endothelial cells and uterine stromal cells. Consequently, the term cytokine is more useful as it refers broadly to any regulatory molecule secreted by cells which modulate the behaviour, function or differentiation state of other cells. Many cytokines which are intimately involved in the regulation of specific and non-specific immune function (for example, as illustrated for IL-1 and IL-2 in Fig. 13.1) probably pre-date adaptive immunity in evolution and have retained important (more important?) roles outside the immune system. Most, if not all, cytokines so far identified have been shown to interact with their target cell via a specific receptor, though the route(s) of signal transduction to the nucleus remain to be defined.

Recombinant DNA technology, protein sequence analysis, the use of monoclonal antibodies and the development of a variety of bioassays has enabled many of the properties of these cytokines to be demonstrated. Interleukins 1–8 have now been described in the literature. In the present context, these molecules can be considered as the molecular messages which convey information between cells of the immune system.

Interleukin 1 (IL-1) is primarily a macrophage product although it is produced by many different cell types. It has a wide range of target tissues but its principal function appears to be macrophage activation. As macrophages have a central role in immune activation, being effectors in the expression of both innate and acquired immunity, IL-1 is clearly centrally placed.

Interleukin 2 (IL-2) is essentially an autocrine immunoregulator as it is a product of T cells which acts primarily on T cells. At least *in vitro*, it maintains growth and proliferation of antigen- or mitogen-activated T-cells and is probably needed to sustain an activated T-cell response *in vivo*. IL-2 therapy is proving beneficial in some forms of cancer, probably through stimulation of the lymphokine-activated killer (LAK) cells (Section 4.15.1). IL-2 is known to maintain the proliferation of activated B cells.

Interleukin 3 (IL-3) is another pan-specific lymphokine which acts on progenitor stem-cell populations and is thus essential to the maintenance of an effective immune system. It is functionally closer to the colony-stimulating factors than the other interleukins.

Interleukin 4 (IL-4), also a T-cell product, appears to be multi-specific, acts on T cells, B cells and macrophages and is probably essential for the maintenance of an activated immune response *in vivo*.

423

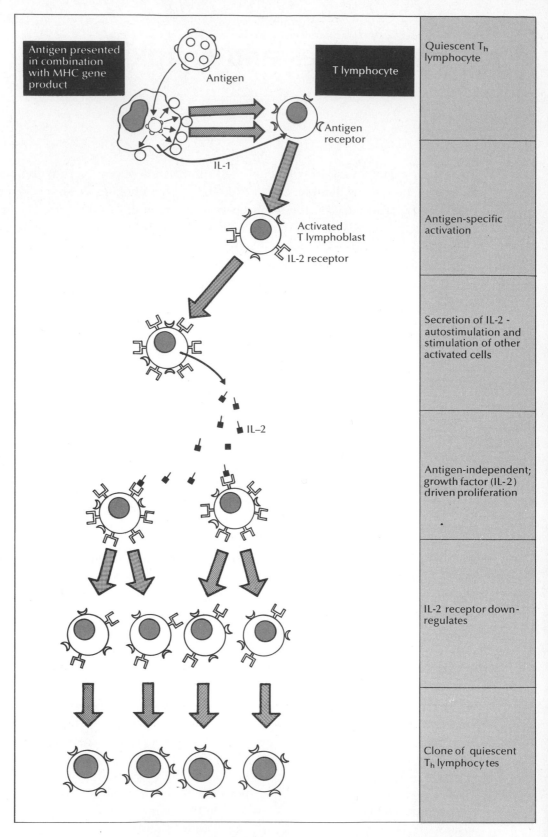

Fig. 13.1 Regulation of antigen-specific clonal proliferation of T lymphocytes by cytokines.
Antigen bridging between the antigen-presenting cell (APC) and T lymphocyte results in secretion
of IL-1 by the APC. Interleukin 1 and antigen activate the T lymphocyte to express its
pre-programmed effector function; in this case secretion of IL-2. At the same time, however, the T
lymphocyte also up-regulates its high-affinity IL-2 receptors and so can respond to extracellular
IL-2, including its own. Whereas the initial activation phase is antigen driven, the later proliferative
phase is largely in response to IL-2.

Feedback control is achieved in turn by the down-regulation of the IL-2 receptor by IL-2 in the
presence of diminishing antigen concentration.

Interleukin 5 (IL-5) is interesting in that it functions specifically to trigger differentiation of eosinophils, which play an important role in response to certain infections (particularly helminth infections). IL-5 also acts on B cells, hence its original name of T cell-replacing factor (TRF).

Interleukin 6 (IL-6) has been relatively recently assigned; human IL-6 was the first to be identified and is known by other names including interferon β_2 (IFN-β_2), and B lymphocyte-stimulating factor 2 (BSF-2). Although it does not have anti-viral activity, it is a multi-specific cytokine and may have a key role in the mediation of inflammatory responses.

Interleukin 7 (IL-7) is the product of stromal cells in the bone marrow and stimulates both pro- and pre-B lymphocytes to proliferate *in vitro*. Other activities will undoubtedly follow.

Interleukin 8 (IL-8) is the most recently assigned interleukin and functions as a neutrophil chemotactic peptide and can be induced in monocytes, fibroblasts, keratinocytes and endothelial cells.

The precise physiological role of a cytokine is often difficult to determine; many have been shown to have several activities *in vitro* and so it is difficult to predict which activity might have *in vivo* relevance. Conversely, several cytokines have been shown to have convergent effects in the immune system; for example, IL-2 and IL-4 both maintain the proliferation of activated T cells, although the molecules are structurally different and presumably act through separate receptors. It seems likely that synergy or inhibition of activity between cytokines may also occur, thus providing opportunities for highly discriminatory fine tuning of the immune system.

As one might imagine, most of the cytokines have been isolated independently in a number of different laboratories throughout the world and so similar or identical molecules are known by a variety of names. Even within the interleukin series, order is more apparent than real; on current evidence the molecules have little sequence or structural homology and even their functional relationships are very loose. Fortunately, it is possible to standardise assays via a growing collection of international and national standard cytokine preparations (Appendix II).

The majority of the cytokines described here are available as recombinant proteins, derived from *in vitro* expression in prokaryotic or eukaryotic systems. Although most recombinant molecules have a comparable activity they are not identical to the native cytokine, especially if derived by prokaryotic expression. In particular, glycosylation patterns may vary quite considerably.

Most cytokines occur in similar or equivalent forms throughout the mammals. However, although nucleotide and amino acid sequence analysis shows considerable homology between the species for some cytokines, the cross-reactivity between species is low or uni-directional. Human IL-2, for example, will stimulate lymphocytes from the rat and the mouse but rodent IL-2 cannot stimulate human lymphocytes.

In order to be sure that a functionally active lymphokine is present in an unknown sample, a bioassay is required. Monoclonal antibodies have been developed into commercially available ELISA and RIA kits. Dot blotting or northern analysis with DNA probes can also be used to define whether a cell is capable of lymphokine production, though this is not as sensitive as a bioassay and not quantitative to any degree of accuracy.

Calculation of results

National/international standards of some cytokines are now available. It is recommended that these are used to calibrate your own laboratory standard which can then be used as a reference for all further assays. Make a bulk preparation of the cytokine of interest, aliquot into convenient samples for storage at $-70°$ and do three or four repeat assays on aliquots of this stored material. The standard preparation should give reproducible results (although there will be some variation due to heterogeneity in the responder-cell population) and a mean of the dose–response curves will enable you to identify the dilution of standard which gives 50% stimulation of activity, cell killing, etc. Assign an arbitrary number of units to this and use as a positive control in all future experiments.

13.1 Interleukin 1 (IL-1)

Also known as endogenous pyrogen, catabolin and haematopoeitin 1. Almost every nucleated cell type can be induced to produce IL-1 but it is produced in greatest amount by activated monocytes and macrophages. IL-1 has stimulatory and regulatory effects in terms of growth and differentiation of numerous cell types and has profound effects on the immune system, regulating both T and B cells, and is a mediator of inflammatory responses.

Two distinct genes have been identified which produce IL-1 activity, referred to as IL-1α and IL-1β. Mature native human IL-1α has an MW_r of 30 000 and IL-1β an MW_r of 17 500. IL-1β is principally a product of monocytes and macrophages and is probably the most important form of IL-1 from an immunological view point.

13.1.1 Thymocyte co-stimulator assay

In this assay thymocytes from young (6–10 weeks) mice are cultured in the presence of a submitogenic concentration of phytohaemagglutinin, PHA which is potentiated by IL-1.

Materials and equipment
Mouse thymocytes
Tissue culture medium
Fetal bovine serum, FBS

Phytohaemagglutinin, PHA (Appendix II)
^{3}H-thymidine
96-well micro-titre plates (Appendix II)
Automated cell harvester (Appendix II)
β spectrometer

Method

1 Remove the thymus from a freshly killed mouse and prepare a single-cell suspension (Section 1.15), using aseptic technique.
2 Wash the cells twice by centrifugation and re-suspend in medium at 1.5×10^7 ml^{-1}.
3 Dispense 100 μl aliquots into individual wells of a 96-well micro-titre plate.
4 Add 50 μl of PHA (diluted 1 : 250 in tissue culture medium containing 10% FBS) to each culture.

The final dilution of 1 : 1000 should be submitogenic, i.e. it should not give a significant proliferative response in the absence of IL-1. If it is does induce a mitogenic response, check that the dilution has been made correctly, then, if you are really sure, dilute the PHA further until it just becomes submitogenic.

5 Add the IL-1 samples under test at a range of dilutions, using 50 μl aliquots of each to triplicate wells.
6 Appropriate controls are:
   cells + medium alone
   cells + PHA alone
   cells + IL−1 alone.
   In each case in a final volume of 200 μl.
7 Incubate the plates at 37° for 48−72 h and pulse with 18.5×10^3 Bq of ^{3}H-thymidine $(74 \times 10^{10}$ Bq mole$^{-1})$ for 4−6 h prior to harvesting.
8 Harvest the plates using an automated cell harvester and process the samples for β scintillation counting

Assessment of results

If a standard IL-1 preparation is available, then a standard curve can be plotted of proliferation (^{3}H-thymidine uptake) against IL-1 concentration and units of activity shown by the unknown samples read off the curve. Alternatively, you may wish to assign an arbitrary number of units to the dilution giving 50% of maximal stimulation.

13.1.2 Calcium ionophore co-stimulation

Interleukin 1 plus calcium ionophore can stimulate certain IL-1 sensitive cell lines to produce IL-2 (see Section 13.2). The IL-2 produced is then measured using an IL-2-dependent T-cell line.

Materials and equipment
EL4.6.1 cell line, (IL-1-sensitive, IL-2 producer) (Appendix III)
IL-2-dependent T-cell line; for example, CT-6, CTLL-D (Appendix III)
Tissue culture medium
Fetal bovine serum, FBS
Calcium ionophore; for example, ionomycin or A6137 (Appendix II)
Dimethyl sulphoxide
96-well micro-titre plates

PREPARATION IN ADVANCE
1 Make a stock solution of calcium ionophore at 1×10^{-3} M in dimethyl sulphoxide (DMSO) and store at $-20°$.
2 Prepare subcultures of the two cell lines to be used 24−48 h in advance of the assay, to ensure that they are in their log phase of growth.

Method
1 Add 100 μl aliquots of IL-1 samples, at a range of dilutions and in triplicate, to 96-well micro-titre plates.
2 Add 50 μl of calcium ionophore diluted to 1×10^{-6} M in complete medium to each well.
3 Harvest EL4 cells from an actively growing culture, wash twice by centrifugation and re-suspend at 4×10^6 ml^{-1}.
4 Add 50 μl of the cell suspension to each well and incubate overnight at 37° in a humidified atmosphere containing 5% CO_2 in air.

Controls should include calcium ionophore plus cells alone, the highest concentration of IL-1 plus cells alone and cells alone.

5 Remove 100 μl of medium from each well and transfer to the corresponding well of a second micro-titre plate.
6 Harvest the CTLL-D (or equivalent) cells from an actively growing culture, wash three times to remove IL-2 from the growth medium and re-suspend the cells at 1×10^5 ml^{-1}.
7 Add a 100 μl aliquot of cell suspension to each micro-titre well containing the transferred supernatants.

Be sure to include cultures containing CTLL-D cells with doubling dilutions of recombinant IL-2, for the construction of a standard curve.

8 Incubate the plates overnight at 37° in a humidified atmosphere of 5% CO_2 in air.
9 Add 18.5×10^3 Bq of ^{3}H-thymidine to each well 4−6 h before harvesting the plates with an automated cell harvester.
10 Process the samples for liquid scintillation counting.

Technical note

The colorimetric MTT assay using the tetrazolium salt, 3−(4,5 dimethylthiazol-2-yl)−2,5-diphenyl tetrazolium bromide (see Section 13.2.1) can also be used to assay for cell proliferation.

13.2 Interleukin 2 (IL-2)

Interleukin 2 was originally known as T-cell growth factor (TCGF) and is produced by activated T cells. For experimental work native IL-2 is usually generated from mitogen-stimulated spleen or lymph-node cells or from an IL-2-producing T-cell line; for example, Jurkat (human IL-2), EL4 (murine IL-2). IL-2 is important for the maintenance and proliferation of a number of cell types in the immune system, including T cells, B cells, NK (natural killer) and LAK (lymphokine-activated killer) cells. It can also induce the secretion of other lymphokines such as interferon γ (IFN-γ) and B-cell growth factor (BCGF).

Assays for IL-2 are based on the maintenance of the proliferation of activated T cells *in vitro*. A number of IL-2-dependent T-cell lines are available which can be used including CT6, CTLL-D and HT-2 (Appendix III). Alternatively, phyto-haemagglutinin- (PHA) or concanavalin A- (Con A) activated T-cell blasts, after extensive washing to remove residual mitogen, can be used as IL-2-dependent cells. The proliferative response to IL-2 is measured by a colorimetric assay or ^{3}H-thymidine uptake.

13.2.1 Colorimetric assay

Materials and equipment

IL-2-dependent T-cell line or mitogen-induced T-cell blasts

Tissue culture medium

Fetal bovine serum, FBS

Phenol red-free tissue culture medium

Phosphate-buffered saline, PBS (Appendix I)

3-(4,5-dimethylthiazol-2-yl)-2,5-diphenyl tetrazolium bromide, MTT (Appendix II); stock solution at 5 mg ml^{-1} in PBS (stored in the dark)

Isopropyl alcohol

96-well micro-titre plates, flat wells

Centrifuge carriers for microplates (Appendix II)

ELISA reader (Appendix II)

Method

1 Wash the cells three times by centrifugation to remove residual mitogen or IL-2 and re-suspend at 1×10^5 ml^{-1} in complete medium (plus 10% FBS).

2 Dispense 100 μl aliquots into individual wells of a micro-titre plate.

3 Add 100 µl aliquots of the IL-2 test samples to individual culture wells and incubate the plates at 37° for 48 h.

Controls should include cells, alone and with a positive standard IL-2 preparation.

4 After 48 h incubation, centrifuge the plates at 90 g for 10 min and remove the medium by rapidly inverting the plates with a firm flick.
5 Add 100 µl of MTT (1 mg ml^{-1} in tissue culture medium without phenol red) and incubate the plates for a further 3−4 h. Centrifuge the plate and remove medium as before.
6 Add 100 µl of isopropyl alcohol to each well to solubilise the formazan dye.
7 Read the plates on an ELISA reader using the following settings: test wavelength 570 nm, reference wavelength 630 nm and calibration setting of 1.99.

Plot a curve of concentration versus optical density (equivalent to cell proliferation) for the standard preparation of IL-2 and use this to determine your unknown samples by interpolation. If a standard preparation of IL-2 is not available, arbitrary units should be assigned to the dilution of IL-2 which gives 50% maximal stimulation.

13.2.2 ^{3}H-thymidine uptake assay

Essentially similar to the colorimetric assay with the following modifications:

1 Use 2×10^4 cells well^{-1} in 100 µl complete tissue culture medium.
2 Add 100 µl aliquots of sample under test.
3 Add 18.5×10^3 Bq of ^{3}H-thymidine in 10 µl medium 4−6 h before the end of the assay.
4 Process the samples for counting in a β spectrometer.

The concentration of IL−2 in the sample can be determined as described above for the colorimetric assay.

Technical note
It is possible to shorten the incubation time to 24 h; although the signal to noise ratio is less favorable the discrimination should still be sufficient for reproducible results.

13.3 Interleukin 3 (IL-3)

Interleukin 3 is a product of monocytes and T cells. It is a chemoattractant for neutrophils, supports the growth of eosinophils, granulocytes, macrophage and mixed pluripotent progenitors, promotes erythroid bursts from normal bone marrow and also promotes colony stimulation of megakaryocytes and mast cells. For experimental purposes it can be derived from the human bladder carcinoma cell line 5637 (Appendix III) and also from the myelomonocytic cell line WEHI-3b (Appendix III).

Interleukin 3 can be detected by its ability to promote the growth and differentiation of cells of monocytic and polymorphonuclear origin in colony-forming assays. It also supports the growth and proliferation of various IL-3-dependent lines; for example, the cloned mast-cell line MC/9 (Appendix III) which can be assayed by ^{3}H-thymidine uptake or colorimetrically using the MTT assay, as described in Section 13.2.

13.3.1 Proliferation assay

Materials and equipment
Mast-cell line; for example MC/9 (Appendix III)
96-well micro-titre plates
3-(4,5-dimethylthiazol-2-yl)-2,5-diphenyl tetrazolium bromide, MTT (Appendix II); stock solution at 5 mg ml^{-1} in PBS (stored in the dark).
Tissue culture medium, with and without phenol red
Fetal bovine serum, FBS
2-mercaptoethanol, 2-ME
ELISA reader (Appendix II)

Method
Essentially the same as the colorimetric assay for IL-2, Section 13.2.1.

1 Dispense 100 μl aliquots of MC/9 cells (1×10^5 ml^{-1} in tissue culture medium containing 4% FBS and 5×10^{-5} M 2-ME) into individual wells of a micro-culture plate.
2 Add test supernatants as 100 μl aliquots in a range of dilutions.
3 Incubate at 37° for 20 h in a humidified atmosphere of 5% CO_2 in air.
4 Centrifuge the plates at 90 g for 10 min, flick off the medium by inverting the plate rapidly, add 100 μl of MTT in indicator-free medium and incubate for a further 3−4 h.
5 Centrifuge the plate as described above, flick off the medium and add 100 μl of isopropyl alcohol to each well.
6 Read the plates on an ELISA reader using a test wavelength of 570 nm, a reference wavelength of 630 nm and a calibration setting of 1.99.

Assessment of results
Plot a curve of concentration versus optical density (equivalent to cell proliferation) for the standard preparation of IL-3 and use this to determine your unknown samples by interpolation. If a standard preparation of IL-3 is not available, arbitrary units should be assigned to the dilution of IL-3 which gives 50% maximal stimulation.

13.4 Interleukin 4 (IL-4)

Also known as B-cell stimulating factor 1 (BSF-1), B-cell growth factor 1 (BCGF-1) and B-cell differentiation factor γ (BCDF γ). Interleukin 4 was originally described in terms of its action on B cells, it induces an IgM to IgE class switch and increases immunoglobulin levels in B cells activated, for example, by treatment with anti-immunoglobulin antibodies. IL-4 also increases IgG1 and IgE release from lipopoly-saccharide (LPS) stimulated murine spleen cells. IL-4 has also been shown to induce class II MHC expression, enhance the proliferation of T cells and the generation of cytotoxic T lymphocytes. It induces Fc receptor expression on B cells, acts as a MAF (macrophage-activating factor) and as a CSF (colony-stimulating factor) for granulocytes and macrophages.

Interleukin 4 is measured by its effect on the proliferation of B cells in a co-stimulator assay.

13.4.1   B-cell co-stimulator assay

Materials and equipment

Purified murine splenic B cells
Anti-murine IgM antibody (conveniently added bound to polyacrylamide beads)
Tissue culture medium
Fetal bovine serum, FBS
96-well micro-titre plates
^{3}H-thymidine
Automated cell harvester
β spectrometer

Method

1   Re-suspend the B cells in tissue culture medium containing 10% FBS and dispense into micro-titre trays at a concentration of 1×10^5 cells well^{-1}.
2   Add anti-IgM antibody at a range of dilutions to determine the stimulatory concentration (this can be replaced by a single dilution in subsequent assays).
3   Dilute the supernatants under test to obtain a range of concentrations and add to triplicate wells to give a final volume of 200 μl. Controls should include:

cells + medium alone
cells + anti-IgM antibody
cells + IL-4 standard
cells + and anti-IgM antibody + IL-4 standard.

4   Incubate the plates at 37° in a humidified atmosphere of 5% CO_2 in air for 72 h.
5   Add 18.5×10^3 Bq of ^{3}H-thymidine during the last 6 h of culture.
6   Harvest the plates using an automated cell harvester and process the samples for β scintillation counting.

Assessment of results

Plot ^{3}H-thymidine uptake (equivalent to proliferative response) against concentration for the IL-4 standard, and determine the units of activity in the unknown samples by interpolation.

Technical note

Interleukin 4 acts on resting B cells and induces them to proliferate, as demonstrated above by enhanced ^{3}H-thymidine uptake. Incubation of resting B cells with IL-4 also causes marked enhancement of expression of class II MHC molecules on the cell surface. This is detectable within 6 h and, by 24 h, can show an increase in antigen density by sixfold or greater. This has been used to assay for active IL-4. It should be borne in mind, however, that other lymphokines, notably IFN-γ also enhance class II antigen expression.

13.5 Interleukin 5 (IL-5)

Also known as TRF (T-cell replacing factor) or EDF (eosinophil differentiation factor), it has B-cell growth factor activity and induces IgM secretion. IL-5 can be derived from some T-cell lines and from the T-cell hybridomas, B151 and NIMP-TH1 (Appendix III) after induction with PMA (phorbol myristate acetate).

13.5.1 Reverse plaque-forming cell assay

IgM secretion by BCL$_1$ cells (Appendix III) is measured using a reverse plaque-forming cell assay for IgM total immunoglobulin.

Materials and equipment

BCL$_1$ cells (Appendix III) growing in a BALB/c mouse
Tissue culture medium
Fetal bovine serum, FBS
96-well micro-titre plates
Protein A-coupled sheep erythrocytes, SRBC (Section 4.5.1)
Rabbit anti-IgM antibody
Other reagents for IgM plaque assay (Section 4.5.1)

Method

1 Prepare BCL$_1$ cells from the spleens of tumour-bearing BALB/c mice (Section 1.15).
2 Deplete the spleen cells of T cells by treatment with anti-Thy-1 monoclonal antibody plus complement (Section 7.5.1).
3 Dispense 1.5×10^5 BCL$_1$ cells into 96-well micro-titre plates in 100 μl aliquots in tissue culture medium.
4 Add a range of dilutions of the samples under test, in 100 μl aliquots.
5 Incubate at 37° in a humidified atmosphere of 5% CO_2 in air for 48 h.
6 Assay the cells for IgM production using a reverse plaque-forming cell assay with protein A-coupled SRBC and anti-IgM antibody (Section 4.5.1).

Assessment of results

Plot plaque number versus concentration of sample. A unit of IL-5 activity is usually represented as that required to induce a half maximal response.

13.5.2 Proliferation assay

Materials and equipment

BCL_1 cells prepared as described above, or, T-cell-depleted normal mouse spleen cells (from C57BL/6×DBA/2 F_1 mice)

Tissue culture medium

Fetal bovine serum, FBS

^{3}H-thymidine

96-well micro-titre plates

Automated cell harvester

β spectrometer

Method

1 Re-suspend the B cells at 1×10^6 ml^{-1} (normal mouse B cells) or 5×10^5 ml^{-1} (BCL_1 cells) and add 100 µl aliquots to individual wells of a 96-well micro-titre plate.

2 Add 100 µl aliquots of a range of dilutions of the supernatant under test to triplicate wells.

3 Incubate at 37° in a humidified atmosphere of 5% CO_2 in air for 72 h.

4 Add 18.5×10^3 Bq of ^{3}H-thymidine and incubate for a further 6 h.

5 Harvest using an automated cell harvester and process the samples for liquid scintillation counting.

Assessment of results

Plot ^{3}H-thymidine uptake (equivalent to proliferative response) against concentration for the IL-5 standard, and determine the units of activity in the unknown samples by interpolation. If a standard preparation of IL-5 is not available, assign an arbitrary number of units to the concentration giving half maximal stimulation.

13.6 Interleukin 6 (IL-6)

Also known as B-cell differentiation factor 2 (BCDF-2) or interferon β_2 (IFN-β_2). This is another lymphokine with several demonstrable activities *in vitro*; for example, when assayed for its ability to induce B-cell differentiation, it increases surface IgM expression and secretion of µ chains. It also enhances cytotoxic T lymphocytes and is a potent growth factor for myeloid cells. IL-6 stimulates hepatocytes to produce acute-phase reactant proteins and therefore has a role in inflammation; it is also said to have nerve growth factor-like activity.

Interleukin 6 can be produced *in vitro* by stimulating human fibroblasts with poly (rI).(rC) or cycloheximide plus actinomycin D and is constitutively produced by the leukaemia virus transformed human T-cell line TCL-Na1 (Appendix III).

13.6.1 ELISA assay for immunoglobulin secretion by an IL-6-responsive cell line

Materials and equipment
IL-6-responsive cell line; for example, SKW6-CL4 or CESS (Appendix III)
Tissue culture medium
Fetal bovine serum, FBS
96-well micro-titre plates
Reagents for anti-IgM (using SKW6-CL4) or anti-IgG (CESS) ELISA (Section 10.6)
ELISA reader (Appendix II)

PREPARATION IN ADVANCE
Subculture the indicator cell of choice 24–48 h before the assay to ensure that it is log-phase growth.

Method
1 Harvest the indicator cells, wash twice by centrifugation and re-suspend in tissue culture medium containing 10% FBS. Adjust the cell concentration to 4×10^4 ml^{-1} (SKW6-CL4) or 6×10^4 ml^{-1} (CESS).
2 Dispense 100 µl aliquots of either cell line into each well of a micro-titre plate.
3 Prepare a range of dilutions of the supernatant under test and add 100 µl aliquots to wells in triplicate.
4 Incubate the plates in a humidified atmosphere of 5% CO_2 in air at 37° for 72 h.
5 Transfer 100 µl aliquots of culture supernatant from each well to the corresponding well in a second micro-titre plate.
6 Assay these supernatants using an anti-IgM or anti-IgG ELISA (Section 10.6) as appropriate for the cell line used.

Assessment of results
The amount of immunoglobulin secreted is proportional to the IL-6 concentration in the sample under test. A plot of concentration of the standard IL-6 versus OD (immunoglobulin secretion) can be used to determine the activity of the sample. If a standard preparation is not available, assign arbitrary units to the concentration which gives half maximal stimulation.

13.6.2 Reverse plaque-forming cell assay

Instead of determining the amount of immunoglobulin (IgM or IgG) secreted by CESS or SKW6-CL4 cells by an ELISA assay, one can assay activation by determining the number of IgM or IgG plaque-forming cells in a reverse plaque assay (Section 4.5.1).

Materials and equipment
As Section 13.6.1 but with reagents for reverse plaque assay (Section 4.5.1)

Method

As Section 13.6.1, but with the following modifications:

1 Incubate the cells for 48 h in a humidified atmosphere of 5% CO_2 in air.
2 Enumerate the antibody-forming cells in a reverse plaque assay (Section 4.5.1), remembering to assay for IgM plaques for SKW6-CL4 cells and IgG plaques for CESS cells.

Assessment of results

The number of plaques is proportional to the IL-6 concentration in the sample under test. A plot of concentration of the standard IL-6 versus the number of plaque-forming cells can be used to determine the activity of the sample. If a standard preparation is not available, assign arbitrary units to the concentration which gives half maximal plaque numbers.

13.7 **The interferons**

The interferons were first described on the basis of their anti-viral activity, even though they are not directly toxic to viruses but instead induce the various host cells to exhibit anti-viral activity.

Interferon α: leucocyte interferon. Induces anti-viral activity and enhances NK cell and mixed lymphocyte reactions; induces increased expression of HLA antigens on lymphocytes; inhibits the growth of human lymphoblastoid cell lines. IFN-α can be prepared from activated lymphocytes (helper T cells, B cells and macrophages) and from Namalva cells (Appendix III).

Interferon β: fibroblast interferon. Enhances NK-cell activity; induces anti-viral activity; inhibits the growth of fibroblasts. IFN-β can be prepared from poly IC-induced fibroblasts, human foreskin cells, fetal muscle cells, epithelial cells, myeloblasts and lymphoblasts.

Interferon γ: immune interferon. Enhances macrophage activation; activates cytotoxic T lymphocytes; enhances class II antigen expression; induces anti-viral activity, but poorly compared with IFN-α and -β. IFN-γ can be prepared from activated lymphocytes and T-cell lines.

The interferons can be assayed using commercially available ELISA or RIA kits which are based on specific antibody. However, anti-viral assays are used to give assessments of units of activity.

Interferon assays

Described below are two assays for determining the anti-viral activity of interferon.

13.8.1 # Inhibition of viral nucleic acid synthesis

Materials and equipment
Indicator cell line; for example, L929 (Appendix III)
Plastic or glass scintillation vials (5 × 1.3 cm) (Appendix II)
Semliki Forest Virus, SFV, at 1×10^7 PFU ml^{-1}
Actinomycin D, AMD (Appendix II)
^{3}H-uridine
Trichloroacetic acid, TCA
Soluene–toluene 1:2 mix
Tissue culture medium
Fetal bovine serum, FBS
β spectrometer

PREPARATION IN ADVANCE
Plate the indicator cells into a 150 cm^2 growth area tissue culture flask and allow to grow to confluence.

Method

1   Harvest the indicator cell line by trypsin treatment, wash twice and re-suspend in 200 ml of tissue culture medium containing 10% FBS.
2   Dispense 1 ml aliquots of cell suspension into the individual vials.
3   Incubate for 24 h at 37° in a humidified atmosphere of 5% CO$_2$ in air.
4   Remove the tissue culture supernatant by aspiration and add 200 µl aliquots (in triplicate) of a range of dilutions of the samples under test, made up in medium containing 2% serum.
5   Incubate overnight under conditions as described in step 3.
6   Add 200 µl of SFV at 1×10^7 PFU ml^{-1} in medium containing 2% FBS and 3 µg ml^{-1}.
7   Incubate for 3 h.
8   Add 100 µl medium containing 2% FBS and 1 µg ml^{-1} AMD and 37×10^4 Bq ml^{-1} ^{3}H-uridine.
9   Incubate for a further 3 h.
10 Aspirate the medium and wash the cell monolayer twice with 1 ml of 5% ice-cold TCA and once with 1 ml ethanol.
11 Aspirate the residual ethanol and dry the vials at 60° for 15 min.
12 Add 500 µl soluene–toluene and 2 ml scintillant. Count the vials in a β spectrometer.

Assessment of results
Plot the mean c.p.m. for replicate cultures against $\log_{10}$ IFN dilution. The inhibition of virus proliferation, measured as inhibition of ^{3}H-uridine uptake into untreated control cells, is proportional to IFN concentration.

13.8.2 Cytopathic effect reduction (CPE)

Materials and equipment
Indicator cell line, usually Hep/2c (Appendix III)
Murine encephalomyocarditis virus, EMCV, 1×10^7 PFU ml^{-1}
96-well micro-titre plates
Gentian violet stain and filter
Tissue culture medium
Fetal bovine serum, FBS

PREPARATION IN ADVANCE
1 Prepare a stock solution of the gentian violet stain at 1% w/v in 20% ethanol in phosphate-buffered saline (Appendix I), warm to 60° and filter to remove insoluble material.
2 Subculture the indicator cell line 24−48 h before use to ensure it is in log-phase growth.

Method
1 Harvest the indicator cells from a culture in log-phase growth and wash twice by centrifugation. Re-suspend in tissue culture medium at 5×10^5 ml^{-1}.
2 Dispense 100 µl aliquots of cell suspension into individual wells of a micro-titre plate.
3 Incubate at 37° in a humidified atmosphere of 5% CO_2 in air for 5 h.
4 Aspirate the medium and add the samples under test to triplicate wells, at a range of dilutions in medium containing 15% serum.
5 Incubate at 37° overnight.
6 Aspirate the medium, add 100 µl formal saline to each well and leave on the bench for 5 min.
7 Aspirate the formal saline and add 3 drops per well of gentian violet stain and leave on the bench for 10 min.
8 Wash gently with running tap water for 3 min.
9 Read the cytopathic effect by counting the number of plaques.

In practice, the results of the experiment can usually be determined by scanning the plate directly by eye to give an end point. Counting plaques will give a more accurate result for determining the titre of the samples. Alternatively the plate can be read by solubilising the stain with 100 µl of 50% ethanol and reading with an ELISA reader at a wavelength of 700 nm.

Assessment of results

As interferon gives a concentration-dependent reduction in virus plaque number compared with untreated virus-infected cells, this may be used to construct a standard curve for the determination of IFN concentration in unknown samples. If a standard preparation of interferon is not available, assign an arbitrary number of units to the dilution giving 50% reduction in plaque number compared with controls.

13.9 Tumour necrosis factors

Tumour necrosis factors α and β (TNF-β is sometimes referred to as lymphotoxin) are distinct and separate gene products but have similar functions and activities *in vitro*, and appear to bind to the same receptor.

TNF-α was originally described as a monocyte/macrophage product derived from certain macrophage-like cell lines, but is also produced by T cells. TNF-α has cytostatic and cytocidal effects on transformed cells; it stimulates bone resorption and inhibits bone reformation; it inhibits lipoprotein lipase activity in adipocytes.

TNF-β is produced by T lymphocytes and has properties similar to TNF-α. The only effective means of distinguishing between the two molecules at present is by the use of appropriate neutralising antibodies.

Identical assays can be used for both TNF-α and TNF-β.

13.9.1 L929 cell-killing assay

Materials and equipment
L929 tumour cells (Appendix III)
Tissue culture medium
Fetal bovine serum, FBS
Actinomycin D, AMD (Appendix II)
96-well micro-titre plates
Phosphate-buffered saline, PBS (Appendix I)
Crystal violet (Appendix II), 1% w/v aqueous solution
ELISA reader (Appendix II)

PREPARATION IN ADVANCE
1 L929 cells can vary in their susceptibility to TNF. It is advisable to work with cell cultures maintained and subcultured for relatively short periods. If TNF assays are to be done on a regular basis, it is recommended that a large number of cells with proven sensitivity to TNF be cryopreserved. Frozen vials can then be used to start up fresh cultures at regular intervals.
2 Subculture the cell line 24 h prior to use to ensure that the cultures are subconfluent.

Method

1 Prepare a suspension of L929 cells, by trypsin treatment of a subconfluent culture, and wash twice by centrifugation.

2 Re-suspend the cells at 4×10^5 ml^{-1} in medium containing 5% serum.

3 Dispense 100 µl aliquots of cells into individual wells of micro-titre plates.

4 Incubate for 4 h at 37° in a humidified atmosphere of 5% CO_2 in air to allow the cells to adhere.

5 Remove the medium by inverting the plate with a rapid flicking motion.

6 Add 100 µl aliquots of a range of dilutions of the samples under test, in medium containing 2% serum and AMP (2 µg ml^{-1} initial concentration).

7 Incubate the plates overnight at 37° in a humidified atmosphere of 5% CO_2 in air.

8 Remove the medium as described and wash the wells once with PBS.

9 Remove the PBS by flicking the plate as described and add 100 µl methanol to each well to fix the cells.

10 Remove excess methanol and dry the plates briefly in air.

11 Add 100 µl of aqueous crystal violet and incubate at room temperature for 5 min.

12 Wash the wells thoroughly with tap water, finally empty the wells by flicking the plate.

13 Solubilise the contents of the wells with 100 µl of 33% acetic acid (in water) and read the plates on an ELISA reader at a test wavelength of 570 nm and a reference wavelength of 420 nm.

Assessment of results

Reduced OD relative to controls without TNF indicates cell killing. Plot OD against sample dilution to determine the dilution of the unknown sample which gives 50% target cell death.

13.9.2 WEHI-164 killing assay

The recently derived subclone 13 of the WEHI-164 murine fibrosarcoma (Appendix III) has provided a highly sensitive assay for TNF/LT activity, it is similar in principle to the standard L929 but has the following modifications:

(a) Actinomycin D is not required in the medium.

(b) The cells are plated at 2×10^4 ml^{-1} in the presence of the test samples.

(c) The culture plates are incubated at 37° for 20 h. Viability can then be assessed using crystal violet staining (Section 13.9.1) or the MTT assay (Section 13.2.1).

Assessment of results

Reduced OD relative to controls without TNF indicates cell killing. Plot OD against sample dilution to determine the dilution of the unknown sample which gives 50% target cell death.

13.10 ELISPOT assay for single-cell production of lymphokine

The ELISPOT assay (Section 4.5.3) may be extended to detect individual cells producing specified lymphokines. A lymphokine-specific monoclonal antibody is coated on to the bottom of a culture well prior to the addition of the cells for assay. Once the cells have settled out of suspension, secreted lymphokine will be bound by the monoclonal antibody and retained after washing away the cells. The bound lymphokine may then be detected by the addition of polyclonal, enzyme-labelled anti-lymphokine antibody. Following washing and addition of substrate, coloured spots are deposited at sites where lymphokine-producing cells have been present.

Materials and method
The materials and method are the same as for the ELISPOT assay (Section 4.5.3) with the exception that the coating layer is replaced by a monoclonal antibody against the lymphokine to be measured, and the detecting antibody is replaced with an enzyme-labelled antibody against the same lymphokine.

13.11 Summary and conclusions

Over the past 5 years a large number of cytokine molecules have been defined and characterised in chemical terms; largely through the application of the techniques of molecular biology. That our knowledge of their biological roles has not kept pace with this advance is not due to lack of application on the part of biologists, but rather is related to the far-reaching, and often apparently unconnected, effects these molecules have on virtually every cell in the body — even dead keratinocytes in heel callus are stuffed full of highly active cytokines. Although more cytokines will undoubtedly be discovered, real progress will only come when we can fit them into a general scheme; the beautifully ordered relationships we can now perceive between the immuno-globulin classes were totally hidden before the elegant work of Rod Porter and Gerry Edelman in the early 1960s.

Although we do not have any depth of understanding, intriguing insights are beginning to emerge when cytokines are used alone and in pairs. It is clear that even though the molecules do not individually possess the refined specificity of immuno-globulin molecules, once used in concert, their potential for fine tuning of biological interactions will reach far beyond the immune system.

13.12 Further reading

Clemens MJ, Morris AG and Gearing AJH (editors) (1987) *Lymphokines and interferons*. IRL Press, Oxford.
Pick E (Series editor) (1980 onwards) *Lymphokines: a Forum for Immunoregulatory Cell Products*, 15 volumes to date. Academic Press, New York.

14 Immunological Techniques in Clinical Medicine

The rapid expansion in knowledge of the immune system has been widely applied in clinical medicine. In fact, reading some textbooks of clinical immunology, one almost gains the impression that virtually all pathology is the result of either a deficiency or hypersensitivity of the immune system. Most of the immunological procedures in this book can be applied to study the human immune system and in this chapter we review the applications which are beginning to give clinically useful information about the status of the immune response.

14.1 Isolation and enumeration of cells involved in the immune response

In the clinical immunology laboratory, examination of cells involved in the immune response is generally performed in cases where immune deficiency or malignancy is suspected. The production of monoclonal antibodies to cell-surface antigens has greatly facilitated these studies. Cells may be examined in anti-coagulant-treated preparations of whole blood after lysis of red cells. Immunofluorescent study (Section 3.5) of blood films is possible but, in laboratories regularly carrying out these studies, flow cytometry (Sections 3.9 and 9.11) is more commonly used. Direct examination of cells is easier following their isolation either in the flow cytometer during analysis (the so-called 'whole blood' technique, Section 3.9) or by density gradient centrifugation (Section 1.13.2).

14.1.1 Lymphocytes and E rosettes

Once lymphocytes have been isolated by density gradient centrifugation (Section 1.13.2), analysis of the various subpopulations is possible using specific monoclonal antibodies to different cell phenotypic markers:

T lymphocytes are frequently assessed as CD4 (T-helper/inducer) and CD8 (T-cytotoxic/ suppressor) positive subpopulations. It is important to report the absolute numbers of cells as a simple ratio might give a misleading impression of normality or disguise information as to which population is varying.

B lymphocytes may be estimated using immunofluorescence with antibodies directed to membrane immunoglobulins.

Different populations of lymphocytes may also be enumerated and isolated by their capacity to form rosettes with various types of red cell (Section 3.5.3). Sheep erythro-

442

cytes adhere weakly to human T cells to form rosettes. Care must be taken to exclude dead cells and monocytes from the count of rosettes. Numbers of rosettes are very dependent upon operator technique and variations in numbers between different laboratories are frequently found.

Different species of red cell will rosette with other cell populations. The interesting CD5 B cells, which are thought to be responsible for producing many autoantibodies, may be isolated by their capacity to bind mouse erythrocytes.

14.1.2   Neutrophils

Neutrophils may be prepared from anticoagulant-treated whole blood by dextran sedimentation to give a leucocyte-rich preparation. The neutrophils may be purified by discontinuous density gradient centrifugation in Percoll A.

Materials and equipment
Leucocytes (from dextran sedimentation, Technical notes)
Centrifuge tube
Percoll, 60% and 80% solutions in tissue culture medium Appendix II

Method
1   Add 5 ml of 80% Percoll to centrifuge tube.
2   Layer on 5 ml of 60% Percoll.
3   Place 5 ml cell suspension on top of gradient.
4   Centrifuge at 240 g for 30 min at 4°.
5   Collect neutrophils from the 60—80% interface.

Technical notes
1   The medium—60% Percoll interface has monocytes, lymphocytes and red blood cells. Total neutrophil yield is generally about 40% with a purity of 90%.
2   Layer 5 ml blood on 10 ml 3.5% w/v T-250 Dextran in 0.14 M saline and incubate for 1 h at 37°. Remove leucocyte-rich supernatant and wash by centifugation.

14.1.3   Monocytes

Monocytes may be prepared as above (Section 14.1.2) by recovering the monocyte-rich fraction from the medium—60% Percoll interface. The monocytes can be separated from the lymphocytes by allowing the monocytes to adhere to a plastic surface for 30 min at 37°. The non-adherent lymphocytes (about 50% of the total population) may then be washed away.

When peripheral blood-derived monocytes are cultured at 37° for 2—3 days in a humidified atmosphere containing 5% CO_2 in air, a large proportion of them transform into macrophage-like cells which can be activated by IFN-γ treatment (Section 13.7).

Phenotypic markers in leukaemias and lymphomas

In this book it is possible to touch only briefly on the subject of the classification of the leukaemias. For detailed information the reader is referred to Janossy *et al.* (1987).

If the morphological appearance of the blood film suggests acute leukaemia, the panel of monoclonal antibodies described in Figs 14.1–14.5 will allow immunophenotyping of the leukaemic clone into one of three major categories: B, T or myeloid. The detection of cytoplasmic expression of CD3, the earliest T-cell marker present in bona fide T cells, and the nuclear enzyme, terminal deoxynucleotidyl transferase (TDT), are valuable criteria for distinguishing lymphoblastic from myeloblastic leukaemias. In

CD designation	Molecular weight (kDa)	Monoclonal antibody	Cellular distribution
CD 10	100	J5 (C) Anti-CALLA (BD)	B cell precursor, common ALL antigen
CD 19	40, 80	B4 (C)	Pan B cells
CD 20	35	B1 (C)	B cells
CD 21	145	B2 (C) Anti CR2 (BD)	Mature B cells C3d and EBV receptor
CD 22	135	Anti-LEU14 (BD)	B cells
CD 23	45	MHM 6	Activated B cells

Suppliers: C — Coulter Electronics Ltd., BD — Becton–Dickinson.

Fig. 14.1 Monoclonal antibodies against B lymphocytes.

CD Designation	Molecular weight (kDa)	Monoclonal antibody	Cellular distribution
CD 2	50	T11 (C) Anti-LEU5 (BD)	Sheep red blood cell receptor
CD 3	19, 29	T3 (C) Anti-LEU4 (BD)	Associated with T-cell receptor
CD 4	64	T4A (C)	Helper/inducer T cells
CD 5	67–71	T1B (C) Anti-LEU1 (BD)	T cells, B cells of B-CLL
CD 7	40	Anti-LEU9 (BD)	T cells, especially T-ALL
CD 8	76	T8A (C) Anti-LEU2 (BD)	Cytotoxic/suppressor T cells
CD 25	55	IL-2R1 (C) Anti-IL-2 receptor (BD)	Activated T and B cells

Suppliers: C — Coulter Electronics Ltd., BD — Becton–Dickinson.

Fig. 14.2 Monoclonal antibodies against T lymphocytes.

CD designation	Molecular weight (kDa)	Monoclonal antibody	Cellular distribution
CD 11b	155, 94	Mol (C) Anti-CR3 (BD)	Monocytes and granulocytes
CD 13	150	MY7 (C)	Granulocytes and monocytes
CD 33	67	MY 9 (C)	Early myeloid progenitors

Suppliers: C — Coulter Electronics Ltd., BD — Becton—Dickinson.

Fig. 14.3 Monoclonal antibodies against myeloid cells and monocytes.

CD designation	Molecular weight (kDa)	Monoclonal antibody	Cellular distribution
—	29, 34	12 (C)	Class II determinants, blasts of myeloid and B-cell lineage, mature B cells, monocytes, activated T cells.

Suppliers: C — Coulter Electronics Ltd.

Fig. 14.4 Monoclonal antibodies against 'Ia-like' antigens (HLA-DR). The HLA-D locus was originally identified purely by the ability of its gene products to stimulate a mixed lymphocyte reaction. Several HLA-D related (hence abbreviation DR) monoclonal and polyclonal typing reagents are now available.

CD designation	Molecular weight (kDa)	Monoclonal antibody	Cellular distribution
CD 16	50—70	Anti-LEU11b (BD)	Large granular lymphocytes

Supplier: BD — Becton—Dickinson.

Fig. 14.5 Monoclonal antibodies against natural killer cells.

cases where a differential diagnosis is difficult, it is possible to use the alkaline phosphatase anti-alkaline phosphatase (APAAP) technique, instead of immuno-fluorescence, and so combine immunocytochemistry with cell morphology and to gain additional information. Marker studies can also contribute to an assessment of the likely prognosis of disease; for example, the presence of immunoglobulin µ heavy chains in the cytoplasm of CD10 positive lymphocytes in common acute lymphoblastic leukaemia (C-ALL) is associated with a poor prognostic outlook.

The typical activity profiles of these monoclonal antibodies with common leukaemias are summarised in Fig. 14.6.

Antibodies (CD numbers in parenthesis)								
J 5 (10)	B 4 (19)	HLA-DR	LEU9 (5)	T11 MY9 (2) (33)	MY7 (13)	CR3 M1 (11)	TdT (TdT)	Cytoplasmic Ig
Early B precursor ALL								
−	+	+	−	−	−	−	+	−
C-ALL +	+	+	−	−	−	−	+	−
Pre-B-ALL +	+	+	−	−	−	−	+	+
B-ALL −	+	+	−	−	−	−	−	−
T-ALL −	−	−	+	+/−	−	−	+	−
AML −	−	+	−/+	−/+	+	−	−/+	−
AMML −	−	+	−	−	+	+	−	−

Fig. 14.6 Typical reactivity of acute leukaemia cells with monoclonal antibody panel.

If a lymphoproliferative disorder is suspected, the panel of monoclonal antibodies employed should include those directed against: CD2, CD5, CD19, surface-membrane immunoglobulin (SMIg), κ and λ light chains. Anti-SMIg staining would define the total B-lymphocyte population; in addition, as the B lymphocytes of B-cell chronic lymphocytic leukaemia (B-CLL) are monoclonal, light-chain staining would detect an abnormal predominance of a single light-chain type. This observation would differentiate B-CLL from a reactive lymphocytosis which would show the approximately equal λ and κ distribution of a polyclonally expanded population.

B-cell chronic lymphocytic leukaemia and B-cell non-Hodgkins' lymphoma (BNHL) may be differentiated on both qualitative and quantitative criteria. The pan T-lymphocyte antigen CD5 is abnormally expressed on the leukaemic B-lymphocyte clone in B-CLL and absent from those of B-NHL. In addition, the light chain-restricted

Monoclonal antibodies (CD number in parenthesis)					
T 11 (2)	LEU 1 (5)	B 4 (19)	κ	λ	SmIg
B-CLL −	+	+	+ (−) Faint fluorescence	− (+)	+
B-NHL −	−	+	+ (−) Bright fluorescence	− (+)	+
T-CLL* +	+	−	−	−	−

* After initial diagnosis with antibodies as above, proceded with T-lymphocyte subset analysis to determine monoclonality, CD4 versus CD8.

Fig. 14.7 Typical reactivity of chronic lymphcytic leukaemias and lymphomas with selected panel of monoclonal antibodies.

B-lymphocyte population in the majority of B-CLL cases shows low intensity SMIg and light-chain immunofluorescence whereas B-NHL B-lymphocytes show bright fluorescence. If T11 staining indicates T-CLL, then T-cell subset analysis should be carried out using antibodies to CD4 (T-helper/inducer) and CD8 (T-cytotoxic/suppressor) antigens: again an abnormal predominance of one phenotype is indicative of monoclonality.

The activity profiles of a panel of monoclonal antibodies used in the diagnosis of lymphoproliferative disorders is summarised in Fig. 14.7.

14.2.1   Storage and transportation of human blood

Ideally samples of blood should be analysed on the day they are taken but, if this is not possible, blood may be stored for short periods. The spectrum of lymphocyte phenotypic markers expected for fresh blood is least altered if whole blood is diluted 1 : 2 in Hank's balanced salt solution and stored in the dark at room temperature in anticoagulant-coated tubes prior to flow cytometer analysis (Sections 3.9 and 9.11). Storage at 4° may change the CD4 (T-helper/inducer) to CD8 (T-cytotoxic/suppressor) ratio. However, if phenotypic analysis is to be carried out on density gradient separated peripheral blood mononuclear cells (PBMC), the blood should not be stored for more than 4 days as granulocytes start to contaminate the lymphocyte fraction on separation. It is best to separate the PBMC as soon as possible and then cryopreserve the cells (Appendix III).

There is little difference between EDTA, acid citrate dextrose or heparin anticoagulants when working with fresh samples of blood; however, EDTA is unsuitable for blood storage as it leads to contamination of the PBMC density gradient fraction with red blood cells.

14.3   Functional analysis

Although estimation of the relative numbers of the lymphoid subpopulations is of obvious value, it begs the next question: do the cells work properly?

14.3.1   Mitogenic response

In vitro assays may be performed to study the functional behaviour of lymphocytes. Mitogenic assays (Section 4.9) may be used with either non-specific stimuli such as lectins — phytohaemagglutinin, concanavalin A or pokeweed mitogen — or specific stimuli such as purified protein derivative of *Mycobacterium hominis*, *Candida*, mumps, tetanus toxoid or streptokinase. The stimulation index in normal subjects is usually greater than 10 for mitogens and more than three for specific antigens. A reduction in this index is indicative of lymphocyte hyporeactivity.

14.3.2   Lymphokine production

Lymphokines are produced by lymphocytes following antigen-specific or non-specific activation. They are most often measured in functional assays (Chapter 13), although an increasing range of commercial immunoassays are becoming available. The functional assays depend upon harvesting culture supernatant from the patient's activated lymphocytes and adding it to indicator cells. The lymphokine effect is quantitated by the degree of change in growth, differentiation or inhibition of function of the treated compared to control population.

14.3.3   Chemotaxis

Neutrophils and monocytes move towards certain chemical stimuli, for example as provided by casein or the peptide f-met-leu-phe. It is possible to test for the ability of a patient's neutrophils or monocytes to respond to a chemotactic signal. Isolated cells to be tested are placed on one side of a chamber and separated by a membrane from medium containing the chemotactic stimulus. After incubation the membrane is stained and examined microscopically to determine how far the cells have migrated towards the stimulus (Fig. 14.8). The same type of assay may be used to investigate the ability of a patient's serum to generate chemotactic activity. Fresh serum is incubated with endotoxin to generate the chemotactic signal.

14.3.4   Phagocytosis and opsonisation

Patients may have defects in the ability of their phagocytic cells to ingest particles or in the capacity of their sera to facilitate the opsonisation of particles via complement. Yeast cells are a convenient particle to use in opsonisation and phagocytosis assays as they activate the alternative complement pathway directly. Yeast cells are incubated with fresh normal serum and added to patients' neutrophils or alternatively patients' sera are incubated with yeast, and then added to normal neutrophils. Following incubation the cells may be examined microscopically for ingested yeast cells. To

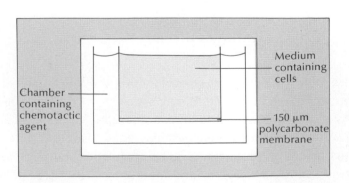

Fig. 14.8 Chamber for testing neutrophil or monocyte chemotaxis.

make visualisation easier the neutrophils can be fixed and stained before counting (Section 3.3). Obviously, control standards must be included in the assay as the 'normal' serum and cells may vary from day to day.

14.3.5 ## Measurement of respiratory burst

Two quantitative techniques are described below for the estimation of the respiratory burst induced by particle ingestion by phagocytes. The second technique offers the distinct advantage that it can be used to assess the distribution of phagocytic activity per cell in an unseparated population of blood cells.

Nitroblue tetrazolium reduction

Phagocytic cells ingest and reduce nitroblue tetrazolium (NBT) dye. The yellow dye is taken up by neutrophils and reduced to a blue derivative. The blue particles may be counted directly under a microscope or the dye extracted and quantitated spectrophotometrically (Section 5.3). The dye is only reduced in activated cells, therefore the number of cells reducing the dye gives an idea of the proportion of activated cells *in vivo*. To assess total function the cells must be activated; for example, with endotoxin.

Continuous-flow cytofluorimetery

Materials
2'7'-dichlorofluorescein diacetate (DCFH-DA) 20 mM in ethanol; store below 0° in the dark
Heparinised whole blood
Dulbecco's phosphate-buffered saline, PBS (free of Ca^{++} and Mg^{++}), containing 5 mM glucose, 1% gelatin, 5 mM sodium azide and DCFH-DA at 250 mM final concentration

Method
1 Dilute 100 µl heparinised whole blood or cell suspension with Dulbecco's PBS containing DCF-DA.
2 Mix 20 min at 37° in shaking water bath.
3 Add 0.5 ml EDTA and 350 ng ml^{-1} phorbol myristic acetate, PMA, in ethanol.
4 Treat with ice-cold distilled water for 20 sec.
5 Centrifuge and re-suspend in PBS—gelatin—glucose.
6 Examine by flow cytometry.

Technical notes
1 Azide inhibits enzymatic decomposition of H_2O_2 by cellular catalase and myeloperoxidase and does not impair H_2O_2 production.

2 Ethanol depresses DCF fluorescence and so should be kept to a minimum concentration.

3 Neutrophils produce between 50 and 70 nmol of superoxide min^{-1} 10^{-7} neutrophils in response to PMA.

Measurement of immunoglobulin

Measurements of immunoglobulin concentration can be useful in patients with a history of recurrent infections, as evidence of immune deficiency. Such measurements can also yield helpful information in patients with inflammatory diseases, particularly in systemic lupus erythematosus (SLE) where IgG is frequently elevated. Quantitation of immunoglobulin is essential where malignancy of the lymphoid system is suspected.

14.4.1 Immunoglobulin quantitation

IgG,IgA and IgM levels are often determined by precipitation with specific antibodies using single radial immunodiffusion (Section 6.6). IgE concentrations must be measured by radio or enzyme immunoassay (Section 10.4 or 10.5). Detection of hypogamma-globulinaemic states usually present no particular problem, but depression of polyclonal immunoglobulin production, can occur in multiple myeloma; the resulting immune deficiency often being fatal. Care must be taken to look for this depression in the presence of abnormally high concentrations of the monoclonal immunoglobulin. In some diseases such as AIDS or malaria there is polyclonal activation of B cells with normal or raised levels of immunoglobulin, but as most of it is not related to infection, the patients may be functionally antibody deficient.

High levels of monoclonal protein as found with plasma-cell malignancies can selectively deplete the detecting antiserum and lead to falsely high values. In both malignancy and some autoimmune diseases 7S as well as 19S IgM may be produced, affecting the accuracy of measurement if 19S standard is used alone.

In body fluids other than serum, for example cerebrospinal fluid (CSF), it is helpful to assess the local synthesis of immunoglobulin against the background of that derived systemically. As albumin is not synthesised in sites such as the brain, the ratio of IgG to albumin can be used as an indirect estimate of the amount of local synthesis. Raised IgG in CSF indicates either local infection or, possibly, multiple sclerosis.

In automated systems, nephelometry (Section 6.8) is frequently used to determine immunoglobulin concentrations. Care must be taken in its use as very high concentrations of immunoglobulin can result in immune complexes formed in gross antigen excess which scatter light less well than complexes formed at or near equivalence and so give falsely low values.

14.4.2 Qualitative examination of immunoglobulinopathies

Abnormalities in immunoglobulin production are often first identified by the detection of an intensely staining band, abnormal in either its position or appearance (Fig. 6.16), on an electrophoretogram of whole serum during routine screening. These abnormal bands would then be typed by immunoelectrophoresis (Section 6.9.2) with specific antisera to each immunoglobulin class, as well as κ and λ light chains. A monoclonal protein will usually be identified by a characteristic bowing in the precipitin line formed with one of the heavy-chain antisera and one of the light-chain types (Fig. 6.19). In general terms, the relative incidence of heavy-chain classes in these immunoglobulinopathies follows the ranking of plasma immunoglobulin concentrations; IgG > IgM > IgA.

Occasionally a patient may have two monoclonal proteins, such as IgG and IgM. This is almost invariably the result of isotype switching, so that both immunoglobulins will have the same light chains and V_H regions (and would therefore react with the same anti-idiotype serum, Section 6.15.1), differing only in their C_H regions. The chance of two independent tumorigenic events in the lymphoid system of the same patient is very small.

Sometimes an abnormal IgA band may be detected without any apparent light chain. This can be the result of masking of the light chains by the heavy chains, presumably owing to steric hindrance. Treatment of the serum with dithiothreitol (Section 8.7) will reveal the light chains. Very rarely, monoclonal heavy chains will be detected in the apparent absence of light chains. These are heavy-chain disease proteins which have deletions within the heavy chain preventing the attachment of light chain.

Not all monoclonal proteins are the result of malignancy. Benign monoclonal gammopathy is frequently seen in older patients, but it should always be followed up, as up to 10% of apparently benign paraproteinaemias progress to malignancy.

14.4.3 Bence-Jones proteins

In normal immunoglobulin synthesis, light chains are synthesised on polyribosomes and then released to form an intracellular pool of free light chains. From here they bind to nascent heavy chains to form complete immunoglobulin molecules (Fig. 14.9). A slight excess of light chains is found in normal individuals and because of their small size these are not retained by filtration in the kidney and so are excreted via the urine. Very sensitive techniques are needed to detect these low levels of light chains. In myeloma a large excess of light chain is frequently produced and can be readily detected in the urine. Bence-Jones, who first discovered these proteins, described their detection by their strange behaviour of first precipitating on heating urine to 56° and then re-dissolving on further heating. This test is no longer used as it is insensitive. Myeloma-derived light chains are now revealed by concentration of the urine by ammonium sulphate precipitation (Section 8.1.1) followed by immunoelectrophoresis against specific antisera (Section 6.9.2). In some patients the malignant plasma cells only produce light chains and no heavy chains.

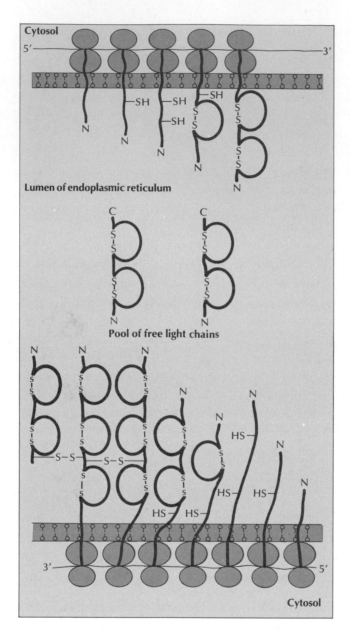

Fig. 14.9 Synthesis of immunoglobulin light and heavy chains. Light chains are synthesised on polyribosomes and released to form a pool of free light chains. Light chains from this pool attach to heavy chains while they are still being formed on their polyribosomes. Complete immunoglobulin molecules are then released from the endoplasmic reticulum.

14.4.4 Oligoclonal proteins in CSF

Immunoglobulin in the CSF is either produced locally or derived from the serum. As an indication of the relative contribution of local synthesis to the immunoglobulin content of CSF, its immunoglobulin : albumin ratio is determined. IgG levels may be raised in several conditions such as neurosyphilis or multiple sclerosis. The diagnostic potential is improved by qualitative examination of the immunoglobulins. This can be performed by polyacrylamide gel electrophoresis (Section 2.10, but without SDS) or isoelectric focusing (Section 6.12). In multiple sclerosis, oligoclonal bands are evident (Fig. 14.10) but the specificity of these antibodies remains to be identified.

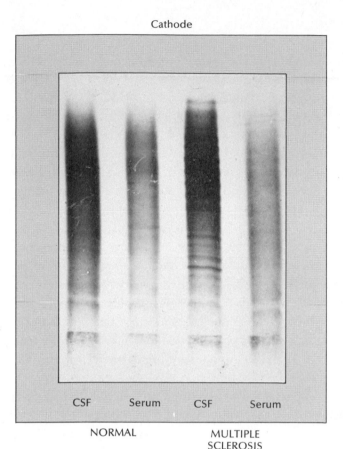

Cathode

CSF   Serum   CSF   Serum

NORMAL   MULTIPLE
SCLEROSIS

Fig. 14.10 Immunoperoxidase staining of isoelectric-focused IgG in samples of cerebrospinal fluid (CSF) and serum. The IgG in the normal samples is so polyclonal that the staining is continuous, whereas in the CSF from the patient with multiple sclerosis clear oligoclonal bands are revealed. (Photograph courtesy of Dr Ed Thompson.)

14.5 Antibody quantitation

14.5.1 Anti-microbial antibodies

Determination of circulating anti-microbial antibodies provides useful information of past or present infections; for instance, with hepatitis B, HIV or rubella. Sensitive techniques such as ELISA (Section 10.6), Western immunoblotting (Section 2.11) or complement fixation (Section 7.2) are used routinely. It is not possible to determine reliably the current status of the infection in the patient from the antibody levels in a single sample of serum; however, if two samples are taken a few days apart, a rising titre of antibody can indicate an acute infection. Similarly, determination of the isotype of the antibody can also be helpful as a high IgM : IgG ratio of antibody, changing in favour of the IgG antibodies between the two samples, can indicate current, primary infection. This principle is crucial to the diagnosis of toxoplasmosis in pregnant females, where antibodies due to a past infection with *Toxoplasma gondii* need not cause alarm. However, a rising titre, and a high IgM : IgG ratio, of anti-*Toxoplasma* antibodies indicates a current infection which may be congenitally acquired by the unborn fetus.

14.5.2 Antibodies in hypersensitivity

IgE antibodies to various antigens can be demonstrated in most patients with atopic allergy by the 'wheal-and-flare' reaction provoked by a skin prick or patch test using the suspected antigen. However, in some individuals, such as those with severe excema, this method of clinical investigation is not applicable so the antibodies are determined using solid-phase immunoassays (Section 10.5). The radio-allergosorbent test (RAST) is a commercially available assay system which uses radiolabeled anti-IgE as the detection reagent. The MAST system utilises allergens bound to cotton threads; antibody bound to the antigen is detected using a chemiluminescent system which allows easy recording and measurement on Polaroid film.

In type III (immune complex-mediated) hypersensitivity, in the presence of large amounts of IgG antibody to extrinsic antigens, immune complexes are formed in the lungs on inhalation of the antigen. This leads to complement activation, polymorph infiltration and the development of extrinsic allergic alveolitis. As high levels of IgG antibody are necessary for this reaction, the antibodies are easily detected by simple and relatively insensitive assays such as precipitation in gel (for example, Ouchterlony immunodiffusion, Section 6.7) or countercurrent immunoelectrophoresis (Section 6.9.3).

Many different inhaled antigens have been implicated in the pathogenesis of type III hypersensitivity reactions and they often result from occupational exposure; for example, *Micropolyspora faeni* from mouldy hay which can cause farmers' lung disease, *Aspergillus claratus* from mouldy barley producing malt workers' lung, and pigeon serum proteins from pigeon droppings which can cause pigeon breeders' disease.

14.5.3 Autoantibodies

Autoantibodies may initiate disease, contribute to pathogenesis and aid diagnosis (Fig. 14.11). It must, however, be remembered that: (a) some autoantibodies are the result of disease rather than its cause; and (b) autoantibodies are sometimes found in the absence of apparent disease, particularly in the elderly. As our understanding of the chemical nature of many autoantigens is poor, they are detected by observing their binding to tissue sections (a very complex antigenic environment!) using immunofluorescence (analagous to Section 4.4) and so the interpretation of the result requires care and experience as it is inevitably subjective.

Many of the tissues employed are obtained from animals, as human and animal tissue antigens are frequently cross-reactive. However, some systems, such as thyroid and pancreas, only work with human tissue. As noted above, immunofluorescence requires skilled observation to recognise the disease relationships of the patterns of tissue reactivity and yields little quantitative data. As the individual antigens are gradually characterised and isolated, immunofluorescence is being replaced by other assays such as Western blotting (Section 2.11), agglutination (Section 6.14), enzyme immunoassays (Section 10.6) and precipitation (Section 6.5).

Disease	Antigen	Test
Rheumatoid arthritis	IgG	Agglutination
Systemic lupus erythematosus	Cell nuclei DNA	Immunofluorescence Immunoassay
Sjögren's syndrome	Salivary ducts	Immunofluorescence
Active chronic hepatitis	Smooth muscle	Immunofluorescence
Primary biliary cirrhosis	Mitochondria	Immunofluoresence
Myasthenia gravis	Acetyl choline receptor	Radioassay with $\alpha-$ bungarotoxin and receptor
Insulin-dependent diabetes	Islet cells	Immunofluoresence
Male infertility	Patient's sperm	Binding assay with labelled anti-IgA
Addison's disease	Cytoplasm of adrenal cells	Immunofluoresence
Pernicious anaemia	Parietal cells Intrinsic factor	Immunofluoresence Vit-B$_{12}$ blocking or binding assay
Thyrotoxicosis	TSH receptors	Bioassay
Hashimoto's thyroiditis	Thyroglobulin	ELISA, agglutination

Fig. 14.11 Tests for autoantibodies in disease.

14.6

Immune complexes

Immune complexes are formed during infection, upon injection of foreign material and in certain autoimmune diseases. Their accurate measurement can be exceedingly difficult (Section 7.4) as it is difficult to discriminate complexed from normal immunoglobulin. Detection is relatively simple in infectious diseases, such as infectious endocarditis, but is fraught with difficulty in autoimmune disease. In systemic lupus erythematosus (SLE), the autoimmune immune complex disease *par excellence*, so many autoantibodies are formed that many of the components of the detection system are themselves recognised. Thus, the use of the RAJI cell assay, which uses a human B-cell line with C3 receptors, can be complicated by the presence of anti-lymphocyte antibodies; these antibodies, as well as immune complexes, may bind to the indicator cell. Assays based on C1q (Section 7.4), now appear to be beset by a similar problem as anti-C1q antibody is frequently found in SLE.

The assays for the detection of immune complexes (in the presence of native immunoglobulin) which rely on differences in relative solubility and molecular weight are probably more reliable, but less sensitive, than the assays described above.

Precipitation of complexes by polyethylene glycol

Polyethylene glycol (PEG) precipitates proteins in proportion to their molecular size and concentration. Thus, free IgG is soluble in 2% w/v PEG, but it is insoluble when part of an immune complex. Although a screening test for complexes could simply involve the measurement of the total protein precipitated from serum by PEG, more accurate information can be obtained by further analysis of the precipitated proteins. For instance IgG may be quantitated in the precipitate and used as a measure of the complexed IgG in the serum. The measurement of complex-bound complement components, particularly C1q and C4, can also give useful information.

Materials and equipment
Test serum samples
Veronal buffered saline, VBS (Appendix I)
Polyethylene glycol, PEG 6000 (20% w/v in VBS) (Appendix II)
0.2 M ethylene diamine tetra-acetic acid, EDTA, disodium salt, titrate to pH 7.6 with 0.1 M NaOH
Plastic test tubes, 3 ml (Appendix II)
Single radial immunodiffusion plate for quantitating IgG (Section 6.6)

Method
1 Adjust PEG solution to its working concentration by mixing 6 ml of 20% PEG with 3 ml 0.2 M EDTA and 1 ml VBS.
2 Add 30 µl PEG working solution to 150 µl of each test serum (in duplicate).
3 Mix and leave overnight at 4°.
4 Centrifuge at 2000 *g* for 20 min at 4°.
5 Place the tubes on ice and carefully remove the supernatants.
6 Re-suspend each precipitate with 2 ml of 2% PEG in 0.01 M EDTA in VBS.
7 Centrifuge at 200 *g* for 20 min at 4°.
8 Remove the supernatants and re-dissolve the precipitates in 150 µl VBS. Incubate at 37° for 1 h to ensure that the precipitated complexes have re-dissolved.
9 Quantitate the precipitated IgG by single radial immunodiffusion (Section 6.6) or nephelometry (Section 6.8).
10 Express the results as µg of IgG precipitated per ml of serum.

Generally up to 100 µg ml^{-1} of IgG will be precipitated from the serum of a healthy individual. Amounts greater than this are indicative of an abnormal amount of circulating immune complexes, which may reach mg ml^{-1} levels in severe cases.

Acute-phase proteins

Acute-phase proteins are a diverse collection of serum proteins whose serum concentrations rise in response to a variety of traumatic states such as bacterial infection, burns, surgery and inflammation. The rise in the concentration of these components may be in the order of 50% (C3, ceruloplasmin) or from two- to three fold (α_1-acid glycoprotein, α_1-anti-proteinase, haptoglobin, fibrinogen) to more than 100-fold (C-reactive protein, serum amyloid protein). Quantitation of these changes may be achieved by precipitation (Section 6.5) or counter-current 'rocket' electrophoresis (Section 6.10) of samples in agar containing specific antiserum. Although the techniques are simple and reproducible, enormous variability is found between different laboratories using acute-phase assays. Why acute-phase protein assays should be so non-reproducible is unclear, but it is hoped that more attention to standardisation (Section 14.10) will improve interlaboratory comparability.

14.8 HLA typing in transplantation and disease associations

The human histocompatibility gene locus is a complex and highly polymorphic region coding for class I and class II major histocompatibility antigens as well as some complement components. The class I antigens A (about 20 allelic types), B (about 40) and C (about 10) are currently typed using cells, usually lymphocytes, in an antibody-based, complement-mediated cytotoxicity assay (Section 7.5). To date, the majority of the typing reagents are polyclonal antibodies (cf. monoclonal anti-HLA programmes, Section 12.12) which are derived from fortuitous immunisation of multi-parous women, in response to HLA differences between fetus and mother, or patients receiving multiple blood transfusions. Before use as typing reagents, the precise specificities of these antisera must be established on cells homozygous at particular HLA loci.

Class II MHC antigens were originally detected by the mixed-lymphocyte reaction (Section 4.10.1) and required standard typing cells, homozygous at the D locus, for stimulation of the cells to be typed (responders). The potential of the stimulator cells to react against the responders was blocked by prior irradiation or mitomycin C treatment. As lymphocytes will not respond to their own HLA antigens because of central tolerance (Section 5.7), the different mixtures of responding and stimulator cells reveal a pattern of reactivity related to HLA differences at the D locus. In each case the mitogenic response is measured by the incorporation of radiolabelled thymidine. Class II, D-related (DR) antigens may also now be recognised serologically (see Fig. 14.4) in complement-mediated cytotoxic assays.

Tissue typing is complicated and expensive, and dependent on having supplies of precious typing sera and cells. However, the success rate of grafting is greatly enhanced by HLA matching. For example, more than 90% of renal allografts matched at two loci survive for >2 years, whereas unmatched donor—recipient pairs have much a much lower success rate (between 40 and 60% graft survival at 2 years depending upon the reporting method).

Typing studies have also revealed associations between particular diseases and certain MHC antigens. This is an interesting research tool but has yet to prove generally useful in clinical immunology. The one notable exception to this is ankylosing spondylitis where more than 95% of patients are HLA-B27 positive (compared to only 8% of the general population). In this disease, HLA typing can be helpful in achieving an accurate differential diagnosis.

The present rate of development of HLA specific gene probes suggests that typing will move from the immunological to the molecular biological arena within the foreseeable future.

Epstein—Barr virus-transformed human lymphoblastoid cell lines

The Epstein—Barr virus (EBV) infects and transforms human B lymphocytes via CD21 (complement receptor 2 for C3d) to produce lymphoblastoid lines which, in some instances, secrete immunoglobulin constitutively. Initially, it was hoped that this technique might provide a route to human monoclonal antibody-producing cell lines or antigen-presenting cells for human T-lymphocyte lines (Section 12.14.2) but these hopes have not been generally realised. We include the technique here as it has been shown to be a useful way of revealing selective B-lymphocyte immunodeficiency states. Lymphocytes are cultured with EBV for 5—10 days (micro-culture technique as Section 4.10) and their immunoglobulin production measured in the supernatant (Section 10.4 or 10.6).

Both EBV and *Staphylococcus aureus*, Cowan strain, are able to drive B lymphocytes into immunoglobulin production in an entirely T lymphocyte-independent manner. Normal B lymphocytes respond by making significant amounts of IgM, IgG and IgA (IgM in a five- to tenfold excess over IgG or IgA). The vast majority of hypo- or agammaglobulinaemic patients produce virtually no IgG or IgA and so the ratio of IgM to the other immunoglobulin classes is enormously increased. In about 5% of immunodeficient patients, however, the ratio of IgM versus IgG or IgA is normal but the absolute amount of each is diminished, suggesting that deficiency is simply the result of a reduced number of normal B lymphocytes rather than a functional deficiency.

Materials and equipment

Heparin, preservative free 1000 U ml^{-1} (Appendix II).

Lymphoprep or similar density gradient (Appendix II)

Tissue culture medium, RPMI-1640 is recommended

Fetal bovine serum, FBS, heat inactivated at 56° for 45 min.

Antibiotics: penicillin, 100 U ml^{-1}, streptomycin 100 µg ml^{-1}, and gentamycin 30 µg ml^{-1} (final concentrations)

24-well tissue culture plates (Appendix II)

Tissue culture flasks, 25 cm^2 growth area (Appendix II)

Cyclosporin A (Appendix II). Stock solution made by dissolving 4 mg cyclosporin A in 10 ml absolute ethanol (Analar grade). This should be stored in the dark (wrapped in aluminium foil) at 4° and this will keep for several months. It is used at 1:200 dilution

Epstein—Barr virus, EBV, from B95—8 marmoset cell line (Appendix III)

Method

1 Prepare peripheral blood mononuclear cells from 5—10 ml of heparinised human blood by density gradient centrifugation (Section 1.14.1).

2   Wash the cells twice, re-suspend in 20 ml RPMI medium and count the number of viable lymphocytes.

3   Centrifuge to pellet the cells (150 g for 10 min at room temperature) and discard the supernatant. Add 1 drop of FBS per 10^6 cells.

4   Add 0.5−1 ml of EBV supernatant (prepared as described in next section), re-suspend the cells by gently tapping the base of the tube. Discard the EBV storage vial into Chloros.

5   Incubate the virus−cell mixture for 60 min at 37°.

6   Prepare the 24-well plate by adding 1.5 ml of medium containing 10% FBS to each well. (See Technical note 2.)

7   Add 1 μl of cyclosporin stock solution to each well (final concentration 0.2 μg.ml^{-1}).

8   Dispense the cells into the culture wells to give 2−4×10^6 per well.

9   Incubate at 37° in a humidified atmosphere of 5% CO_2 in air for 1 week.

10 Remove 1 ml of medium from each well and replace with 1 ml of fresh medium containing 10% FBS (cyclosporin A is no longer needed).

Observe the plates every week or so, but ignore cell clumps appearing during the first week; these are not EBV transformed cells.

11 After 3−4 weeks assess each well for clumps of viable cells using an inverted microscope and transfer those which appear to be growing into 25 cm^2 tissue culture flasks containing 10 ml of RPMI with 10% FBS. As you will inevitably leave some cells in the original wells, add fresh medium as an insurance against accidental loss of the transferred cells.

12 The cells often grow in clumps as well as in single-cell suspension and should be subcultured weekly, or as required.

Technical notes

1   Use a category 2 hood throughout these procedures to protect both the operator and the cultures. The hood should have a UV light for decontamination after experimental use (EBV is very sensitive to UV irradiation).

2   In the 24-well plates, use the wells diagonally across and down the plate to minimise cross-contamination during long-term culture.

3   It is advisable to store samples of actively growing cells in liquid nitrogen (see Appendix III).

4   Cyclosporin A is added to kill anti-EBV cytotoxic T lymphocytes which may have been present in the lymphocyte donor.

14.9.1   EBV transformation of human B cells

Human B lymphocytes can be immortalised by transformation *in vitro* with EBV. Such transformed cell lines have been used for the production of human monoclonal antibodies. Transformed B lymphocytes can also be used as antigen-presenting cells

(APC) for T cells *in vitro* (Section 12.14.2). However, it should be borne in mind that B lymphocytes are not efficient APC for all types of antigen, particularly complex antigens which require considerable 'processing' to give epitopes which will stimulate T cells.

PREPARATION OF EBV

Materials and equipment
B95−8 marmoset cell line (Appendix III)
RPMI-1640 tissue culture medium, without HEPES buffer
Fetal bovine serum, FBS
Tissue culture flasks (25 cm^2, 75 cm^2, 150 cm^2 growth area) (Appendix II)
Screw-cap freezing vials (Nunc, Appendix II)

Method
1 Wash an aliquot of the marmoset cells and re-suspend in tissue culture medium containing 10% FBS, transfer to a 25 cm^2 culture flask containing 10 ml tissue culture medium.
2 Subculture the cells into new flasks and expand as required. A large (150 cm^2) flask in log-phase growth is required.

The cells grow in suspension, but a few may become attached and have a macrophage-like appearance.

3 As the pH of the medium begins to fall in a log-phase culture, the virus yield can be increased by stressing the cells.
4 To stress the cells, place the flask in an incubator at 33° for 2 days, or place the flask at 4° overnight.
5 Transfer the contents of the flask to 50 ml sterile centrifuge tubes and centrifuge at 150 *g* for 10 min to pellet the cells. Recover and keep the supernatant — it contains the virus.
6 Centrifuge the supernatant again at 2000 *g* for 10 min.
7 Aspirate the supernatant and filter through a 0.45 μm membrane to remove any residual cell debris.
8 Dispense in 1 ml aliquots into screw-capped freezing vials and store at −70° or in liquid nitrogen (cryopreservation as for cells, Appendix III).

Technical notes
1 If required, use 5×10^6 of the cell pellet from step 5 to initiate fresh cultures, alternatively discard the whole into chloros.
2 Do not use a 0.22 μm membrane to filter the virus suspension in step 7 as it might hold back some of the virus which is large and can form clumps.
3 One 1 ml vial stored in liquid nitrogen is sufficient for one transformation experiment. The vials should not be re-frozen as the potency of the virus drops by at least 50% each time.

4 The virus remains viable for at least 1 year at $-70°$ and probably indefinitely in liquid nitrogen.

14.9.2 ## Titration of EBV-transforming units

The EB virus will stimulate neonatal human B cells, obtained from cord blood, to transform and produce IgM. Neonatal T cells will not interfere with this because they have no immunity to the virus and so no cyclosporin A is required in these cultures.

Cord blood is obtained from maternity units and should be collected after clamping of the cord or after delivery of the placenta. 10 ml of blood is adequate, though a placenta can yield up to 70 ml. The blood should be collected sterile by venepuncture and care should be taken to avoid contamination with maternal blood (and thus possibly with immune T cells) or with 'Wharton's jelly' expressed from the cut end of the cord, which is viscous and can hinder separation of the lymphocytes.

Materials and equipment
Heparinised cord blood
Lymphoprep or similar density gradient (Appendix II)
RPMI-1640 tissue culture medium
Fetal bovine serum, FBS
Micro-culture plates, U-shaped wells (Appendix II)

Method
1 Isolate the peripheral blood mononuclear cells by density gradient centrifugation (Section 1.14.1).

The leucocytes at the plasma—density gradient interface will contain many nucleated red cells. These are difficult to remove, but will not interfere with the assay.

3 Wash the cells three times in medium.
4 Re-suspend in medium plus 10% FBS at 2×10^6 lymphocytes ml^{-1}.
5 Thaw an aliquot of EBV preparation from liquid nitrogen.
6 Make 10 $\log_2$ dilutions of the virus suspension in medium containing 10% FBS and dispense 100 μl aliquots into replicate micro-titre wells (four replicates per dilution).
7 Add 50 μl aliquots of the cell suspension (1×10^5 cells per well) to each well.
8 Incubate the culture plates at $37°$ in a humidified atmosphere of 5% CO_2 in air for 4—6 weeks.

Examine the plates for transformed cells which appear as clumps of viable cells among the cell debris. The end point is determined from the dilution which produces no transformation. Alternatively, results can be obtained after 1 week of culture by assaying the supernatants for IgM production (Section 10.6).

14.10 Standards and quality control

Immunological assays are notoriously variable, partly because the cells and antisera are difficult to obtain or produce uniformly and to characterise fully. Antibodies are biological materials and not chemical reagents — unexpected cross-reactions may appear even when using monoclonal antibodies. It is essential, in laboratory work, that: (a) all reagents are checked for specificity; and (b) known standards are incorporated into each assay. A major problem with many assays using serum samples from patients is the presence of rheumatoid factor, autoantibodies to IgG. These occur in normal individuals (especially in older people) as well as in rheumatoid arthritis. They can be induced following infection or vaccination. These antiglobulins will bind on to IgG antibodies used in immunoassays and, depending upon the system, may cause inhibition or enhancement.

Many molecules of immunological interest are now available as national or international standards. These include immunoglobulins, specific autoantibodies such as rheumatoid factor and anti-nuclear antibody, and cytokines (Appendix II). Introduction of standards can make for dramatic improvements in the reproducibility and reliability of results. For instance, when the World Health Organisation introduced a standard for immune complexes, variation between laboratories, which had ranged between 1400 μg ml^{-1} and 30 μg ml^{-1} for a test sample of 40 μg ml^{-1}, was virtually abolished when results were normalised in terms of the 'in-test' standard.

External quality control programmes are also available and laboratories should use these; not only for verification of their own accuracy, but also to reveal problems or to permit compatibility between centres in assay methodology. It soon becomes apparent, when scrutinising these results, which assays are likely to be more reliable for particular applications.

14.11 Summary and conclusions

Although immunological techniques may be used over virtually the whole field of medicine, their two major uses are to investigate immune deficiency and hypersensitivity. In a basic evaluation of immune deficiency, the cells involved in the immune response, lymphocytes, monocytes, neutrophils, etc. may be quantitated. Further information is gained by using the wide variety of specific antibodies for different cell phenotypes. Monoclonal antibodies have greatly enriched these studies, and improved reproducibility and accuracy.

14.12 Further reading

Bryant NJ (1986) *Laboratory Immunology and Serology*. WB Saunders and Co, London.
Chapel H and Haeney M (1988) *Essentials of Clinical Immunology*, 2nd edition. Blackwell Scientific Publications, Oxford.

Grieco MH and Mariney DK (editors) (1983) *Immunodiagnosis for Clinicians Interpretation of Immuno-assays*. Year Book Medical Publishers, Chicago.

Janossy *et al.* (1987) Monoclonal antibodies. In *Methods in Hematology*, Beverley PCL (editor). Churchill Livingstone, Edinburgh.

Pruzanski W and Keystone EC (1985) *Paraproteins in Disease. Investigation of Plasma Cell Dyscrasias*. Churchill Livingstone, Edinburgh.

Reeves WG (series editor) (1986 onwards) *Immunology and Medicine*. MTP Press, Lancaster

Rose NR, Freidman H and Fahey JL (editors) (1986) *Manual of Clinical Laboratory Immunology*, 3rd edition. American Society for Mircobiology, Washington.

Thompson RA (editor) (1981) *Techniques in Clinical Immunology*, 2nd edition. Blackwell Scientific Publications, Oxford.

Wells JV and Nelson DS (editors) (1986) *Clinical Immunology Illustrated*. Williams and Wilkins, London.

Appendices

Appendices

1 Buffers and Media

All solutions must be made up in distilled water which has been prepared by an endosmosis purification system (Appendix II) or double glass distillation.

Acetate–acetic acid buffer, pH 4.0, ionic strength 0.1

Materials
0.6 M sodium acetate (49.2 g litre^{-1})
0.6 M acetic acid (34.4 ml glacial acetic acid in 1000 ml distilled water)

Method
1 Mix 435 ml 0.6 M acetic acid with 130 ml 0.6 M sodium acetate.
2 Adjust to 1000 ml with distilled water.

0.001 M acetate–acetic buffer, pH 4.4

Materials
Sodium acetate, CH$_3$COONa (8.20 g litre^{-1})
Acetic acid (6.0 g litre^{-1})

Method
1 Mix 1/3 sodium acetate solution with 2/3 acetic acid solution.
2 Dilute 1 : 1000 to give 1 mM.

Balanced salt solution (BSS)

Materials
Calcium chloride (0.14 g litre^{-1})
Sodium chloride (8.00 g litre^{-1})
Potassium chloride (0.40 g litre^{-1})
0.8 mM magnesium sulphate, MgSO$_4$·7H$_2$O (0.20 g litre^{-1})
1.0 mM magnesium chloride, MgCl$_2$·6H$_2$O (0.20 g litre^{-1})
0.4 mM potassium dihydrogen phosphate (0.06 g litre^{-1})
1.4 mM disodium hydrogen phosphate, Na$_2$HPO$_4$·2H$_2$O (0.24 g litre^{-1})

Method
1 If required, 1 g litre^{-1} of glucose may be added.
2 Dissolve all components in 1000 ml.
3 Membrane filter, if required sterile.

Barbitone buffer, pH 8.2, ionic strength 0.08

Materials
Barbital sodium (5'5-diethyl barbituric acid, Na salt)
Barbital (5'5 diethylbarbituric acid)
5 M sodium hydroxide
Merthiolate

Method
1 Dissolve 12.00 g sodium barbital in 800 ml distilled water.
2 Dissolve 4.40 g barbital in 150 ml distilled water at 95°.
3 Mix solutions 1 and 2 and adjust pH to 8.2 with concentrated sodium hydroxide.
4 Add 0.15 g merthiolate (preservative) and adjust final volume to 1000 ml.

Technical note
For electrophoresis on cellulose acetate membranes use 0.05–0.07 M barbitone buffer, pH 8.6. The exact buffer composition and concentration can be adjusted according to requirements. At lower concentrations, the protein bands are wider and their mobility increased. A higher buffer concentration produces the reverse effect with crowding of the bands.

0.15 M barbitone-buffered saline, pH 7.6 (for complement fixation test)

Materials
Sodium chloride
Barbital (5'5 diethylbarbituric acid)
Barbital sodium (5'5 diethylbarbituric acid, Na salt)

Magnesium chloride
1.0 M calcium chloride (111.1 g l^{-1})

STOCK SOLUTIONS
A 85.0 g sodium chloride + 2.75 g sodium diethylbarbiturate in 1400 ml of distilled water.
B 5.75 g diethylbarbituric acid in 500 ml hot distilled water.
C 20.3 g $MgCl_2{\cdot}6H_2O$ (2.0 M) dissolved in 50 ml distilled water + 30 ml 1.0 M calcium chloride solution. Adjust to 100 ml with distilled water. Final concentrations 1.0 M $MgCl_2$, 0.3 M $CaCl_2$.

Method
1 Mix solutions A and B and cool to room temperature.
2 Add 5 ml of C.
3 Adjust final volume to 2 litres with distilled water and store at 4°.

Technical note
This buffer is five times the concentration used in the text. Dilute just before use.

0.1 M borate buffer, pH 7.4

Materials
Disodium tetraborate $Na_2B_4O_7{\cdot}10H_2O$ (9.54 g in 250 ml distilled water)
Boric acid (24.73 g in 4 litres distilled water)

Method
Add approximately 115 ml borate solution to 4 litres boric acid solution until pH reaches 7.4.

Borate–saline buffer, pH 8.3–8.5, ionic strength 0.1

Materials
Boric acid (6.18 g litre^{-1})
Sodium tetraborate (borax) (9.54 g litre^{-1})
Sodium chloride (4.38 g litre^{-1})

Make up to 1000 ml with distilled water

0.15 M borate–succinate buffer, pH 7.5 (for tanning erythrocytes)

Materials
Solution A – 0.05 M sodium tetraborate $Na_2B_4O_7{\cdot}10H_2O$ (19.0 g litre^{-1})
Solution B – 0.05 M succinic acid (5.9 g litre^{-1})
Sodium chloride
Horse serum (Appendix II)

Method
1 Take 1000 ml of A and add B until pH 7.5.
2 Add sodium chloride to 0.14 M and 1% horse serum (final concentration) previously heat inactivated (56° for 45 min).

0.28 M cacodylate buffer, pH 6.9

Materials
Sodium cacodylate
3 M hydrochloric acid

Method
1 Dissolve sodium cacodylate (60 g litre^{-1}) in distilled water.
2 Titrate to pH 6.9 with 3 M HCl.
3 Adjust to 1000 ml with distilled water.

Carbonate–bicarbonate buffer

Stock solution A – 0.2 M solution of anhydrous sodium carbonate (21.2 g in 1000 ml)
Stock solution B – 0.2 M solution of sodium hydrogen carbonate (16.8 g in 1000 ml)

For use: x ml of A + y ml of B, diluted to a total of 200 ml will yield the approximate pH shown. If an accurate final pH is required, titrate the two solutions on a pH meter using the volumes given below as a guide.

x	y	pH
5.0	45.0	9.2
7.5	42.5	9.3
9.5	40.5	9.4
13.0	37.0	9.5
16.0	34.0	9.6
19.5	30.5	9.7

(Cont.)

x	y	pH
22.0	28.0	9.8
25.0	25.0	9.9
27.5	22.5	10.0
30.0	20.0	10.1
33.0	17.0	10.2
35.5	14.5	10.3
38.5	11.5	10.4
40.5	9.5	10.5
42.5	7.5	10.6
45.0	5.0	10.7

Adjust volume to achieve the required molarity using distilled water

0.1 M citrate buffer, pH 3.0–7.0

Materials
0.1 M citric acid, $C_6H_8O_7 \cdot 1H_2O$ (21.01 g l^{-1})
0.1 M disodium hydrogen phosphate, $Na_2HPO_4 \cdot 2H_2O$ (17.80 g litre^{-1})

Method
1 pH 5.0: is approximately a 50:50 mixture of citric to phosphate.
2 Below pH 5.0: titrate pH of citric acid with phosphate.
3 Above pH 5.0: titrate pH of phosphate with citric acid.

C1q buffers

Buffer 1

Materials
Ethyleneglycol-bis-(β-amino-ethyl ether)-N, N'-tetra-acetic acid, EGTA (19.76 g)
11 M sodium hydroxide solution

Method
1 Add 1500 ml distilled water to the EGTA.
2 Slowly add strong NaOH (about 8 ml of 11 M NaOH) to both dissolve the EGTA and adjust to pH 7.5.
3 Add distilled water to a total volume of 2 litres.

Buffer 2

Materials
0.02 M sodium acetate (1.64 g in 1000 ml distilled water)
Acetic acid 0.02 M, 1.14 ml glacial acetic acid in 1000 ml distilled water
Ethylene diamine tetra-acetic acid EDTA, disodium salt (1.79 g)
Sodium chloride (21.91 g)

Method
1 Add the EDTA and sodium chloride to 300 ml of the acetic acid.
2 When dissolved, add further acetic acid and sodium acetate solution to attain pH 5.0 and a volume of 500 ml.

Buffer 3

Materials
EDTA, trisodium salt (86 g)
Concentrated HCl

Method
1 Dissolve EDTA in 3.5 litres of water
2 Adjust to pH 5.0 with HCl and add distilled water to 4 litres, final volume

Buffer 4

Materials
Potassium dihydrogen phosphate (0.34 g in 500 ml distilled water)
Sodium chloride (21.91 g)
EDTA, trisodium salt (1.79 g)

Method
1 Dissolve the sodium chloride and EDTA in about 200 ml of the disodium hydrogen phosphate solution.
2 Add further disodium hydrogen phosphate and potassium dihydrogen phosphate solution to pH 7.5 and a volume of 500 ml.

Buffer 5

Materials
EDTA, trisodium salt (50.15 g)
Concentrated HCl

Method

1 Dissolve the EDTA in 3.5 litres distilled water.
2 Titrate to pH 7.5 with concentrated HCl.
3 Make up the volume to 4 litres with distilled water.

Buffer 6

Materials
As for buffer 2

Method

1 Dissolve EDTA and the sodium chloride in 300 ml sodium acetate solution.
2 Adjust to pH 7.5 and a volume of 500 ml with further sodium acetate and acetic acid solutions.

Diamino ethane—acetic acid buffer, pH 7.0, ionic strength 0.1

Materials
Diamino ethane
1 M acetic acid (57.3 ml glacial acetic acid in 1000 ml distilled water)

Method

1 Mix 2.88 g diamino ethane with 73.0 ml 1 M acetic acid.
2 Adjust to 1000 ml with distilled water.

0.05 M diethylamine—HCl buffer, pH 11.5

Materials
Diethylamine
1.0 M HCl

Method

1 Dissolve 365.5 mg diethylamine in 50 ml distilled water.
2 Titrate to pH 11.5 with 1.0 M HCl.
3 Adjust to 100 ml final volume with distilled water.

ELISA conjugate buffer

To 9 ml of phosphate-buffered saline (as below) add:

100 µl sheep serum
10 mg casein
10 µl Tween 20
5 µl antibody—enzyme conjugate.

Make up to a final volume of 10 ml.

Giemsa buffer (for May—Grünwald/Giemsa staining)

Materials
0.1 M citric acid (21.01 g litre^{-1})
0.2 M disodium hydrogen phosphate Na$_2$HPO$_4$ (28.39 g litre^{-1})

Method

1 Mix 85 ml 0.1 M citric acid with 115 ml 0.2 M disodium hydrogen phosphate and adjust pH to 5.75.
2 Make up to 1000 ml.

0.1 M glycine—HCl buffer, pH 2.5 or 2.8 (for acid elution of antibodies from immunoadsorbents)

Materials
0.2 M glycine (15.01 g litre^{-1})
0.2 M HCl

Method

1 Titrate 500 ml of 0.2 M glycine to pH2.5—2.8 as required, with 0.2 M HCl.
2 Make up to 1000 ml with distilled water.

0.5 M glycine—saline buffer, pH 8.6 (for immunofluorescence mountant and latex agglutination)

Materials
Glycine (14.00 g)
Sodium hydroxide, solid (0.7 g)
Sodium chloride (17 g)
Sodium azide (preservative) (1 g)

Method

1 Dissolve components in 500 ml of distilled water and adjust to pH 8.6 with alkali, as required.
2 Make up to 1000 ml with distilled water.

Mounting medium made as follows: 30 ml above buffer plus 70 ml glycerol.

Hank's saline (there are other formulations for this medium)

Materials
Sodium chloride (8.00 g litre^{-1})
Calcium chloride (0.20 g litre^{-1})
Magnesium sulphate (0.20 g litre^{-1})
Potassium chloride (0.40 g litre^{-1})
Potassium dihydrogen phosphate, KH$_2$PO$_4$
    (0.10 g litre^{-1})
Sodium bicarbonate (1.27 g litre^{-1})
Glucose (2.00 g litre^{-1})

Method
1 Dissolve in 1000 ml of distilled water.
2 Sterilise by membrane filtration.
   (Concentrated Hank's saline is sold commercially, but often has phenol red added as a pH indicator. This makes visualization of haemolytic plaques difficult.)

Jacalin storage buffer

Materials
10 mM HEPES
150 mM sodium chloride
100 mM calcium chloride
20 mM galactose
0.08% sodium azide as preservative

Mix together:

4.38 g NaCl
5.55 g CaCl$_2$
1.80 g galactose
1.19 g HEPES
0.4 g sodium azide

and adjust to 500 ml with water.

0.5 M phosphate buffers

Materials
Sodium dihydrogen phosphate 1 hydrate,
    NaH$_2$PO·4H$_2$O (69.0 g l^{-1})
Disodium hydrogen phosphate, anhydrous,
    Na$_2$HPO$_4$ (71.0 g litre^{-1})

Method
Prepare stock solutions of each salt in water and add 1 drop of chloroform as a preservative. Store at room temperature. Mix the two solutions to obtain the required pH using a pH meter and then adjust to the desired molarity. Take care not to add too much chloroform especially if the buffer is to be used with plastic chromatography columns.

0.15 M phosphate-buffered saline (PBS), pH 7.2

Materials
Sodium chloride (8.00 g litre^{-1})
Potassium chloride (0.20 g litre^{-1})
0.008 M disodium hydrogen phosphate,
    Na$_2$HPO$_4$ (1.15 g litre^{-1})
Potassium dihydrogen phosphate (0.20 g
    litre^{-1})

Method
Dissolve in 1000 ml of distilled water.

Technical notes
1 It is convenient to make up a ×10 solution for storage and dilute as required.
2 Sterilise by autoclaving or add 20 mM (final concentration) sodium azide as a preservative.
3 Remember that azide is not compatible with many experimental systems (not only cell culture) — it will inactivate lactoperoxidase, bind to ion-exchangers, etc.

0.20 M phosphate—saline buffer, pH 7.2 (for tanning erythrocytes)

Materials
0.02 M potassium dihydrogen phosphate,
    KH$_2$PO$_4$ (12.2 g)
0.06 M disodium hydrogen phosphate,
    Na$_2$HPO$_4$ (40.4 g)
0.12 M sodium chloride (36.0 g)

Method
Dissolve in 5 litres of distilled water.

Polyacrylamide running buffer

Stock solution

Tris—glycine buffer ×10:

$\left.\begin{array}{l}\text{144 g glycine} \\ \text{30 g Tris}\end{array}\right\}$ in 1000 ml water, pH 8.3.

Dilute stock solution ×10 then add: 3 ml 20% SDS to 600 ml of diluted stock solution.

Polyacrylamide sample buffer

Materials
20% SDS (in water) (6.0 ml)
Glycerol (3.0 ml)
1 M Tris–HCl, pH 6.8 (2.4 ml)
Distilled water (15.6 ml)
Bromophenol blue, few grains

Method
Mix the above quantities together to prepare the final sample buffer.

Technical notes
1 Prepare Tris solution on each occasion; the others may be kept as stock solutions.
2 Glycerol is added to increase the density of the solution and so aid loading of the polyacrylamide gel. It can be replaced by a 60% w/v sucrose solution.
3 Bromophenol blue dye is used as a marker to monitor the progress of the protein front during electrophoresis.
4 Prepare 2 M dithiothreitol as a stock solution and store at −20°. Add to sample dissolved in sample buffer just before boiling, if the separation is to be performed under reducing conditions.

0.14 M saline — physiological or 'normal' saline

Sodium chloride (8.5 g litre^{-1}). Store at a ×10 concentration and dilute as required. Sterilise by autoclaving

Scintillation fluid

Materials
2,5-diphenyloxazole, PPO (6 g)
2,2'-*p*-phenylene-bis (5-phenyloxazole), POPOP (0.05 g)
Toluene (1000 ml)

Tissue culture media (see also information on general *in vitro* culture techniques in Appendix III)

Many different culture media are available, each usually in an 'old' and 'new' or 'improved' formulation. For general use we suggest Eagle's minimal essential medium (EMEM) and Dulbecco's modification of Eagle's minimal essential medium (DMEM) or RPMI 1640 for culture under more demanding conditions.

Tris–ammonium chloride (for erythrocyte lysis)

Materials
0.17 M Tris (hydroxymethyl) aminomethane (20.60 g l^{-1})
0.16 M ammonium chloride (8.30 g litre^{-1})

Method
Add 10 ml of 0.17 Tris to 90 ml of 0.16 M ammonium chloride and adjust to pH 7.2.
This buffer induces red-cell lysis without reducing lymphocyte viability, unlike 1.0% acetic acid which is also used to lyse erythrocytes during white cell counts

Tris–HCl buffers

Materials
Tris (hydroxy methyl) aminomethane (12.1 g)
1 M HCl

Method
1 Dissolve Tris in 100 ml distilled water to prepare a 1.0 M stock solution.
2 Titrate to desired pH with HCl, then dilute to the required molarity.

Technical note
To measure and adjust the pH of a Tris solution, it is necessary to purchase a special Calomel Tris electrode — the electrochemistry of the normal electrode does not apply to Tris.

3.0 M Tris–HCl, pH 8.7

Dissolve 181.65 g Tris in 450 ml distilled

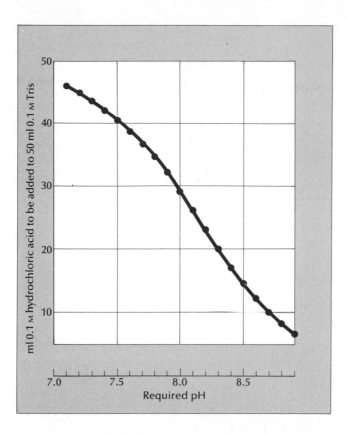

Fig. AI.1 Tris buffer. Variation in pH of Tris buffer obtained by adding 0.1 M hydrochloric acid to 50 ml 0.1 M Tris base. Dilute the resulting mixture to the required molarity.

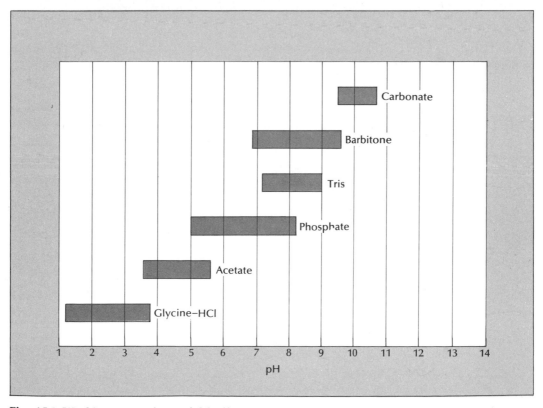

Fig. AI.2 Working ranges for useful buffers.

water, titrate to pH 8.7 with 1 M HCl, finally adjust to 500 ml with distilled water.

0.1 M Tris-buffered saline, pH 8.0
(for IgM preparation)

Materials
Tris (hydroxy methyl) aminomethane (12.1 g)
Sodium chloride (29.22 g)
Glycine (0.75 g)
Sodium azide (0.2 g)
1 M HCl

Method
1 Dissolve ingredients in 800 ml distilled water and adjust to pH 8.0 with HCl.
2 Make volume up to 1000 ml with distilled water.

Tris–glycine buffer, pH 8.3; 0.25 M Tris, 1.92 M glycine

Materials
Tris (hydroxymethyl) aminomethane (30.3 g)
Glycine (134.6 g)
Sodium dodecyl sulphate (10 g)

Method
Dissolve materials in water and make up to 1000 ml.

Veronal buffered saline (for PEG precipitation)

Materials
Sodium chloride (85.0 g)
Sodium barbitone (3.75 g)
Barbitone (5.75 g)

Method
Dissolve and make up to 2 litres with distilled water.

This buffer is 5 times the concentration used in the text, as it is more stable as a concentrated stock solution. Dilute just before use.

II Equipment Index and Manufacturers Index

Equipment index

Numbers indicate listing in address index.

Manufactures address index

USA suppliers are given below the UK supplier where appropriate. Telephone numbers in italic.

1   Abbot Laboratories Ltd
Queenborough Road
Kent ME11 5EI
0795 580099

Laboratories Abbot Limitée
Montreal
Canada H4P 1A5

2   Aldrich Chemical Co.
The Old Brickyard, New Road,
Gillingham, Dorset SP8 4JL
07476 2211

See Sigma, Fluka, Biorad, Baxter Health Care

3   American Type Culture Collection
Sales and Marketing Department
12301 Parklawn Drive
Rockville, MD, USA 20852

4   Amersham International p.l.c.
Lincoln Place Green End
Aylesbury, Bucks HP20 2TP
0296 35222

Amersham Corporation
Arlington Heights, USA
312 364 7100

5   Amicon Ltd.
Upper Mill
Stonehouse, Gloucestershire GL10 2BJ
045 382 5181

Amicon Division, W. R. Grace and Co.
24 Cherry Hill Drive
Danvers, MA, USA 01923
617 777 3622

6   Anderman and Co. Ltd.
145 London Road
Kingston upon Thames
Surrey KT2 6NH
01 541 0035

Schleicher and Schuell
10 Optical Avenue
Keene, New Hampshire,
03431 USA

7   Baxter Health Care
Wallingford Road
Compton,
nr. Newbury, Berks RG 16 0QW
0635 200020

Baxter Health Care, Scientific Products Division,
1430 Waukegan Road
Mcgaw Park, IL USA 60085
312 689 8410

8   BDH Ltd.
Broom Road
Poole, Dorset BH12 4NN
0202 745520

See Sigma, Fluka, Biorad, Baxter Health Care

9   Becton–Dickinson
Between Towns Road
Cowley, Oxford OX4 3LY
0865 777722

Becton–Dickinson, Clay Adams Division,
299 Webro Rd
Parsippany, NJ, USA 07054
201 887 4800

10 Biorad Laboratories
Caxton Way, Watford Business Park
Watford, Herts WD1 8RP
0923 240322

Biorad Chemical Division
1414 Harbour Way So
Richmond, CA, USA 94804
415 232 7000

11 British Biotechnology
Brook House, Watlington Road
Cowley, Oxford OX4 5LY
0865 718817

R and D Systems
614 Mckinley Place NE
Minneapolis, MN, USA 55413
800 328 2400

12 Calbiochem-Behring
Novabiochem (UK) Ltd, 3 Heathcoat
Building, Highfields Science Park
University Boulevard, Nottingham
NG7 2QL
0602 430840

Calbiochem Brand Biochemicals
10933 North Torrey Pines Road
La Jolla, CA, USA 92037
800 854 3417

13 Cambridge Bioscience
Newton House
142 Devonshire Road
Cambridge CB1 2BL
0223 316855

See Sigma, Flow

14 DAKO Ltd.
22 The Arcade, The Octagon
High Wycombe, Bucks HP11 2HT
0494 452016

DAKO Corporation
22 North Milpas Street
Santa Barbara, CA, USA 93103
805 963 9881

15 Difco Laboratories Ltd.
PO Box 14b Central Avenue
East Molesey KT8 0SE
01 979 9951

Difco Labs
PO Box 1058
Detroit, MI, USA 48232
313 961 0800

16 Distillers
Cedar House, 39 London Road
Reigate, Surrey RH2 9QE
07372 41133

17 Dynatech Laboratories Ltd.
Daux Road
Billingshurst, West Sussex RH14 9SJ
0403 813381

Dynatech Labs Inc.
14340 Sullyfield Circle
Chantilly, VA, USA 22021
800 336 4543

18 Elkay Lab Products UK Ltd.
Unit 2, Crockford Lane
Basingstoke, Hants RG24 0NA
0256 475727

See BDH, Becton–Dickinson

19 European Collection of Animal Cultures
PHLS Centre for Applied Microbiology
and Research Porton Down
Salisbury, Wiltshire SP9 OJG

20 Flow Laboratories Ltd.
Woodcock hill, Harefield road
Rickmansworth, Herts WD3 1PQ
0923 774666

Flow Laboratories Inc.
PO Box 1065
Dublin, Va, USA 24084
703 674 8861

21 Fluka Chemicals Ltd.
Peakdale road
Glossop, Derbyshire SK13 9XE
04574 62518

Fluka Chemical Corporation
980 South Second St
Ronkonkoma, NY, USA 11779
516 467 0980

22 Froxfield Farms (UK) Ltd.
Unit 3, Broadway Cottage, Kings Lane,
Froxfield
Petersfield, Hants GU32 1DR
0730 63821

Harlan Sprague Dawley Inc.
PO Box 29176
Indianapolis, IN, USA 46229
317 894 7521

23 Gallenkamp
Belton Road West
Loughborough LE11 0TR
0509 237371

Schott America
3 Odell Plaza
Yonkers, NY, USA 10701
914 968 8900

Or try Flow, Biorad

24 CBI Labs Ltd.
Northgate
Pontefract, West Yorkshire WF8 1HJ
0977 708155

See Gelman Sciences Inc.

25 Gelman Sciences Ltd.
10 Harrowden Road
Brackmills, Northampton NN4 0EZ
0604 65141

Gelman Sciences Inc.
Laboratory Diagnostics, 600 South
Wagner Road
Ann Arbor, MI, USA 48106
313 665 0651

26 Gibco Ltd.
Unit 4, Cowley Mill Trading Estate,
Longbridge Way
Uxbridge UB8 2YG
0895 36355

Gibco Laboratories, Department of Life
Technologies Inc.
3175 Staley Rd
Grand Island, NY, USA 14072
716 773 0700

27 Griffin and George
Bishops Meadow Road
Loughborough, Leicestershire LE11 0RG
0903 772071

See Gelman Sciences Inc.

28 Harlan Olac Ltd.
Shaw Farm, Blackthorn
Bicestor, Oxon OX6 0TP
086 9243241

Harlan Sprague Dawley Inc.
PO Box 29176
Indianapolis, IN, USA 46229
317 894 7521

29 Phillip Harris Scientific
618 Western Avenue, Park Royal
London W3 0TE
01 992 5555

30 Arnold R Horwell (Reagents) Ltd.
73 Maygrove Road, West Hampstead
London NW6 2BP
01 328 1551

Becton–Dickinson, Clay Adams Division
299 Webro Road
Parsippany, NJ, USA 07054
201 887 4800

31 Houghton Poultry
The Institute For Animal Health,
Houghton Laboratory
St Ives, Cambridge P17 2DA
0480 64101

Harlan Sprague Dawley Inc.
PO Box 29176
Indianapolis, IN, USA 46229
317 894 7521

32 VA Howe and Co. Ltd.
12—14 St Annes Crescent
London SW18 2LS
01 874 0422

33 ICN Biomedicals
Free Press House, Castle Street
High Wycombe, Bucks HP13 6RN
0494 443 826

ICN Biomedicals Inc.
PO Box 19536
Irvine, CA, USA 92713
714 545 0133

34 Ilford Scientific Products
Town Lane, Mobberley
Cheshire WA16 7HA
0565 50050

Polysciences Inc.
400 Valley Rd
Warrington, PA, USA 18976
215 343 6484

35 Janssen Pharmaceuticals
Life Sciences Products Division,
Turnhoutseweg 30, B-2340
Beerse, Belgium

36 Jencons (Scientific) Ltd.
Cherrycourt Way, Industrial Estate,
Stanbridge Road
Leighton Buzzard, Bedfordshire LU7 8UA
0525 372010

Baxter Health Care, Scientific Products
Division
1430 Waukegan Road
Mcgaw Park, IL, USA 60085
312 689 8410

37 Koch Light Ltd.
163 Dixons Hill Road
North Mymms
Hatfield, Herts AL9 7JE
07072 75733

38 E. Leitz Instruments Ltd.
48 Park St
Luton LU1 3HP
0582 404040

E. Leitz Inc. Instruments Division
24 Link Drive
Rockleigh, NJ, USA 07647
201 767 1100

39 LKB
Pharmacia LKB Ltd., Midsummer
Boulevard
Milton Keynes, Bucks MK9 3HP
0908 66101

40 Lorne Diagnostics
PO Box 6, Twyfords
Reading, Berks RG10 9NL
0734 342400

41 Luckham Ltd.
Victoria Gardens
Burgess Hill, Sussex RH15 9QN
044 46 5348

Denville Scientific
PO Box 304
Denville, NJ, USA 07834

42 Medicell International Ltd.
239 Liverpool Road
London N1 1LX
01 607 2295

43 Miles Laboratories Ltd.
Stoke Court, Stoke Poges
Slough SL2 4LY
02814 5151

See Sigma

44 Millipore UK Ltd.
11—15 Peterborough Road
Harrow, Middlesex HA1 2IH
01 864 5499

Millipore Corporation
80 Ashby Rd
Bedford, MA, USA 01730
617 275 9200

45 MSE
Sussex Manor Park
Crawley, West Sussex RH10 2QQ
0293 31100

46 National Diagnostics
Unit 3, Chamberlain Rd
Aylesbury, Bucks HP19 3D7
0296 436177

National Diagnostics Inc.
1013–1017 Kennedy Boulevard
Manville, NJ, USA 08835
201 722 8600

47 Nordic Immunologicals
PO Box 544
Maidenhead, Berks SC6 2PW
0628-24978

Nordic
Drawer 2517
Capistrano Beach, CA, USA 92624
714 661 1188

48 Novabiochem UK Ltd.
3 Heathcoat Building, Highfields Science
Park, University Boulevard
Nottingham NG7 2QL
0602 430840

Calbiochem Brand Biochemicals
10933 North Torrey Pines Road
La Jolla, CA, USA 92037
800 854 3417

49 National Institute for Biological Standards
and Control
Blanche Lane
South Mimms
Herts
ENG 3QG
0707 54753

50 Nycomed UK Ltd.
Nycomed House, 2111 Coventry Road
Sheldon, Birmingham B26 3EA
021 742 2444

51 Organon Teknika Ltd.
Science Park, Milton Road
Cambridge CB4 4BH
0223 313650

52 Ortho Diagnostic Systems
Enterprise House, Station Road,
Loudwater
High Wycombe, Bucks HP10 9UF
0494 442211

Ortho-Diagnostic Systems Institute
Route 202
Raritan, NJ, USA 08869
201 524 0400

53 Oxford Scientific Instruments
Osney Mead
Oxford

54 Pharmacia LKB Ltd.
Pharmacia House, Midsummer Boulevard
Milton Keynes, Bucks MK9 3HP
0908 66101

Pharmacia LKB Biotechnology Inc.
800 Centennial Ave
Piscataway, NJ, USA 08854
414 347 7442

55 PHLS Centre for Applied Microbiology
and Research
Porton Down
Salisbury SP4 0JG
0980 610391

American Type Culture Collection
12301 Parklawn Drive
Rockville, MD, USA 20852

56 Pierce And Warriner UK Ltd.
44 Upper Northgate Street Chester, CH1
4EF
0244 382525

Pierce Chemical Co.
PO Box 117
Rockford, IL, USA 61105
815 968 0747

57 Porvair Ltd.
Riverside Industrial Estate, Estuary Road
Kings Lynn, Norfolk NE30 2HS
0553 76111

58 Scientific Supplies Co.
Scientific House, Vine Hill
London EC1 5EB
01 278 8241

59 Serotec
22 Bankside Station Approach
Kidlington, Oxford OX5 1JE
08675 79941

Bioproducts For Science Inc.
PO Box 29176
Indianapolis, IN, USA 46229
317 997 7536

60 Unipath
Norse Road
Bedford MK41 0QG
0234 47161

Oxoid USA
9017 Red Branch Road
Columbia, MD, USA 21045
301 997 2216

61 Shandon Southern Products
Chadwick Road, Astmoor
Runcorn, Cheshire WA7 1PR
0928 566611

62 Sigma Chemical Co.
Fancy Road
Poole, Dorset BH17 7NH
0202 733114

Sigma Chemical Co.
3050 Spruce Street, PO Box 14508
St Louis, MO, USA 63178
314 771 5750

63 Sterilin Ltd.
Lampton House, Lampton Road
Hounslow, Middlesex TW3 4EE
01 572 2468

Bellco Glass Inc.
PO Box B, 340 Edrudo Road
Vineland, NJ, USA 08360
609 691 1075

64 Vector Laboratories
16 Wulfric Square
Bretton, Peterborough PE3 8RF
0733 265530

Vector Laboratories
30 Ingold Road
Burlingame, CA, USA 94010
415 697 3600

65 Wellcome Diagnostics Ltd.
Temple Hill
Dartford, Kent
0322 77711

Wellcome Triangle Park Diagnostics
Division
North Building, 3030 Cornwallis Road,
Research Triangle Park
North Carolina, USA 27709
919 248 3000

66 Whatman Lab Sales Ltd.
PO Box 6, Twyfords
Reading, Berks RG10 9NL
0734 342400

Whatman Inc.
9 Bridewell Place
Clifton, NJ, USA 07014
201 773 5800

67 X O-GRAPH Ltd.
Malmesbury, Wiltshire
4641 06662

Further reading

Coombs J and Alston YR (1988) *International Biotechnology Directory 1989*. Macmillan, London.
Haugland RP (1988) *Handbook of Fluorescent Probes and Research Chemicals 1989–1991*. Molecular Probes Inc., PO Box 22010, Eugene, Oregon 97402, USA.
Linscott's Directory of Immunological and Biological Reagents. PO Box 55, East Grinstead, Sussex RH17 3YL.

III Laboratory Safety, Tissue Culture Techniques and Useful Data

Laboratory safety

Work in the laboratory environment is closely regulated by legislation; usually reinforced and exemplified by institutional and local codes of practice. The notes given here draw attention to hazardous procedures or chemicals described in the book.

Many of the requirements for 'good laboratory practice' rely on common sense; for example, it is essential that there is no eating, drinking, smoking or application of cosmetics in laboratory areas; disposable paper tissues should be provided for nose blowing; protective clothing with side or rear fastening should be worn in laboratory areas but removed before entry into areas such as offices and coffee rooms; disposable rubber gloves must be worn when handling radioactive materials, carcinogens, corrosive or toxic chemicals, human tissue and pathogens. In other instances, however, the recommendations are based on a thorough knowledge of the likely risks and their avoidance. For example, both insulating gloves and a protective visor should be used when handling samples frozen in liquid nitrogen, thus guarding against frost bite and possible eye damage resulting from an exploding vial; genetic manipulations carry maximum risk when self replicating pathogenic sequences are expressed, partial sequences require lower levels of protection and containment.

Human material

Invariably, blood and human tissue samples should be treated as though they were a source of potential hepatitis or HIV infection — wear a laboratory overall, latex gloves and eye protection; do not use glass pipettes, avoid creating aerosols, work in a class II lamina flow hood and disinfect all equipment after use (1:10 freshly diluted bleach (Chloros)

or other suitable disinfectant). Transformation of human cells by viruses or by transfection should only be carried out in designated areas with suitable protection. *Never* transform your own lymphocytes; a histocompatibility barrier provides the only effective protection against tumour growth following accidental self inoculation.

Bleeding human volunteers

Blood should be taken only by trained staff in designated areas. To minimise blood leakage during venesection, we recommend the use of Becton—Dickinson Vacutainers. To avoid needle stick injuries, care must be taken in re-sheathing needles; insert the needle into a sheath held in a mechanical holder not in the hand. Blood must not be taken if the volunteer gives a *positive* answer to *any* of the following questions:
(a) For male volunteers, have you had sex with another man on any occasion since 1978?
(b) If you have visited or lived in Africa (south of the Sahara) since 1978, did you have sex with any man or woman living there?
(c) If you are a drug abuser, have you injected drugs intravenously since 1978?
(d) Are you a haemophiliac and have you received untreated blood products since 1978?
(e) Have you had sexual contact with anyone in the above groups?

Disinfection

Tissue culture flasks or any container that has been in contact with human tissue should be disinfected, for example with 5% hycoline, before disposal. Anything containing viruses or bacteria should be disinfected with hypochlorite solution (1:10 freshly diluted bleach). Work surfaces should be disinfected with a 1% solution of hycoline. Lamina flow hoods may be disinfected by evaporating 25 ml of formaldehyde in the hood while it is running, use a hot plate or add minute amounts of potassium permanganate to the formaldehyde solution. As formaldehyde is toxic and a potential carcinogen; this procedure should be carried out 'after working hours', warning notices displayed, the vapour contained during disinfection and finally ventilated directly to atmosphere.

Hazardous chemicals

Hazardous reagents must be stored in a locked area. These chemicals include many of the substances mentioned in this book; for example, known and potential carcinogens, poisons, drugs, venoms, bacterial toxins, azides, acrylamide, iodoacetamide, enzyme inhibitors, formic acid, phenyl diamine, thiomersal and cyanogen bromide. Flammable liquids must be stored in small volumes, in a metal safety cabinet and mutually reactive chemicals must be stored separately. Incorrect disposal of laboratory chemicals can also create an environmental hazard; the Aldrich Chemical Catalogue (free upon request, Appendix II) contains information for the safe disposal of each chemical offered for sale.

Carcinogens

A large number of commonly used laboratory chemicals are potentially carcinogenic or mutagenic, including the following mentioned in this book: benzidine, benzene, 2-naphthylamine, phorbol esters (for example, PMA) diphenylamine, O-toluidine, acridine orange, trypan blue, DNP, TNP, toluene, xylene, formaldehyde, glass fibre, chloroform, carbon tetrachloride, diaminobenzidine and propidium iodide. Handle them with care.

Radiochemicals

There are defined legal requirements for the handling of radioisotopes — see further reading at the end of this section for regulations applying to the UK.

The work area should be specially designated for the use of radioisotopes. The design of the apparatus and experimental procedure should seek to minimise the handling of the radioactive material and avoid exposure to radiation. Appropriate shielding and distance reduces the radioactive dose received (inverse square law); move away from radioisotopes during incubation periods. All work with volatile materials — including radioiodine and isotopes in organic solvents — should be carried out in a fume hood.

Laboratory benches and trays should be lined with a water-impermeable absorbent material — such as Benchcote — to facilitate decontamination. Containers of a decontamination solution (for example, Deconex) should be readily available for immediate immersion of contaminated apparatus, thus minimising irreversible binding of the isotope. All radioactive waste must be discarded in the manner specified by local guidelines and its total radioactive content recorded.

Monitor the work area and your person regularly and systematically and record the results. Although direct monitoring with a scintillation probe is possible for the detection of γ emitters, monitoring for β emitters requires that a swab of the area be taken and the radioactivity measured using scintillation fluid and a β spectrometer. Contamination must be kept to the lowest possible level; in any case personal contamination must be less than 30 Bq cm^{-2} body surface for ^{125}I and less than 3 Bq cm^{-2} for ^{32}P.

Tissue culture techniques

Modern immunology uses many of the techniques previously confined to the cell biology laboratory. Tissue culture should be carried out in a sterile environment (usually a lamina flow hood where the air is filtered to remove airborne bacteria and fungi) using aseptic technique. If the cells being cultured constitute a potential biohazard, for example human clinical specimens or virus-infected cell lines, then a class II hood should be used so that both operator and culture are protected.

Tissue culture media

Many different culture media are available, each usually in an 'old', 'new' and 'improved' formulation. For general use we suggest a simple medium such as Eagle's minimal essential medium (EMEM) for growth of 'robust' cell lines. For cell growth under more demanding conditions, for example during cell cloning or for the growth of more fastidious lines, we recommend a more complex medium, such as Dulbecco's modification of Eagle's medium (DMEM) or RPMI 1640.

Buffers for culture media

A good argument can be made for using sodium bicarbonate (26 mM) buffered by CO_2 in air, as this is at least physiological under closed-culture conditions (5% CO_2 in air in a gassed incubator). Although its buffering capacity is low, it is relatively cheap and has a low toxicity. Recently double-buffering systems have been used to good effect; for example, RPMI containing bicarbonate, 24 mM and HEPES, 50 mM (N-2-hydroxyethylpiperazine N-2-ethanesulphonic acid) (In general, the HEPES concentration must be double that of the bicarbonate for good buffering). In this case, under low CO_2 tension, the pH is maintained by the interaction of the bicarbonate with the HEPES; and in the culture, under high CO_2 tension (5%), the bicarbonate also acts as a buffer, as described above. Although 20 mM HEPES alone can control the pH of the culture medium within physiological limits, cells grow better in the presence of CO_2 and HCO_3^-. Oxygen tension is also important for the growth of cells — in static culture the depth of medium should not be greater than about 5 mm.

To avoid the expense of large volumes of relatively expensive media, cells may be prepared from the animal in PBS and washed into medium immediately before culture. For *in vitro* handling of lymphocytes, not involving culture, we have used DMEM containing HEPES, 20 mM, adjusting to pH 7.4 with 1 M sodium hydroxide.

Most cells grow well at pH 7.4. At this pH the most commonly used indicator, phenol red, is red, becoming blue—red at pH 7.6 and purple at pH 7.8; on the acidic side it is orange at pH 7.0 and yellow at pH 6.5.

Antibiotics for culture media

Again many workers have their own recipe. We suggest penicillin 200 units ml^{-1} and streptomycin 100 μg ml^{-1} or gentamycin 30 μg ml^{-1}. If there is persistent yeast contamination it is possible to add Fungizone (amphotericin B) at up to 10 μg ml^{-1} (final concentration); cell lines vary in their sensitivity, so start at 2 μg ml^{-1}.

Serum supplements

For murine cells: 10% fetal bovine serum (FBS). It is necessary to select a 'good' batch of serum, i.e. giving acceptable cell survival, without a high background of incorporation of the DNA analogue due to mitogenic stimulation by the FBS. The proportion of FBS required may be reduced by adding 2 mercaptoethanol. The medium listed below was developed for murine mixed-lymphocyte cultures, but it may be used for the maintenance of mouse cell lines (including hybridoma lines).

Dulbecco's modification of EMEM containing:

arginine (200 mg $litre^{-1}$)
folic acid (12 mg litre $^{-1}$)
asparagine (36 mg $litre^{-1}$)
2-mercaptoethanol (5×10^{-5} mol $litre^{-1}$)
HEPES (1×10^{-2} mol $litre^{-1}$)
FBS 5% v/v.

Horse or calf serum can be used as a cheaper alternative to fetal bovine serum for the maintenance of some cell lines; for example, the hybridoma parent lines X-63. However, a period of 'adaptation' (probably resulting in cell selection) is required, during which the concentration of one supplement is decreased while the other is increased.

Serum-free media are available and can offer advantages if secreted products, such as antibodies or cytokines, are to be purified

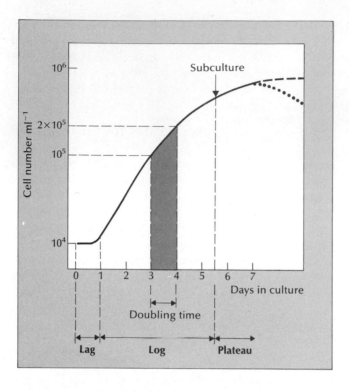

Fig. III.1 Typical growth curve of a continuous cell line. The data shown above was obtained from a cell line growing in suspension culture. Growth of adherent cells follows the same curve but cell density values are approximately 10-fold lower.

There are three distinct phases to cell growth *in vitro*: lag, log and plateau.

In the *lag phase*, there is little increase in cell numbers as this is a period of recovery and adaptation; for example, the cell may need to re-synthesise elements of its glycocalyx after trypsinisation. This process is often cell-density dependent; if cells are subcultured at too low an initial density they may never escape into log phase.

Log phase is the optimum time for cell use as the population is phenotypically at its most homogenous and has high viability. As cell numbers increase exponentially the time taken for the cell number to increase two-fold is equal to the cell doubling time. This should not be confused with the cell cycle time, which is a measure of the time taken for a population of synchronised cells to traverse the cell cycle and return to the starting point. Cells growing in log phase are not normally synchronous but instead are uniformly distributed throughout the stages of the cell cycle (G1 → S → G2 → M → return to G1, etc.).

The *plateau phase* occurs towards the end of log phase and is evidenced by a rapid reduction in growth rate. Growth eventually ceases, after one or two divisions, to terminate in the G1 phase of the cell cycle. Normal cells, for example fibroblasts, stop growing at high density and remain viable for several weeks (dashed line). Cultures of transformed cells and cell lines deteriorate rapidly (dotted line) and so should be subcultured as described in the text.

from the culture supernatant. However, in general these media still contain high concentrations of added proteins and are relatively expensive.

Subculture of cell lines

The growth curve of a typical line is shown in Fig. III.1. This curve should be determined for every cell type in long-term culture, as it yields essential information on the growth characteristics and requirements of the line. Most cultures have an optimum lower cell density at initiation and tend to die at plateau

densities, when nutrients or toxic waste become limiting. To maintain high viability, cells should be 'fed' by changing the medium once the indicator dye turns orange−yellow and the cell density should be reduced by dilution of the culture before the plateau phase is reached.

Subculture of non-adherent cells

Shake the culture vessel gently to bring all the cells into suspension and count the cell number using a haemocytometer. Either remove and discard a fraction of the suspension, before adding fresh medium, or transfer an aliquot of suspension to a fresh flask containing medium, in each case the intention is to reduce the cells back to their optimum inoculation density (Fig. III.1).

Subculture of adherent cells

Materials and equipment
Phosphate-buffered saline, PBS (Appendix I)
Trypsin 0.25% in PBS, with or without 1 mM EDTA
Tissue culture medium containing a serum supplement

Method
1 Pour the spent medium off the culture and wash with PBS to remove all traces of serum (this would inhibit the action of the trypsin).
2 Add 3.0 ml of trypsin solution per 25 cm² growth area of cells, tip the flask to cover the culture and leave for 30 sec at room temperature.
3 Pour off the trypsin solution and incubate the culture at 37° until the cells are seen to detach, usually 5–15 min.
4 Add tissue culture medium containing serum (this inhibits the residual trypsin so there is no need to wash the cells), disperse the cells by gentle aspiration with a pipette and count using a haemocytometer.
5 Withdraw an aliquot containing an appropriate seeding number of cells and transfer to a fresh flask containing medium.

Technical notes
1 EDTA should only be used if treatment with trypsin alone fails to release the adherent cells.
2 Cross contamination between cell lines can lead to overgrowth by the fastest grower. Never use the same pipette for different cell lines and work out a routine in which only one line at a time is subbed in the lamina flow hood.

Cryopreservation of cells

Cells may be stored for an indefinite period in a frozen state under liquid nitrogen. Freeze viable, actively growing cells whenever possible; they are your insurance against accidental loss.

Materials
Cryoprotective solution; by volume:
Fetal bovine serum, FBS, 50%
Dimethyl sulphoxide, DMSO, 20%
Tissue culture medium 30%

Method
1 Harvest the cells by centrifugation (150 *g* for 10 min at 4°), count and adjust to 1×10^7 ml^{-1}.
2 Add cell suspension dropwise to an equal volume of cryoprotective solution.
3 Dispense convenient volumes into ampoules suitable for storage in liquid nitrogen.
4 Freeze slowly (at about 1° min^{-1}) down to at least −50° and then immerse in liquid nitrogen.

Technical notes
1 DMSO (or alternatively, glycerol) allows water to go from a liquid to a solid state without the formation of ice crystals.
2 Use a fresh bottle of DMSO every 2–3 months to avoid the accumulation of toxic peroxides. Alternatively, re-distill with care.
3 DMSO must be handled with care, it can penetrate the skin and carry with it any harmful substance in regular use; for example, carcinogens

THAWING
Cells may be recovered from liquid nitrogen storage by thawing rapidly to 37° (in a water bath) and washing three times in tissue culture medium by centrifugation (150 *g* for 10 min at room temperature).

Cell lines

Most of the cell lines described in this book are generally available in laboratories throughout the world, for which they may be begged, borrowed but hopefully not stolen. In addition many are available from commercial suppliers; for example, Flow Laboratories, Appendix II), the American Type Culture Collection (ATCC), or the European Collection of Animal Cell Cultures (ECACC). If all else fails, the originator of the cell line will often respond positively to a polite request for a starter culture.

When you import a cell line, it is always advisable to screen it for *Mycoplasma* infection. *Mycoplasma* does not necessarily slow down cell growth, but can play havoc with the results of *in vitro* bioassays. If a culture is contaminated, discard it and start again. Although, it is possible to have cell lines 'cured' of the infection, but this is rarely complete.

In the list below, we have indicated availability through the ECACC or ATCC as the first point of contact, otherwise, original references are quoted. References are also given for the less well-known cell lines.

American Type Culture Collection,
Sales and Marketing Department,
12301 Parklawn Drive,
Rockville, MD 20852, USA.

European Collection of Animal Cell Cultures,
PHLS Centre for Applied Microbiology,
Porton Down,
Salisbury, Wiltshire SP4 OJG.

Chapter 4

Daudi	ATCC.
K-562	ATCC.
Me-180	ATCC.
P-815	ATCC.
T-24	ATCC.

Chapter 12: B-cell hybridomas

MOPC 21	ATCC.
NS1-Ag4-1	ECACC and ATCC.
P3/X63-Ag8	ECACC and ATCC.
Sp2/O-Ag14	ECACC and ATCC.

Chapter 12: T-cell hybridomas

BW-5147 ATCC.

FS6-14.13 Kappler *et al.* (1981; *J. Exp. Med.* **153**: 1198.

MOLT-4 ECACC and ATCC.

Chapter 12: T-cell clones

MLA-144 ATCC. Rabin *et al.* (1981) *J. Immunol.* **127**: 1852. Gibbon cell line with constitutive production of a mixture of growth factors, including IL-2. *Like all primate lines, assume that it contains xenotropic viruses and handle accordingly.*

Chapter 13

2.19 Sideras *et al.* (1985) Secretion of IgG1 induction factor by T cell clones and hybridomas. *Euro. J. Immunol.* **15**: 585−593.

5637 ATCC.

B151 Takatsu *et al.* (1980) Antigen-induced TR cell-replacing factor (TRF). III. Establishment of T hybrid clone continuously producing TRF and functional analysis of released TRF. *J. Immunol.* **125**: 2646.

BCL₁ ATCC. Slavin S and Strober S (1977) Spontaneous murine B-cell leukaemia. *Nature* **272**: 62−626.

CESS Muraguchi *et al.* (1981) T cell-replacing factor (TRF)-induced IgG secretion in a human B blastoid cell line and demonstration of acceptors for TRF. *J. Immunol.* **127**: 412−416.

CT-6 Ho *et al.* (1987) Differential bioassay of interleukin 2 and interleukin 4. *J. Immunol. Methods* **98**: 99−104.

CTLL-D Gearing *et al.* (1987) A simple sensitive bioassay for interleukin 1 which is unresponsive to 10^3 U ml^{-1} of interleukin 2. *J. Immunol. Methods* **99**: 7−11.

EL4.6.1 ATCC. Luscher *et al.* (1985

Cell-surface glycoproteins involved in the stimulation of interleukin 1-dependent interleukin 2 production by a subline of EL4 thymoma cells. *J. Immunol.* **135**: 3951—3957.

Hep/2c ECACC and ATCC.

HT-2 Ho *et al.* (1987) Differential bioassay of interleukin 2 and interleukin 4. *J. Immunol. Methods* **98**: 99—104.

Jurkat Gillis S and Watson J (1980) Biochemical and biological characterization of lymphocyte regulatory molecules. V. Identification of an interleukin 2 producer human leukaemia T-cell line. *J. Exp. Med.* **152**: 1709.

L929 ATCC and ECACC.

MC/9 ATCC. Nabel *et al.* (1981) Inducer T lymphocytes synthesise a factor that stimulates proliferation of cloned mast cells. *Nature* **291**: 332—334.

NIMP-TH1 Warren D and Sanderson CJ (1985) production of a T cell hybrid producing a lymphoid stimulating eosionophil differentiation factor. *Immunol.* **54**: 615—623.

Namalwa ATCC.

SKW6-CL4 ATCC. Saiki O and Ralph P (1981) Clonal differences in response to T cell-replacing factor for immunoglobulin M secretion and T cell-replacing factor receptors in a human B lymphoblastoid line. *Eur. J. Immunol.* **13**: 31.

TCl-Na1 Shimizu *et al.* (1985) Immortalization of BGDF and BCDF-producing T cells by human T cell leukaemia virus and characterization of human BGDF. *J. Immunol.* **134**: 1728—1733.

WEHI-3 ATCC and ECACC. Luqer *et al.* (1985) Epidermal cells synthesise a cytokine with interleukin 3-like properties. *J. Immunol.* **134**: 915—919.

WEHI-164 ATCC. **Clone 13** Espevik T and Nissen-Meyer J (1986) A highly senstive cell line, WEHI-164 clone 13, for measuring cytotoxic factor and tumour necrosis factor from human monocytes. *J. Immunol. Methods* **95**: 99—105.

Useful data

Element (mass number)	Radiation	Half life
^{3}H	β	12.26 years
^{14}C	β	5730 years
^{22}Na	β, γ	2.6 years
^{32}P	β	14.3 days
^{51}Cr	κ, γ	27.8 days
^{60}Co	β, γ	5.26 years
^{125}I	γ	60 days
^{131}I	β, γ	8.1 days

Class	Concentration (mg ml^{-1})
IgG	8—16
IgA	1.4—4
IgM	0.5—2
IgD	0—0.4
IgE	17—450 ng ml^{-1}

Subclass	% of total in class
IgG 1	70
IgG 2	18
IgG 3	8
IgG 4	3
IgA 1	80
IgA 2	20

Serum concentration of human immunoglobulins and distribution of subclasses

Protein	Molecular weight	$E_1^{1\%}{}_{cm}$	Wavelength (nm)	Solvent
IgG	160 000	14.3	280	0.2 M NaCl pH 7.5
IgA	170 000	10.6	280	
IgM	900 000	11.85	280	0.2 M NaCl pH 7.5
IgD	184 000			
IgE	188 000			
μ chain	73 814			
α chain	59 582	10.6	280	5 M guanidine HCl
γ chain	50 179	13.7	280	0.01 N HCl
light chain	25 170	11.8	280	0.01 N HCl
Fab$_\gamma$	50 000	15.3	278	PBS
F(ab$_\gamma$)$_2$	104 000	14.8	280	PBS
Fc$_\gamma$	50 000	12.2	278	PBS
pFc'$_\gamma$	26 000	13.8	280	PBS
Ovalbumin	43 500	7.35	280	PBS
Human serum albumin	68 460	5.3	279	PBS
Bovine serum albumin	67 000	6.67	279	Water
Fowl γ-globulin		13.5	280	—
Keyhole limpet haemocyanin	3 000 000 (*Megathura crenulata*)			
Squid haemocyanin	611 800 (*Ommatostrephes sloani pacificus*)			
Murex haemocyanin		18.1	278	Water
Limulus haemocyanin		11.2	278	Water
2,4-dinitrophenyl (DNP)	184	14 900 ($E_M^{1\,cm}$)	358	0.5 M phosphate pH7.4
4-hydroxy-3-nitro-5-iodo phenacetyl azide (NIP azide)	348	—	—	—
Fluorescein	389	53 000 ($E_M^{1\,cm}$)	490	0.15 M NaCl, p.02 M K phosphate pH 7.4

Molecular weights and spectral properties of immunoglobulins and antigens of immunological interest

	Approximate molarity (M)	% by weight	Specific gravity
Acetic acid	17.4	99.6	1.05
Hydrochloric acid	11.6	36.0	1.18
Nitric acid	15.7	70.0	1.42
Phosphoric acid	16.0	90.0	1.75
Sulphuric acid	18.3	98.0	1.835

Common acids.

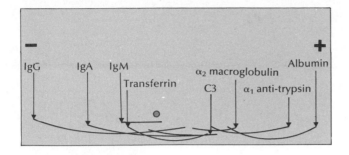

Immunoelectrophoresis of human serum in agar, sodium—barbitone buffer, pH 8.2. The main immunoglobulin classes are shown together with several other major proteins.

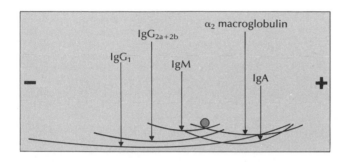

Immunoelectrophoresis of normal BALB/c serum in agar, sodium—barbitone buffer PH 8·6. Proteins visualised with a rabbit antiserum to mouse immunoglobulin. Such antisera invariably contain antibodies to 2-α-macroglobulin.

Further reading

The Ionising Radiations Regulations (1985) HMSO.

The Protection of Persons Against Ionising Radiations Arising from any Work Activity (1985) HMSO.

Guidance Notes For the Protection of Persons Against Ionising Radiations Arising From Medical and Dental Use (1988) National Radiological Protection Board, HMSO.

Ballance PE, Day LR and Morgan J (1987) *Phosphorus-32: Practical Radiation Protection*. Occupational Hygiene Monograph Number 16. Science Reviews, Northwood.

Barnes DW, Sirbasku DA and Sato GH (editors) (1984). Cell Culture Methods for Molecular and Cell Biology, 4 volumes. Alan R Liss Inc, New York.

Freshney RI (1987) *Culture of Animal Cells — a Manual of Basic Technique*. Alan R Liss, New York.

Prime D (1985) *Health Physics Aspects of the Use of Radioiodines*. Occupational Hygiene Monographs Number 3. Science Reviews, Northwood.

Index

Page references in *italics* refer to figures or the legends accompanying them.

497